Communications
in Computer and Information Science   515

Commenced Publication in 2007
Founding and Former Series Editors:
Alfredo Cuzzocrea, Dominik Ślęzak, and Xiaokang Yang

Editorial Board

Simone Diniz Junqueira Barbosa
  Pontifical Catholic University of Rio de Janeiro (PUC-Rio),
  Rio de Janeiro, Brazil
Phoebe Chen
  La Trobe University, Melbourne, Australia
Xiaoyong Du
  Renmin University of China, Beijing, China
Joaquim Filipe
  Polytechnic Institute of Setúbal, Setúbal, Portugal
Orhun Kara
  TÜBİTAK BİLGEM and Middle East Technical University, Ankara, Turkey
Igor Kotenko
  St. Petersburg Institute for Informatics and Automation of the Russian
  Academy of Sciences, St. Petersburg, Russia
Ting Liu
  Harbin Institute of Technology (HIT), Harbin, China
Krishna M. Sivalingam
  Indian Institute of Technology Madras, Chennai, India
Takashi Washio
  Osaka University, Osaka, Japan

More information about this series at http://www.springer.com/series/7899

Habib M. Fardoun · Victor M.R. Penichet
Daniyal M. Alghazzawi (Eds.)

ICTs for Improving
Patients Rehabilitation
Research Techniques

Second International Workshop, REHAB 2014
Oldenburg, Germany, May 20–23, 2014
Revised Selected Papers

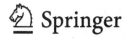 Springer

Editors
Habib M. Fardoun
King Abdulaziz University
Jeddah
Saudi Arabia

Daniyal M. Alghazzawi
King Abdulaziz University
Jeddah
Saudi Arabia

Victor M.R. Penichet
University of Castilla - La Mancha
Albacete
Spain

ISSN 1865-0929   ISSN 1865-0937 (electronic)
Communications in Computer and Information Science
ISBN 978-3-662-48644-3   ISBN 978-3-662-48645-0 (eBook)
DOI 10.1007/978-3-662-48645-0

Library of Congress Control Number: 2015951800

Springer Heidelberg New York Dordrecht London
© Springer-Verlag Berlin Heidelberg 2015
This work is subject to copyright. All rights are reserved by the Publisher, whether the whole or part of the material is concerned, specifically the rights of translation, reprinting, reuse of illustrations, recitation, broadcasting, reproduction on microfilms or in any other physical way, and transmission or information storage and retrieval, electronic adaptation, computer software, or by similar or dissimilar methodology now known or hereafter developed.
The use of general descriptive names, registered names, trademarks, service marks, etc. in this publication does not imply, even in the absence of a specific statement, that such names are exempt from the relevant protective laws and regulations and therefore free for general use.
The publisher, the authors and the editors are safe to assume that the advice and information in this book are believed to be true and accurate at the date of publication. Neither the publisher nor the authors or the editors give a warranty, express or implied, with respect to the material contained herein or for any errors or omissions that may have been made.

Printed on acid-free paper

Springer-Verlag GmbH Berlin Heidelberg is part of Springer Science+Business Media
(www.springer.com)

Preface

Rehabilitation, both its motor and cognitive forms, is a complex universe, or should I say, a complex multiverse. It gathers several disciplines, a multitude of approaches, a myriad objectives, and a swarm of cultural and (pre)defined ideas and praxis. The rise of information and communication technologies (ICT) has added a new layer to this field. New exercises and new forms of interaction with the equipment, and with the caregivers, are slowly becoming an option in rehab clinics. They include motion capture, hardware and software, and 3D interactive and immersive applications that try to substitute real-life exercises in a more pleasant and motivating way.

Hardware, such as Microsoft's Kinect or Nintendo's Wii, although not designed nor developed with a rehab aim in mind, are being used since their first release, especially by research and development groups, for rehab purposes. The main reason for this rests behind the idea (or wishful thought) that motion capture could be used as a natural way to interact with the exercise.

3D worlds have long been used for clinical purposes and are a way to provide a natural and meaningful environment that intends to mimic real-life events while being fully controlled by the therapist. 3D digital environments, with or without the motion capture systems, are being developed and tested to assist patients with a wide range of disabilities. Some researchers are using virtual reality (VR) systems to help patients with chronic back pain to overcome their kinesiophobia through the manipulation of visual feedback. Others are using multilevel exercises to stimulate a wide range of cognitive functions that were compromised by acquired brain impairments. Such platforms are based on instrumental activities of daily life where the patients exercise activities, and the cognitive functions required to complete them, that they usually perform on a regular basis on a normal day. And yet others are using VR for both cognitive and motor rehab, as an attempt to offer a holistic approach that encapsulates the interdependency of motor and cognitive functionalities. The common ground of all these approaches is that they try to reduce costs and time, by working with off-the-shelf software and hardware that offer top-notch graphic and interaction quality.

Rehab is all about repetition, repetition, repetition, motivation, and feedback. Only with an almost endless repetition of the impaired functionality it is possible to totally, or partially, regain the lost function. But whereas repetition is not much of a problem for computers, in fact they are quite good at it, human beings are not that keen on repeating the same process over and over again, especially if it causes any pain or discomfort, as happens with rehab exercises. One strategy to overcome this problem is to keep the patients motivated so that they can endure the boring and repetitive process of executing the same exercise repeatedly. Another strategy is to keep the patients up to date with the success or failure of their actions, while executing the exercises. Feedback is, therefore, paramount to keep the patients in the loop of their performance.

The feedback (and monitoring) theme played a major role in REHAB 14. A majority of the papers published in this book are about ways of getting data out of the performance of the rehab exercise, so as to be used by the therapists and the patients alike. The widespread use of sensors and motion capture devices, alongside VR, helps to improve the performance through the collection and assessment of data from the exercise while it is ongoing, delivering better insight into the outcomes of the therapy.

The rest of the studies presented at REHAB 14 comprised work reporting on some of the latest advances in motor rehab. Several studies of gait and of upper limb rehab illustrate how technologies are being applied in this context. These studies reflect the mainstream use of VR for rehab purposes.

The rest of the studies were split into areas that are now emerging as clients of ICT-based rehab. Several studies of the use of VR to stimulate cognitive functioning are now available opening new possibilities for the use of VR in the context of rehab. Also, reports on the contribution of ICT on speech and navigational problems were discussed.

These examples of the studies that got podium time at Rehab 14 illustrate the overall tendency of ICT-based rehab solutions. Nevertheless, some groups are looking for additional opportunities. For example, avatars are being investigated to be used as surrogates of clinicians to help assist patients when caregivers are not around, or to train clinicians with virtual IA-enabled patients. Another trend is to couple the existing platforms with pervasive and continuous monitor valences, which are able to collect ongoing data from the patient's physiology and behavioral status. This trend also includes the use of mobile systems so that the assessment can be made anytime and anywhere.

May 2014   Habib M. Fardoun
                                                    Victor M.R. Penichet
                                                 Daniyal M. Alghazzawi

Organization

King Abdulaziz University and ISE Research group (UCLM)

Chairs and Program Co-chairs

Habib M. Fardoun	King Abdulaziz University, Saudi Arabia
Victor M.R. Penichet	University of Castilla-La Mancha, Spain
Daniyal M. Alghazzawi	King Abdulaziz University, Saudi Arabia

Organizing Committee

Pedro Gamito	COPELABS, Lusophone University, Portugal
Sergio Albiol Pérez	University of Zaragoza, Spain

Technical Coordination

D. Mª Elena de la Guia	University of Castilla-La Mancha, Spain

Program Committee

Belinda Lange	Institute for Creative Technologies, University of Southern California, USA
Willem-Paul Brinkman	Delft University of Technology, The Netherlands
Mariano Luis Alcañiz	Instituto Interuniversitario de Investigación en Bioingeniería, Spain
Beatriz Rey	Universidad Politécnica de Valencia, Spain
Christos Bouras	University of Patras, Greece
Imre Cikajlo	Univerzitetni rehabilitacijski inštitut Republike Slovenije, Slovenia
Roberto Lloréns	Instituto Interuniversitario de Investigación en Bioingeniería, Spain
José Antonio Gil	Universidad Politécnica de Valencia, Spain
Mónica Cameirão	University of Madeira, Portugal
Sergi Bermudez	University of Madeira, Portugal
Emily Keshner	Temple University, USA
Hermenegildo Gil	Universidad Politécnica de Valencia, Spain
Kjartan Halvorsen	Uppsala University, Sweden
Thalmann Daniel	University of Paul Sabatier, France
Rosa Maria E. Moreira	Universidade do Estado do Rio de Janeiro, Brasil
Georgina Cárdenas-López	Universidad Nacional Autónoma de México, Mexico

Evelyne Klinger   French National Research Agency, France
Ben Challis   Cardiff School of Creative & Cultural Industries, UK
Guillermo Palacios   University of Zaragoza, Spain

Contents

Assessing Cognitive Functions with VR-Based Serious Games that Reproduce Daily Life: Pilot Testing for Normative Values

Pedro Gamito[1,2(✉)], Jorge Oliveira[1,2], Rodrigo Brito[1,2],
Paulo Lopes[1,2], Diogo Morais[1,2], Ludmila Pinto[2], Luís Rodelo[2],
Fátima Gameiro[1,2], and Beatriz Rosa[1,2]

[1] COPELABS, Universidade Lusófona,
Edifício U, 1º Andar, 388 Campo Grande,
1749-024 Lisbon, Portugal
pedro.gamito@ulusofona.pt
[2] School of Psychology and Life Sciences,
Universidade Lusófona, Lisbon, Portugal

Abstract. Acquired brain impairments are responsible for cognitive dysfunctions that affect daily life activities. Promoting recovery via exercises stimulating cognitive functions through ecologically valid interactive media such as virtual reality (VR) is a fast-emerging option. However, assessment still relies largely on non-ecological measures such as pencil-and-paper protocols. We propose that an effective alternative to those protocols is to assess patients while they execute exercises that mimic real-life tasks in a VR scenario (e.g. shopping, dressing, or preparing breakfast). For this, normative data is required. We describe a VR scenario-based assessment tool and report a study to define normative (non-clinical sample) performance levels in daily-life exercises with that tool. We discuss the results on task performance and effects of prior experience with video-games.

Keywords: Virtual reality · Cognitive rehabilitation · Normative data

1 Introduction

Acquired brain impairments may result from a variety of causes, ranging from infectious diseases (for example, herpetic encephalitis) to traumatic brain injuries (from, e.g., motor vehicle accidents) or even substance abuse (e.g. alcohol or heroin). These often impact on cognitive functioning, including on attention, memory, and decision-making, thus compromising the regular performance of daily life activities [1–5]. The most common way to assess such deficits, as well as the impact of training, stimulation and rehabilitation programs, is through paper-and-pencil evaluation measures such as memory and attention tests. However, these tests do not reproduce people's actual daily tasks. It is quite possible that the validity of their results may be somewhat limited to performance on those specific exercises that appear in the questionnaire, and that the generalization of improved performance onto daily life functioning may be quite limited. Standardized evaluation measures that diagnose and assess the impact of

© Springer-Verlag Berlin Heidelberg 2015
H.M. Fardoun et al. (Eds.): REHAB 2014, CCIS 515, pp. 1–10, 2015.
DOI: 10.1007/978-3-662-48645-0_1

intervention programs in daily life contexts are thus required. This work is an extended version of [25] in which the descriptive data on task performance and effects of prior experience with video-games are discussed. In this chapter, we propose that a virtual reality (VR) platform where patients could fulfill daily-life activities compromised by cognitive impairments and where, at the same time, data from the performance of such activities could be drawn from, could be a viable solution for this problem [6].

VR-Based Psychological Treatments. VR, with its ability to reproduce several aspects of daily life, due to such characteristics as interactivity and immersion, has been long used as a surrogate of reality to treat anxiety disorders through exposure in a controlled and non-threatening environment, as well as to engage cognitively impaired patients in safe and appealing VR-based rehab games (for a review, see [7, 8]). These VR-based rehab games are a type of serious games (SGs), which are an offshoot of realistic videogames used for entertainment. These are called 'serious' in order to highlight their serious purposes, in contrast to games designed purely for entertainment purposes. This does not mean that the games themselves are not fun or entertaining for users. Indeed, part of their appeal lies in the fact that they share 'entertaining' features with video-games. Rather, it means that SGs use these entertaining features for training, education, health, communication, and treatment purposes [9]. VR/SG-based psychological treatments are mostly of two kinds: treatments of anxiety disorders, and cognitive rehabilitation treatments.

Typically, anxiety disorders are treated with two very different approaches: a pharmacological approach, and a cognitive-behavioral therapy approach. The pharmacological approach, in which serotonin- and serotonin-norepinephrine reuptake inhibitors are generally used as first-line agents, in conjunction with more targeted agents for second- and third-line strategies, is used for a wide variety of anxiety disorders (including panic-, social anxiety-, generalized anxiety-, posttraumatic-, and obsessive-compulsive disorders). However, many patients with anxiety disorders fail to respond adequately to these pharmacological treatments [10]. Conversely, the cognitive-behavioral approach to the treatment of anxiety disorders is based on con-fronting patients with anxiety-inducing situations but within a safe and controlled environment, thereby reeducating their erroneous beliefs about those situations by learning to dissociate those situations with negative outcomes. This can be done by imagination (following instructions to imagine a situation), by watching pictures or clips associated to the situation, or by actually reliving the situation associated to the anxiety. For example, arachnophobic patients face images of spiders or even live spiders repeatedly, until the phobic fear of spiders is abated through learned dissoci-ation between spiders and actual danger [11].

A VR/SG approach to the treatment of anxiety disorders builds on the principles of cognitive-behavioral therapy, but provides an even more controlled and safe envi-ronment, which offers patients a number of advantages of real live stimuli, without many of the drawbacks. Thus, on the one hand, patients are aware that the images are not real, therefore feeling safer than in real-life environments. However, on the other hand, the rich interactive simulation in VR produces a more life-like situation, in which patients actually participate, and thus inducing a greater degree of immersion (i.e. feeling that one is living the actual situation). Furthermore, VR tools allow therapists to develop scenarios with ecological validity (i.e. that reproduce most aspects of a type of setting that patients associate with an anxiety-inducing situation). VR/SG therapies have been successfully developed to treat a diversity of anxiety disorders. In sum, VR/SG therapies for anxiety disorders can be defined as masked exposure therapy techniques under the guise of games, with embedded features such as novelty, playfulness, control, and security. These characteristics are ideal to deliver the key therapeutic outcome of desensitization to anxiety-inducing stimuli.

VR also seems to be a viable option to conduct cognitive stimulation exercises on impaired populations [12–16]. Traditional (non-computer based) cognitive therapies involve direct interaction between therapists and patients and include direct attention training, training in metacognitive strategies to increase awareness (with feedback), visuospatial cuing for visuospatial functioning, and training in formal problem-solving abilities for remediation of executive functioning. The effects of these techniques are ambivalent. A major problem seems to be lack of generalization of specific training to daily life situations. A VR/SG approach overcomes this problem by training people directly in real-life situations.

An Argument for Extending VR Tools to Cognitive Assessment. Although VR-based solutions are often perceived as paradigmatically innovative, the assessment techniques used in VR-based interventions are still based on traditional pencil-and-paper tests. This is somehow awkward in our view. The ecological and immersive advantages of the VR applications find no correspondence in the paper-and-pencil evaluations. The common evaluation methods are focused on specific cognitive domains, which do not necessarily produce an insight on the ability of participants to maintain a functional daily life. This inability of traditional assessment methods to produce data from which daily life behavior could be inferred has been well described elsewhere [see 17, 18].

We argue here that traditional assessment methods should be complemented by approaches able to measure patients' ability to perform real life tasks rather than only improvements in pencil-and-paper exercises, in particular if the choice of cognitive rehabilitation program can be considered a surrogate of a real-life approach. In other words, the assessment strategy should follow the same principles of the rehabilitation program.

Furthermore, the digital nature of VR applications make it relatively easy to assess what is going on in the virtual world. The system can be programmed to record everything that happens: trajectories, execution times, errors, and indecisions, among many other indicators. The VR environment can be assumed to reflect in a more truthful way the actual obstacles that an impaired individual has to overcome in his/her daily routine. Improvements on indicators of overcoming these obstacles (e.g. less errors, lower execution times, less indecisions and shorter trajectories) may indicate that the cognitive functions to perform the required tasks were improved. Although it is not possible to assure the direct translation to a real world situation, improvements on VR tasks that mimic real life are probably more reliable than non-ecologically-based pencil-and-paper test results.

Establishing Normative Data with VR-Based Tools. If we assume the above, it becomes necessary, in order to develop reliable measures for VR-based cognitive rehabilitation, to establish standard values from a non-clinical population (i.e. not impaired by trauma or substance abuse) so that deviations from normal functioning can be assessed. The study reported in this paper represents this first step.

One of the first signs of cognitive decline is the difficulty in performing instrumental activities, which specifically reflects executive and memory dysfunctions [19]. Our main concern in developing a VR platform for cognitive training and assessment was therefore to create tasks that require the use of these cognitive functions during the execution of real-life activities. We thus created a number of tasks based on activities of daily living that are usually assessed with functionality self-report scales (shopping, food preparation, etc.) administered to patients or caregivers, but that not always reflect the real impairments in daily function.

These exercises were designed to not only exercise, but also to assess executive and memory dysfunctions that are often associated with loss of functional independence, such as planning and sequencing (executive functioning), working, and short-term memory abilities.

In order to be able to assess both cognitive impairments and cognitive recovery, however, we first needed to establish the normative data from non-clinical samples in performance on these tasks. Our aim was to produce normative data for the daily tasks we had created in our VR platform.

2 Method

2.1 Participants

59 participants (28 males) were recruited from the general population (universities and companies in Lisbon region, Portugal). They were asked to participate in a study designed to evaluate cognitive abilities. Their mean age was 27 yrs (SD = 10.69) and 69.5 % had previous experience in using a PC for gaming purposes. Education levels ranged from 9 years of formal education to post-graduate education, with an average of 13 years of education (SD = 2.05).

2.2 Measures

The VR application scenario consisted of several daily life activities designed to train cognitive functions. Our aim was to collect normative data concerning performance in each of the tasks. The dependent variables were based on hit rates and execution time during each of the tasks. A total execution time was also estimated as a global indicator of task performance. These data were automatically saved on a *.txt file for further analysis.

2.3 Procedure

The VR platform consisted of a small town populated with digital robots (bots). The town consisted of streets and buildings arranged in eight square blocks, along with a 2-room apartment and a mini-market in its vicinity, where participants were able to

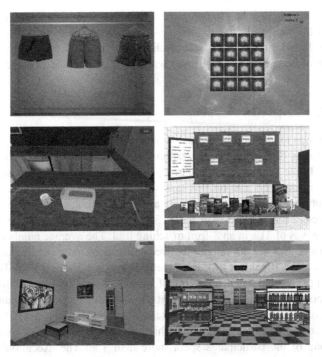

Fig. 1. Examples of the VR platform. On the top, the Wardrobe and Memory game; in the middle, the Breakfast and Virtual Kitchen; and the Recall and Shopping tasks in the bottom panel.

move freely around and to pick up objects, if they so wished (Fig. 1). The platform was developed using Unity 2.5.

Each participant underwent a short training in a 3D scenario in order to ensure a minimum ability to move around and to interact with 3D objects. After this training session, the participant's avatar was spawned in the apartment, where it had to complete a number of tasks in the following order: Wardrobe – Task 1; Memory Game – Task 2; Breakfast – Task 3; Virtual Kitchen Test – Task 4; Recall – Task 5; Shopping – Task 6. In the Wardrobe task the participants were instructed to choose 3 pieces of clothing according to their gender (e.g. shirt, pants and shoes). In the Memory Game task, a matching game, participants had to complete an 8-fruits matching trial to assess memory. In the Breakfast Preparation task the participants had to perform three movements in pre-determined order: pick up bread and butter; use a toaster; and make the movement to drink from a cup. The Virtual Kitchen Test used a 3D-kitchen scenario, which we have previously developed, and the participants' task involved planning and executing a sequence of steps in the preparation of a breakfast and the baking of a cake [20]. This task requires that the participant drag sequentially, from a kitchen cabinet, the ingredients for a cake that are displayed on a list. In the Recall Task, participants' were exposed to an LCD screen in the virtual apartment with 15 video clips of TV news. After a 60-seconds period, they were asked to recall each of the video clips. Once outside the apartment, the avatar had to find its way to the mini-market store where it had to complete a shopping task with a predefined amount of money. In the final task, the participants were instructed to buy 7 products (i.e., 1 milk bottle, 1 pack of sugar, 1 bottle of olive oil, 1 package of crackers, 1 bottle of soda, 1 bottle of beer, and 1 can of tuna) with the least possible expense (25€ max).

3 Results

Our main aim was to identify the normative values for each of the tasks: (1) Wardrobe; (2) Memory game; (3) Breakfast preparation; (4) Virtual Kitchen Test (5) Recall task; (6) Shopping. In the Wardrobe Task, participants were instructed to choose 3 pieces of clothing. The average hit rate on this task was 81.4 % for 3 correct pieces, and the average execution time was 1.02 min. Only a small percentage of participants failed to choose 3 pieces (2 pieces, 15.3 %, 1 piece, 3.4 %). In the Memory Game, the average execution time was of 31 s in an 8-fruit matching trial. The average number of attempts was 14.79 moves (SD = 2.80; ranging between 10 and 26 moves), with an average hit rate of 94.5 %. The Breakfast task took participants on average 13 s (SD = 21 s) to complete, and the Virtual Kitchen (baking of a cake) 14 s (SD = 11 s), with a hit rate of 98.3 % in choosing the required 5 ingredients. In the Recall task, participants correctly recalled an average of 7 out of 15 news items. In the shopping task, 58.5 % of the participants accomplished the main goal, which was to spend the least possible money (12.05€). None of the participants spent more than 15€. The execution time in the shopping task ranged from about 2 min to 14 min with an average of 6.9 min (SD = 3.90). The overall execution time of the aggregated tasks was on average 19.79 min (SD = 2.43) (Table 1).

Performance on each task was measured by two different variables (execution time and correct responses). In order to compute Pearson r correlations with most representative variables of each task, we chose variables more adjusted to normal distribution (i.e., skewness and kurtosis equal to < 1). Thus, the bivariate correlations were computed for execution time in the Wardrobe, Memory game, Breakfast, and Virtual Kitchen, and the Shopping task, whereas the correct responses were used for the Recall task. According to Table 2, the most significant correlations (p < .05) were obtained for the Shopping task (Task 6), that correlated positively (p < .05) with the Wardrobe, Memory game, Breakfast and Virtual Kitchen tasks. However, this task was negatively correlated with the Recall task, which was not expected because both of theses tasks were proposed for memory abilities.

Following this analysis, our intent was to study the possible influence of the sociodemographic data on each of these outcomes. Thus, Multiple Linear Regression analyses with stepwise method were carried out using 4 predictors: gender, age, education level, and video-game experience. With the exception of age, the remaining categorical variables were transformed into dummy variables with binary coding (male VS female; secondary education VS high education; without VS with video-game experience). Table 3 depicts the r² for each model and the respective standardized Beta scores for the predictors.

Regarding the Wardrobe task (Task 1) and Memory Game (Task 2), larger execution times in these tasks were predicted exclusively by the absence of video-game experience

Table 1. Descriptive data

	Min.	Max.	M	SD	Skewness	Kurtosis
Task 1 (execution time)	.3	3.51	1.02	.74	1.29	1.62
Task 1 (hits)	1	3	2.78	.49	−2.23	4.40
Task 2 (execution time)	.18	.49	.31	.07	.68	−.31
Task 2 (no. moves)	10	26	14.79	2.80	1.39	3.35
Task 2 (hits)	6	8	7.96	.27	−7.55	.57
Task 3 (execution time)	.01	1.53	.13	.21	5.34	33.45
Task 3 (hits)	3	3	3	0	–	–
Task 4 (execution time)	.03	.47	.14	.11	1.13	.83
Task 4 (hits)	4	5	4.98	.13	−7.68	.59
Task 5 (hits)	4	11	7.41	1.57	.01	−.48
Task 6 (money spent)	12.05	12.95	12.19	.22	1.49	1.76
Task 6 (execution time)	95.19	846.56	341.36	191.34	1.13	0.41
Total execution time	16.53	28.48	19.79	2.43	1.22	1.88

Legend: Task 1 – Wardrobe; Task 2 – Memory Game; Task 3 – Breakfast Preparation; Task 4 – Virtual Kitchen; Task 5 – Recall test; Test 6 – Shopping.

Table 2. Correlations among the VR-based tests

	Task 1 (execution time)	Task 2 (execution time)	Task 3 (execution time)	Task 4 (execution time)	Task 5 (hits)	Task 6 (hits)
Task 1 (execution time)	1	.48**	.30*	.53**	−29*	.63**
Task 2 (execution time)	.48**	1	.21	.33*	−.11	.47**
Task 3 (execution time)	.30*	.21	1	.23	−.09	.55**
Task 4 (execution time)	.53**	.33*	.23	1	−.23	.55**
Task 5 (hits)	−.29*	−.11	−.09	.23	1	−.26*
Task 6 (execution time)	.63**	.47**	.55**	.55**	−.26*	1

Legend: Task 1 – Wardrobe; Task 2 – Memory Game; Task 3 – Breakfast Preparation; Task 4 – Virtual Kitchen; Task 5 – Recall test; Test 6 – Shopping. (** $p < .01$; * $p < .05$)

(both Beta scores are positive: .49 and .30, respectively). As for the Breakfast Preparation in the VR (Task 3), the best predictors of execution times were absence of video-game experience (B = .34), age (B = .41) and secondary education (B = .29). These Beta scores were positive which indicates that absence of video game experience, age and secondary education predicted larger execution times in this task. In the Kitchen Test (Task 4), execution times were predicted negatively by previous video-game

Table 3. Multivariate linear regression analysis for eachVR-based test

DVs	Adjusted r2	Predictors	β
Task 1 (execution time)	.23	Absence of VGE	.49
Task 2 (execution time)	.07	Absence of VGE	.30
Task 3 (execution time)	.23	Absence of VGE Age Secondary ed.	.34 .41 .29
Task 4 (execution time)	0.24	VGE	−.33
Task 5 (hits)	–	–	–
Task 6 (execution time)	0.17	Absence of VGE Age	.54 .23

Legend: Task 1 – Wardrobe; Task 2 – Memory Game; Task 3 – Breakfast Preparation; Task 4 – Virtual Kitchen; Task 5 – Recall test; Test 6 – Shopping; VGE – Video game experience.

experience (B = −.33). In this sense, higher video-game experience predicted shorter execution times in this task. On the other hand, no significant predictors were found for hits in the Recall task (Task 5), whereas execution time in the Shopping task (Task 6) was also predicted by the absence of video-game experience (B = .53) and age (B = .23). These variables were associated with larger execution times in the Shopping task.

4   Conclusion

The aim of this study was to evaluate a set of cognitive exercises for neuropsychological assessment and rehabilitation and to produce normative data for these measures. Our assessment was based on the performance on several daily life tasks from a VR-based serious games approach designed to improve specific cognitive abilities and overall functionality in patients with cognitive impairments. The overall results of a descriptive analysis showed no floor or ceiling effects in each of the tasks performed, which supports the suitability of the tasks. The linear regressions indicated that the execution of these tasks in a VR setup is affected mainly by previous computer experience. Even with an initial session of training, most of the dependent measures were influenced by video-game practice. This result suggests previous video-game experience is an important confounder of task execution in VR-based setups and would suggest a distinction in normative values as a function of video-game practice. On the other hand, the lack of influence of education on task execution measures is also interesting and suggests these exercises are robust measures not affected by education level, which is not the case of the validated traditional paper-and-pencil tests [21–24]. It is worth noting, however, that sample size and sample characteristics may have limited these results. Although we found no impact of age and education, larger and more representative samples, in particular with a broader range of age and education levels, would give us more solid evidence for older and less educated populations.

Acknowledgments. We would like thank the technicians involved in the development of the VR applications: Felipe Picareli, Marcelo Matias and Filipa Barata.

References

1. Hoffmann, M.: Higher cortical function deficits after stroke: an analysis of 1,000 patients from a dedicated cognitive stroke registry. Neurorehabil. Neural Repair. **15**(2), 113–127 (2001)
2. Connor, B., Wing, A.M., Humphreys, G.W., Bracewell, R.M., Harvey, A.: Errorless learning using haptic guidance: research in cognitive rehabilitation following stroke. In: Proceedings of the 4th International Conference on Disability Virtual Reality & Associated Technology, The University of Reading, Hungary, p. 77, 18–20 Sept 2002
3. Moselhy, H.F.: Frontal lobe changes in alcoholism: a review of the literature. Alcohol Alcohol. **32**, 357–368 (2001)
4. Oscar-Berman, M., Marinkovic, K.: Alcohol: effects on neurobehavioral functions and the brain. Neuropsychol. Rev. **17**, 239–257 (2007)
5. Gruber, S.A., Silveri, M.M., Yurgelun-Todd, D.A.: Neuropsychological consequences of opiate use. Neuropsychol. Rev. **17**, 299–315 (2007)
6. Pugnetti, L., Mendozzi, L., Attree, E., Barbieri, E., Brooks, B., Cazzullo, C.L., Motta, A., Rose, F.D.: Probing memory and executive functions with virtual reality: past and present studies. CyberPsychol. Behav. **1**(2), 151–161 (1998)
7. Rizzo, A., Buckwalter, J.G.: Virtual reality and cognitive assessment and rehabilitation: the state of the art. Stud. Health Technol. Inform. **44**, 123–145 (1997)
8. Gamito, P., Oliveira, J., Morais, D., Rosa, P., Saraiva, T.: Serious games for serious problems: from Ludicus to Therapeuticus. In: Kim, J.J. (ed.) Virtual Reality, pp. 527–548. InTech Publishing, Croatia (2011). doi:10.5772/12870
9. Zyda, M.: From visual simulation to virtual reality to games. Computer **38**(9), 25–32 (2005)
10. Ravindran, L.N., Stein, M.B.: The pharmacological treament of anxiety disorders: a review of progress. J. Psychiatry **71**(7), 839–854 (2010)
11. Garcia-Palacios, A., Hoffman, H.G., Carlin, A., Furness, T.A., Botella, C.: Virtual reality in the treatment of spider phobia: a controlled study. Behav. Res. Ther. **40**, 983–993 (2001)
12. Gamito, P., Oliveira, J., Lopes, P., Morais, D., Brito, R., Saraiva, T., Bastos, M., Cristóvão, S., Caçôete, C., Picareli, F.: Assessment of frontal brain functions in alcoholics following a health mobile cognitive stimulation approach. Stud. Health Technol. Inf. **191**, 110–114 (2013)
13. Gamito, P., Oliveira, J., Pacheco, J., Morais, D., Saraiva, T., Lacerda, R., Baptista, A., Santos, N., Soares, F., Gamito, L., Rosa, P.: Traumatic brain injury memory training: a virtual reality online solution. Int. J. Disabil. Hum. Dev. **10**(2), 309–315 (2011)
14. Lange, B., Requejo, P., Flynn, S., Rizzo, A., Valero-Cuevas, F., Baker, L., Winstein, C.: The potential of virtual reality and gaming to assist successful aging with disability. Phys. Med. RehabilClin. N. Am. **21**(2), 339–356 (2010)

15. Zhang, L., Abreu, B., Seale, G., Masel, B., Chrisiansen, C., Ottenbacher, K.: A virtual reality environment for the evaluation of a daily living skill in brain injury rehabilitation: reliability and validity. Arch. Phys. Med. Rehabil. **84**, 1118–1124 (2003)

16. Edmans, J., Gladman, J., Hilton, D., Walker, M., Sunderland, A., Cobb, S., Pridmore, T., Thomas, S.: Clinical evaluation of a non-immersive virtual environment in stroke rehabilitation. Clin. Rehabil. **23**, 106–116 (2009)

17. Chaytor, N., Schmitter-Edgecombe, M.: The ecological validity of neuropsychological tests: a review of the literature on everyday cognitive skills. Neuropsychol. Rev. **13**(4), 181–197 (2003)

18. Spooner, D., Pachana, N.: Ecological validity in neuropsychological assessment: a case for greater consideration in research with neurologically intact populations. Arch. Clin. Neuropsychol. **21**, 327–337 (2006)

19. Soto, M.E., Vellas, B.: Medical factors interfering with competence in dementia. In: Stoppe, G. (ed.) Competence Assessment in Dementia 2008, pp. 35–40. Springer, NewYork (2008)

20. Oliveira, J., Gamito, P., Morais, D., Brito, R., Lopes, P., Norberto, L.: Cognitive assessment of stroke patients with mobile apps: a controlled study. Stud. Health Technol. Inform. **199**, 103–107 (2014)

21. Saykin, A.J., Gur, R.C., Gur, R.E., Shtasel, D.L., Flannery, K.A., Mozley, L.H., Malamut, B.L., Watson, B., Mozley, P.D.: Normative neuropsychological test performance: effects of age, education, gender and ethnicity. Appl. Neuropsychol. **2**(2), 79–88 (1995)

22. Manly, J.J., Jacobs, D.M., Sano, M., Bell, K., Merchant, C.A., Small, S.A., Stern, Y.: Effect of literacy on neuropsychological test performance in nondemented, education-matched elders. J. Int. Neuropsychol. Soc. **5**(3), 191–202 (1999)

23. Wiederholt, W.C., Cahn, D., Butters, N.M., Salmon, D.P., Kritz-Silverstein, D., Barrett-Connor, E.: Effects of age, gender and education on selected neuropsychological tests in an elderly community cohort. J. Am. Geriatr. Soc. **41**(6), 639–647 (1993)

24. Ostrosky-Solís, F., Ramirez, M., Ardila, A.: Effects of culture and education on neuropsychological testing: a preliminary study with indigenous and nonindigenous population. Appl. Neuropsychol. **11**(4), 186–193 (2004)

25. Gamito, P., Oliveira, J., Pinto, L., Rodelo, L., Lopes, P., Brito, R., Morais, D.: Normative data for a cognitive VR rehab serious games-based approach. In: Proceedings of the 8th International Conference on Pervasive Computing Technologies for Healthcare (PervasiveHealth '14). ICST (Institute for Computer Sciences, Social-Informatics and Telecommunications Engineering), ICST, Brussels, Belgium, pp. 443–446 (2014). http://dx.doi.org/10.4108/icst.pervasivehealth.2014.255277, doi:10.4108/icst.pervasivehealth.2014.255277

Validation of the Balance Board™ for Clinical Evaluation of Balance Through Different Conditions

Bruno Bonnechère[1,2(✉)], Bart Jansen[3,4], Lubos Omelina[3,5],
Marcel Rooze[1], and Serge Van Sint Jan[1,2]

[1] Laboratory of Anatomy, Biomechanics and Organogenesis (LABO),
Université Libre de Bruxelles,
Lennik Street 808, CP 610, 1070 Brussels, Belgium
bbonnech@ulb.ac.be
[2] Faculty of Medicine, Center for Functional Evaluation,
Université Libre de Bruxelles, Brussels, Belgium
[3] Department of Electronics and Informatics – ETRO,
Vrije Universiteit Brussel,
Pleinlaan 2, 1050 Brussels, Belgium
[4] Department of Future Health, iMinds,
Gaston Crommenlaan 8,
Box 102, 9050 Ghent, Belgium
[5] Institute of Computer Science and Mathematics,
Slovak University of Technology,
Bratislava, Slovakia

Abstract. The quantitative assessment of balance still needs to be performed in a laboratory equipped with force plates because there is, currently, no other validated tool available. The Wii Balance Board™ (WBB) could be used as a portable, easy-to-use and inexpensive tool to assess balance. Before being used in clinics such kind of tool must go through an important validation process. In clinics not only the total displacement of Center of Pressure (CP) is relevant but other parameters can be derived from CP. The aim of this study was to validate the use of the WBB, compared to FP, in different balance testing conditions (standing and sitting) for multiple parameters derived from CP displacement (CP velocities, area of 95 % prediction ellipse, dispersion of CP from the mean position…). Fifteen subjects participated in this study and performed a combination of single and double legs standing balance tests and a sitting balance test. Bland and Altman plots, paired-sample T-Tests and Pearson's coefficient correlations were computed. For the nine studied parameters excellent correlations were found for each different task (mean correlation = 0.97). Unlike previous work on the WBB these excellent results were obtained without using any calibration procedure. Therefore, the WBB could be used in clinics to assess balance through different conditions.

Keywords: Balance · Force plate · Biomechanics · Motor control

© Springer-Verlag Berlin Heidelberg 2015
H.M. Fardoun et al. (Eds.): REHAB 2014, CCIS 515, pp. 11–23, 2015.
DOI: 10.1007/978-3-662-48645-0_2

1   Introduction

The evaluation of balance and postural control is an important field in various domains such as health (e.g. preventions of falls in elderly people) [1], rehabilitation (e.g. balance training after stroke) [2] and sports (e.g. to increase athlete's performance or decrease injuries' risk) [3]. Even though this wide potential field of application, it appears that balance assessment using a force plate (FP) (i.e., during quantitative functional evaluation) in laboratory is not as used as it should be in clinics for patients' evaluation or follow up [4]. Despite this the measurement of the center of pressure (CP) using FP is considered as gold standard to assess balance [5]. This is probably due to the fact FPs are, most of the time, not transportable due to their embedment in the laboratory floor. Their relatively high price is also probably blocking their widespread use outside the laboratory. Access to this kind of tool is therefore limited and does not allow regular measurement for patient follow up or evaluation of a treatment if a specially-equipped laboratory is not available. In daily clinics evaluation of balance is performed using scales such as the qualitative Berg Balance Scale [6]. Despite the fact that these scales have been validated for various neurological conditions [7] they are not sensitive enough to detect small clinically relevant changes [6]. There is thus a need in clinics for portable, easy to use and cost-effective quantitative balance assessment tools. The Wii Balance Board™ (WBB) (Nintendo®, Kyoto, Japan), originally developed for video game control using CP displacements, meets the above criteria. Before being used in clinics such kind of devices must go through a strict validation process. Several works have been done to validate the WBB: estimation of CP path length during standing [8, 9] and force estimation [11]. In clinics, the WBB has been used to assess patients suffering from various diseases such as Parkinson's disease [12] or other conditions as for instance anterior cruciate ligaments injuries [13], and with elderly patients [14, 15]. The scope of these previous studies [8, 9, 12–14] was limited to the analysis of the CP path length during various conditions (double and single limb standing, eyes open or closed, simple or double tasks). However, more reliable and clinically-relevant parameters, such as the Total Mean Velocity (TMV), can be obtained from CP data [16]. The above studies are using a force calibration procedure prior to measurement. An important question that still needs to be answered is whether such a kind of calibration procedure is required in order to get clinically-meaningful results with the WBB. To the best of our best knowledge, no study has evaluated the possibility of the WBB for assessing posture in sitting position, although the study of postural control of patients unable to stand (e.g. paraplegia patients) is clinically of interest [17].

This paper is a complement to a publication presented in the workshop of the 8th International Conference on Pervasive Computing Technologies for Healthcare (PervasiveHealth '14) on the use of serious games to improve balance of cerebral palsy children [18].

The aim of this study was to validate a broad range of parameters derived from CP using the WBB without any calibration to assess posture during several conditions including sitting position what has, to our best knowledge, never been done in previous studies.

2 Material and Method

2.1 Participants

Fifteen young healthy adults (age = 24 (2) years, height = 172 (12) cm, weight = 66 (12) kg, 4 women) participated in this study. This study was approved by the Ethical Committee of the Erasme Hospital (CCB: B406201215142) and written informed consent was obtained from all subjects prior to their participation. No participants presented any neurological or orthopedic disorders and none of the subjects was taking medication at the time of the study that may have influenced balance or posture.

2.2 Procedures

A WBB (size 45 cm × 26.5 cm) was placed on the top of FP (AMTI model OR6-6, Watertown, MA, U.S.A., size 50 cm × 46 cm) that was embedded within the laboratory floor. This setting allows simultaneous measurement in order to eliminate bias introduced by subject variability if measurements were performed sequentially [9]. The WBB was connected to a laptop (Intel Core I5, Windows 7, 6 GB RAM) via Bluetooth connection, data were retrieved using a custom-written software based on the wiimotelib software [10]. WBB and FP data collection frequency were 100 Hz and 1000 Hz, respectively. The FP was calibrated before measurement. For the WBB no calibration procedure was used although some methods have been proposed [8, 9, 12–14]. Such calibration-free methodology was adopted because one of the purposes of this study was to evaluate the clinical WWB usability without the practical constraint of systematic calibration.

Participants performed a series of twelve balance tasks in a single session distributed as follows: three repetitions of double limb standing in the middle of the WBB (experimental condition called "Standing" in this study), four repetitions of double limb standing on four different locations on the WBB surface (right, left, front and back sides) ("Positions"), two repetitions of single limb standing (right and left respectively) ("Single Leg") and three repetitions of sitting in the middle of the WBB ("Sitting"). All these repetitions were performed eyes open. Subjects were instructed to stand as still as possible, arms aligned along the body and the eyes fixing a target on the wall in front of them (distance = 2.5 m, height = 1.8 m). The optimal trial duration during balance analysis is still controversial. To assess the body sway in adults 30 s was previously recommended [19]. Data were thus collected during 30 s for each trial. Multiple repetitions were asked in order to fight against inter-trial variability (e.g. positions of the foot on the WBB…).

2.3 Data Processing

Data processing was done using a custom-made Matlab code (The Mathworks, Natick, RI, USA) based on [22]. Previous works have shown that the time interval between samples of WBB were inconsistent [9] therefore linear interpolation of the raw signals of WBB sensors was applied to get a regular sample rate of 1000 Hz [20]. Both data from WBB and FP were then filtered using a second order Butterworth low-pass filter with a cutoff frequency of 12 Hz [8, 9]. For WBB CP, anterior-posterior (CP AP) and medio-lateral (CP ML) displacements were obtained from the 4 four strain gauge loads located at the four corners of the plate using Eqs. 1 and 2 respectively:

$$CPap = FL - PL + PR \tag{1}$$

$$CPml = PL - PR + PR + FL + FR \tag{2}$$

Where PL, PR, FL and FR are the force values from the posterior left, posterior right, anterior left and anterior right WBB sensors respectively [8].

For the FP, CP AP and CP ML displacements were obtained using Eqs. 3 and 4 respectively [21]:

$$CPap = \frac{-5.5 \times Fy - Mx}{Fz} \tag{3}$$

$$CPml = \frac{-5.5 \times Fx + My}{Fz} \tag{4}$$

CP was analyzed during 20 s (between the 5th and the 25th s of each trial).

Most of the papers comparing WBB and FP are only focusing on the total length of CP displacement during the trial [6–12] to analyze balance instability. In this paper, supplementary variables were processed from the available CP data [22]: - the total displacement of sway (DOT); - the area of the 95 % prediction ellipse (often referred to as the 95 % confidence ellipse [23, 24]) (Area); - the dispersion of CP displacement from the mean position (SD ap and SD ml); - the distance between the maximum and minimum CP displacement (AdCP ap and AdCP ml); - the mean velocity of CP displacement (MV ap and MV ml); - and the AP and ML displacements of the total CP sway divided by the total duration of the trial (TMV).

In summary, this study computed 9 variables from the data captured in four different conditions (i.e., "Standing", "Positions", etc.) resulting in 36 features to be compared between WBB and FP.

2.4   Statistical Analysis

Several statistical tests were performed as follows. All dependent variables were normally distributed (Kolmogorov-Smirnov test); therefore parametric tests were applied. For every parameter Pearson's correlation coefficients (R), a two-way - random effects - single measure (mean of the trials) intra-class correlation coefficient (ICC) [25] and paired-sampled t-test were computed. Agreement between both devices was examined using Bland and Altman (B&A) plots [26]. After correlation analysis, linear regressions were used to correct results of WBB based on FP data (regression equations are available from Fig. 1); a leave-one-out method was used to evaluate these equations [27]. Those corrected WBB results were compared with FP using paired-sampled t-test,

Pearson's correlation and the normalized root-mean square error ($NRMSE = \frac{RMSE}{(WBB+FP)/2} \times 100$). All statistical analysis was conducted using Matlab.

3 Results

Table 1 presents the mean results and statistics of the variables for the four different conditions before applying regressions on WBB data. Linear regression equations and correlations for the four conditions are presented in Fig. 1. Bland & Altman plots are presented in Fig. 2. In order to avoid any bias, due to the fact that for some conditions four trials were recorded and for others one only two, mean values of the conditions were plotted.

Only 4 out of the 36 variables studied did not present statistically significant differences between WBB and FP (paired sampled t-test). However, high correlations were found for every parameter: mean R values were 0.97 for total results (not taking into account the task performed) and 0.92, 0.90, 0.79 and 0.89 for Standing, Single leg, Sitting and Positions respectively.

Those high correlations allow correcting results of the WBB in order to have similar results as those obtained with FP. Equations used to correct these results and codes to calculate these variables in Matlab are presented in Table 2. Results before and after corrections (using leave-one-out method) are presented in Table 3. After correction mean values were similar for correlation (R = 0.97 and 0.96 before and after regression, respectively), very highly significantly increase for P-value (p < 0.001 before and p = 0.97 after regressions) and the NRMSE is decreased from 25 to 20 %. Results for the different conditions are presented in Table 4.

4 Discussion

Our results are comparable with previous studies concerning CP path length (DOT) in standing position. We also found good correspondence (mean R values = 0.97) between results obtained with WBB and FP in standing positions (double or single leg stance) [8, 9, 12]. Additional to DOT we computed 8 variables that are clinically relevant for posture analysis. According to the FP literature, approximately 40 parameters can be derived from CP including the mean velocity that is considered as the variable offering the highest reliability among different trials [16]. Another FP-based study underlined the importance of the speed by reporting that peak velocity showed the highest reliability [28]. One previous study has shown that WBB and FP show similar results for CP path velocity during single or double legs stance [9]. In this study, the highest correlations were found for TMV during Standing and Single leg compared to correlation for DOT (ICC = 0.96 and R = 0.86 for Standing, ICC = 0.96 and R = 0.92 for Single leg) (values obtained before regression correction, see Table 1). Sitting correlation was found higher for DOT (R = 0.88) than for TMV (R = 0.78). Measurement of velocity of the displacement of CP during single or double legs stance have been found comparable with WBB and FP, similar results were found after

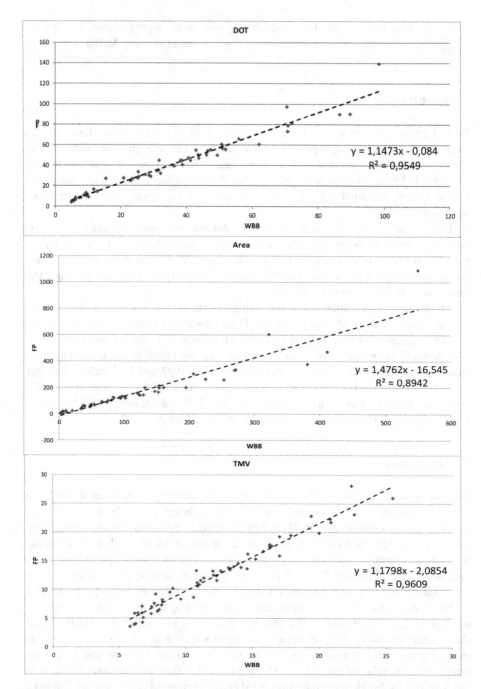

Fig. 1. Scatter plots, correlation lines and equations for three features (DOT, Area and TMV). For each of the four conditions, the mean value over the different conditions was plotted (4 conditions × 15 subjects).

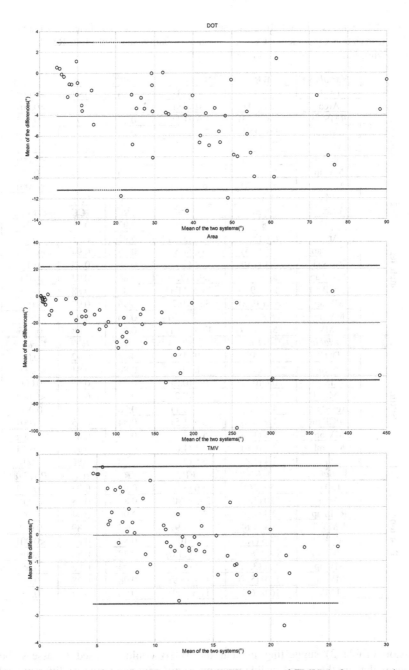

Fig. 2. Bland & Altman plots for three features (DOT, Area and TMV) before regression. For each different condition the mean values were computed (4 × 15 = 60 trials). Red lines (middle one) represent the mean difference between the devices. Blue lines (extremities) indicate upper and lower agreements (1.96 SD).

Table 1. Mean (std) results for the processed variable, Pearson's coefficient correlation (R), IntraClass Correlation Coefficient (ICC) and P-value of paired-sampled t-test. Results obtained before applying linear regression on the WBB results.

	Variable	WBB	FP	R	ICC	P-value
Standing	DOT	32 (11)	37 (13)	0.86	0.92	<0.001
	Area	64 (34)	81 (38)	0.95	0.97	<0.001
	RMS ap	1.4 (0.63)	1.6 (0.74)	0.95	0.97	<0.001
	RMS sl	2.6 (0.84)	3.0 (0.91)	0.84	0.91	<0.001
	AdCP ap	7.2 (3.2)	8.4 (3.7)	0.92	0.95	<0.001
	AdCP ml	12.1 (3.8)	13.8 (4.1)	0.87	0.93	<0.001
	MV ap	6.3 (1.9)	5.9 (3.1)	0.96	0.93	0.07
	MV ml	8.0 (2.4)	8.5 (2.7)	0.96	0.98	<0.001
	TMV	11.3 (3.3)	11.6 (4.5)	0.96	0.96	0.2
	Variable	*WBB*	*FP*	*R*	*ICC*	*P-value*
Single leg	DOT	118 (29)	125 (31)	0.92	0.96	0.004
	Area	730 (333)	828 (378)	0.91	0.95	0.003
	RMS ap	5.5 (1.5)	6.0 (1.5)	0.89	0.94	<0.001
	RMS sl	7.1 (1.9)	7.4 (2.1)	0.88	0.93	0.14
	AdCP ap	26.6 (7.1)	29.3 (7.3)	0.86	0.92	<0.001
	AdCP ml	35.1 (9.3)	36.2 (11.1)	0.80	0.88	0.39
	MV ap	31.1 (9.3)	32.9 (9.7)	0.96	0.97	0.002
	MV ml	26.8 (7.8)	27.7 (7.9)	0.96	0.97	0.06
	TMV	45.1 (12.7)	47.3 (13.1)	0.96	0.98	0.005
	Variable	*WBB*	*FP*	*R*	*ICC*	*P-value*
Sitting	DOT	8 (3)	9 (4)	0.88	0.92	<0.001
	Area	5 (5)	8 (9)	0.80	0.81	<0.001
	RMS ap	0.8 (0.5)	0.9 (0.5)	0.74	0.85	0.006
	RMS sl	0.4 (0.2)	0.4 (0.2)	0.90	0.92	<0.001
	AdCP ap	4.7 (2.7)	5.8 (3.1)	0.70	0.82	0.004
	AdCP ml	1.9 (0.9)	2.6 (1.5)	0.84	0.85	<0.001
	MV ap	5.9 (1.7)	5.1 (2.1)	0.79	0.87	<0.001
	MV ml	3.2 (0.6)	3.1 (1.0)	0.66	0.72	<0.001
	TMV	7.4 (1.8)	6.5 (2.4)	0.78	0.86	0.001
	Variable	*WBB*	*FP*	*R*	*ICC*	*P-value*
Positions	DOT	59 (26)	66 (32)	0.92	0.95	<0.001
	Area	220 (187)	292 (290)	0.88	0.88	0.001
	RMS ap	2.9 (1.5)	3.3 (1.8)	0.90	0.94	<0.001
	RMS sl	3.8 (1.6)	4.2 (1.9)	0.83	0.89	0.004
	AdCP ap	14.3 (7.3)	17.3 (10.8)	0.82	0.86	<0.001
	AdCP ml	18.9 (8.4)	21.5 (11.0)	0.78	0.86	0.008
	MV ap	9.3 (3.7)	9.4 (4.8)	0.94	0.96	0.65
	MV ml	11.9 (5.3)	12.6 (5.9)	0.96	0.98	0.01
	TMV	16.9 (6.6)	17.5 (7.9)	0.96	0.97	0.08

regression (Table 3) suggesting us that the WBB could be used to assess these parameters that are the more sensible to compare different age group or different health conditions [29]. Unlike the other previous studies, no calibration procedure was used before measurements. However, results were highly correlated using directly the WBB without any previous step. In order to get similar results with WBB and FP regression equations, were directly integrated into the code used to process these variables from

Table 2. Variables obtained from CP and codes, including correction by regression, to calculate these variables in MATLAB (adapted from [22]). Before using these codes the tendency of the CP signal must be removed (using "detrend" function).

	Code	Regression
DOT	`DOT = sum(sqrt(CPap.^2 + CPml.^2)`	1.1473*DOT-0.084
Area	`[vec,val] = eig(cov(CPap,CPml));` `Area = pi * prod(2.4478 * sqrt(svd(val)))`	1.4762*Area-16.545
RMS ap	`RMSap = sqrt(sum(CPap.^2) / length` `(CPap))`	1.149*RMS ap +0.0196
RMS sl	`RMSml = sqrt(sum(CPml.^2) / length` `(CPml))`	1.1289*RMS ml +0.0255
AdCP ap	`AdCPap = max(CPap) - min(CPap)`	1.2667*AdCP ap-0.7107
AdCP ml	`AdCPml = max(CPml) - min(CPml)`	1.1464*AdCP ml-0.03
MV ap	`MVap = sum(abs(diff(CPap))) * freq /` `length(CPap)`	1.2533*MV ap-2.1774
MV ml	`MVml = sum(abs(diff(CPml))) * freq /` `length(CPml)`	1.1104*MV ml-0.5389
TMV	`TMV = sum(sqrt(diff(CPap).^2 + diff` `(CPml).^2)) * freq / length(CPap)`	1.1798*TMV-2.0854

Table 3. Mean (std) differences (WBB-FP), Pearson's coefficient correlation, P-value of paired-sample t-test and NRMSE for the different variables before and after correction of the WBB results using linear regression.

	PRE				POST			
	Diff.	R	P	NRMSE	Diff.	R	P	NRMSE
DOT	−5 (7)	0.98	<.001	22	0 (6)	0.97	.97	16
Area	−34 (80)	0.95	.002	69	−1 (73)	0.92	.88	51
RMS ap	−0.3 (0.3)	0.98	<.001	21	0 (0.2)	0.97	.99	14
RMS ml	−0.3 (0.5)	0.96	<.001	23	0 (0.5)	0.96	.96	19
AdCPap	−1.7 (2.3)	0.96	<.001	28	0 (1.9)	0.95	.98	19
AdCPml	−1.7 (3.1)	0.95	<.001	27	0 (3.0)	0.94	.98	24
MV ap	0.3 (1.1)	0.96	.02	15	0 (0.9)	0.96	.97	12
MV ml	−0.4 (0.9)	0.99	.003	11	0 (0.8)	0.98	.99	10
TMV	−0.1 (1.4)	0.98	0.52	12	0 (1.2)	0.98	.98	10
MEAN	/	0.97	<.001	25	/	0.96	.97	20

CP. This approach is hence more user-friendly compared to an approach where a calibration procedure is required prior to the use of the WBB.

The use of the WBB to assess balance in sitting position was not tested before despite the fact that the quantitative evaluation of sitting balance is being studied for patients that cannot stand (independently) [17]. Results of our study suggest that the

Table 4. Pearson's coefficient correlation, P-value of paired-sample t-test and NRMSE for the different variables after correction of the WBB results.

	Variable	R	P-value	NRMSE
Standing	DOT	0.85	0.97	20
	Area	0.95	0.97	17
	RMS ap	0.95	0.92	15
	RMS sl	0.82	0.99	18
	AdCP ap	0.91	0.93	19
	AdCP ml	0.86	0.97	16
	MV ap	0.96	0.95	15
	MV ml	0.95	0.98	10
	TMV	0.95	0.97	12
	Variable	**R**	**P-value**	**NRMSE**
Single	DOT	0.91	0.93	11
	Area	0.90	0.93	21
	RMS ap	0.87	0.93	13
	RMS sl	0.86	0.88	15
	AdCP ap	0.81	0.82	15
	AdCP ml	0.77	0.96	19
	MV ap	0.95	0.92	10
	MV ml	0.95	0.97	9
	TMV	0.95	0.93	9
	Variable	**R**	**P-value**	**NRMSE**
Sitting	DOT	0.87	0.95	25
	Area	0.72	0.97	92
	RMS ap	0.68	0.86	44
	RMS sl	0.85	0.92	33
	AdCP ap	0.64	0.93	47
	AdCP ml	0.82	0.90	37
	MV ap	0.76	0.84	25
	MV ml	0.65	0.97	23
	TMV	0.75	0.84	23
	Variable	**R**	**P-value**	**NRMSE**
Positions	DOT	0.92	0.97	21
	Area	0.86	0.95	59
	RMS ap	0.89	0.99	27
	RMS sl	0.81	0.97	28
	AdCP ap	0.80	0.98	40
	AdCP ml	0.75	0.98	35
	MV ap	0.94	0.99	17
	MV ml	0.96	0.98	14
	TMV	0.95	0.99	14

WBB provides results that are correlated with results of the FP even if those correlations are lower than for standing conditions (R = 0.79 compared to R = 0.92 for double legs and R = 0.90 for single legs). This lower correlation could be due to the hardware configuration of the WBB, as it is composed of four strain gauge load sensors.

A previous study has estimated dead weight noise and how this noise can affect the measurements [30]. The same study suggested that the noise can be increased when CP velocities are low [30]. Our results obtained in the sitting condition confirm this; the WBB seems less sensitive when CP amplitudes and velocities are low.

Due to the hardware configuration and the low price of the WBB it might be expected that the position of the subject relative to the sensors could influence the results. Subjects were asked to stand at the four extreme positions of the WBB, results were compared to FP and expressed in percentage (100 % is the results of FP). An ANOVA was applied to compare differences between WBB and FP for the four positions and the position in the middle of the WBB. No difference was found for the five positions. A graphical representation of these results is presented in Fig. 3. It is interesting to note that for the different positions CP displacements are higher than for the centered positions. Since these results are higher for both WBB and FP we can assume that it is not due to the WBB. These results are probably due to the fact that when the subject is standing at the side of the WBB, his balance is less stable, inducing an increase in the base of support. In clinics it is not possible to ensure that all subjects always stand on exactly the same spot on the balance board, but it is expected that subjects stand more or less in the middle of the WBB. Our results show that small position changes on the WBB do not influence the results.

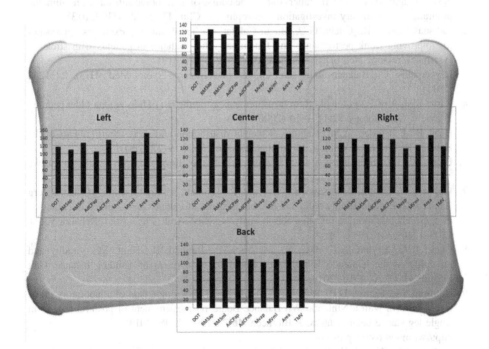

Fig. 3. Influence of the position of the body related to the WBB on the results. Results of the WBB are expressed in percentage of FP's value. No significant statistical difference was found between the different positions (ANOVA).

5 Conclusion

This study confirms the good results previously presented of the WBB compared to gold standard laboratory FP. This study provides relevant additional data. The first aspect is that it is not required to perform any calibration procedure prior to using the WBB to assess balance. Instead of a calibration procedure we directly applied regression equations within the code used to provide clinical parameters derived from CP displacement. The WBB provides comparable data for displacements and velocities derived from CP in standing (double or single legs) and sitting positions. The position of the subject relative to the WBB does not have influence on the results. Therefore the WBB can be used to assess and to follow in a quick and inexpensive way the patients' evolution.

Acknowledgments. This study is a part of the ICT4Rehab project and RehabGoesHome (www. ict4rehab.org). Those projects are funded by Innoviris (Brussels Capital Region).

References

1. Carette, P., Kemoun, G., Watelain, E., Dugué, B.: Concomitant changes in clinical and posturographic data in elderly fallers during the course of an in-home anti-falling multimodal program - a preliminary investigation. Neurophysiol. Clin. **43**(4), 229–236 (2013)
2. Cabanas-Valdés, R., Cuchi, G.U., Bagur-Calafat, C.: Trunk training exercises approaches for improving trunk performance and functional sitting balance in patients with stroke: a systematic review. NeuroRehabilitation **33**(4), 572–592 (2013)
3. Hrysomallis, C.: Balance ability and athletic performance. Sports Med. **41**(3), 221–232 (2011)
4. Piirtola, M., Era, P.: Force platform measurements as predictors of falls among older people - a review. Gerontology **52**(1), 1–16 (2006)
5. Haas, B.M., Burden, A.M.: Validity of weight distribution and sway measurements of the Balance Performance Monitor. Physiother. Res. Int. **5**(1), 19–32 (2000)
6. Blum, L., Korner-Bitensky, N.: Usefulness of the Berg Balance Scale in stroke rehabilitation: a systematic review. Phys. Ther. **88**(5), 559–566 (2008)
7. La Porta, F., Caselli, S., Susassi, S., Cavallini, P., Tennant, A., Franceschini, M.: Is the Berg Balance Scale an internally valid and reliable measure of balance across different etiologies in neurorehabilitation? a revisited Rasch analysis study. Arch. Phys. Med. Rehabil. **93**(7), 1209–1216 (2012)
8. Clark, R.A., Bryant, A.L., Pua, Y., McCrory, P., Bennell, K., Hunt, M.: Validity and reliability of the Nintendo Wii Balance Board for assessment of standing balance. Gait Posture **31**(3), 307–310 (2010)
9. Huurnink, A., Fransz, D.P., Kingma, I., van Dieën, J.H.: Comparison of a laboratory grade force platform with a Nintendo Wii Balance Board on measurement of postural control in single-leg stance balance tasks. J. Biomech. **46**(7), 1392–1395 (2013)
10. http://wiimotelib.codeplex.com
11. Bartlett, H.L., Ting, L.H., Bingham, J.T.: Accuracy of force and center of pressure measures of the Wii Balance Board. Gait Posture **39**(1), 224–228 (2014)
12. Holmes, J.D., Jenkins, M.E., Johnson, A.M., Hunt, M.A., Clark, R.A.: Validity of the Nintendo Wii® balance board for the assessment of standing balance in Parkinson's disease. Clin. Rehabil. **27**(4), 361–366 (2013)

13. Howells, B.E., Clark, R.A., Ardern, C.L., Bryant, A.L., Feller, J.A., Whitehead, T.S., Webster, K.E.: The assessment of postural control and the influence of a secondary task in people with anterior cruciate ligament reconstructed knees using a Nintendo Wii Balance Board. Br. J. Sports Med. **47**(14), 914–919 (2013)

14. Koslucher, F., Wade, M.G., Nelson, B., Lim, K., Chen, F.C., Stoffregen, T.A.: Nintendo Wii Balance Board is sensitive to effects of visual tasks on standing sway in healthy elderly adults. Gait Posture **36**(3), 605–608 (2012)

15. Young, W., Ferguson, S., Brault, S., Craig, C.: Assessing and training standing balance in older adults: a novel approach using the 'Nintendo Wii' Balance Board. Gait Posture **33**(2), 303–305 (2011)

16. Cornilleau-Pérès, V., Shabana, N., Droulez, J., Goh, J.C., Lee, G.S., Chew, P.T.: Measurement of the visual contribution to postural steadiness from the COP movement: methodology and reliability. Gait Posture **22**(2), 96–106 (2005)

17. Serra-Añó, P., Pellicer-Chenoll, M., Garcia-Massó, X., Brizuela, G., García-Lucerga, C., González, L.M.: Sitting balance and limits of stability in persons with paraplegia. Spinal Cord **51**(4), 267–272 (2013)

18. Bonnechère, B., Omelina, L., Jansen, B., Rooze, M., Van Sint Jan, S.: Balance training using specially developed serious games for cerebral palsy children, a feasibility study. In: Proceedings of the 8th International Conference on Pervasive Computing Technologies for Healthcare (PervasiveHealth 2014), pp. 302–304. ICST (Institute for Computer Sciences, Social-Informatics and Telecommunications Engineering), Brussels (2014). doi:10.4108/icst.pervasivehealth.2014.255332

19. Le Clair, K., Riach, C.: Postural stability measures: what to measure and for how long. Clin. Biomech. **11**(3), 176–178 (1996)

20. Pua, Y.H., Clark, R.A., Ong, P.H., Bryant, A.L., Lo, N.N., Liang, Z.: Association between seated postural control and gait speed in knee osteoarthritis. Gait Posture **37**(3), 413–418 (2013)

21. Winter, D.: Biomechanics and Motor Control of Human Movement, 4th Revised edn. Wiley, Hoboken (2009)

22. Duarte, M., Freitas, S.M.: Revision of posturography based on force plate for balance evaluation. Rev. Bras. Fisiother. **14**(3), 183–192 (2010)

23. Rocchi, M., Sisti, D., Ditroilo, M., Calavalle, A., Panebianco, R.: The misuse of the confidence ellipse in evaluating statokinesigram. Int. J. Sports Sci. **12**, 169–171 (2005)

24. Schubert, P., Kirchner, M.: Ellipse area calculations and their applicability in posturography. Gait Posture **39**(1), 518–522 (2014)

25. Müller, R., Büttner, P.: A critical discussion of intraclass correlation coefficients. Stat. Med. **13**(23–24), 2465–2476 (2004)

26. Bland, J.M., Altman, D.G.: Statistical methods for assessing agreement between two methods of clinical measurement. Lancet **1**(8476), 307–310 (1986)

27. Ripley, B.D.: Pattern Recognition and Neural Networks. Cambridge University Press, Cambridge (1996)

28. Doyle, T.L., Newton, R.U., Burnett, A.F.: Reliability of traditional and fractal dimension measures of quiet stance center of pressure in young, healthy people. Arch. Phys. Med. Rehabil. **86**(10), 2034–2040 (2005)

29. Raymakers, J.A., Samson, M.M., Verhaar, H.J.: The assessment of body sway and the choice of the stability parameter(s). Gait Posture **21**(1), 48–58 (2005)

30. Pagnacco, G., Oggero, E., Wright, C.H.: Biomedical instruments versus toys: a preliminary comparison of force platforms and the nintendo wii balance board – biomed 2011. Biomed. Sci. Instrum. **47**, 12–17 (2011)

A Mobile Solution to Improve
the Rehabilitation Process

Habib M. Fardoun[✉] and Daniyal M. Alghazzawi

Information Systems Department,
King Abdulaziz University (KAU), Jeddah, Saudi Arabia
{hfardoun,dghazzawi}@kau.edu.sa

Abstract. Rehabilitation of patients is a process aimed at enabling them to reach and maintain their optimal physical, sensory, intellectual, psychological and social functional levels. However, rehabilitation process is complex and patients need to be diagnosed, receive therapy, manage therapy sessions, be monitored and also obtain direct instructions by personal assistant. In this chapter, we present a project based on mobile devices and cloud computing which provides a new rehabilitation process. In this way, the interconnectivity of both the patient and the therapist in the field of psychological therapy is improved. The proposed solution is a mobile application that has several features taking advantage of the extensive technological utilization in the area of psychological rehabilitation. Its basic functionality is to assist people with stress or anxiety so that they can evaluate the degree of professional assistance acquisition using this application. In case they do not require professional assistance, the application would help them by suggesting appropriate relax aspects, providing them theoretical material and an available assistant for such purposes. As a cloud computing application, the system functionalities aim at providing direct communication and active contact with a therapist.

1 Introduction

Nowadays, people live in a world where instability and uncertainty govern aspects of labour, economic, political and social life. This uncertainty can sometimes cause a person to suffer from confusion in which the search for balance and stability becomes a life priority. This uncertainty and confusion becomes a problem for a person when he feels overwhelmed and generates a physical response, which is commonly known by the term anxiety [1].

Anxiety is one of the most common disorders in the society we live. Many people suffer from anxiety or stress without any knowledge of what their symptoms are or what the consequences might cause. Anxiety can be related to stress, panic, eating disorders [2] or leading to depression. It mainly affects women [3] and children.

Usually, anxiety can be treated by specialists who are fully trained in mental health problems such as psychiatrists, psychologists or counselors who can provide some ideas on methods and techniques in order to manage anxiety disorders.

This chapter is a complement to a publication presented in the rehab workshop of the 8th International Conference on Pervasive Computing Technologies for Healthcare

© Springer-Verlag Berlin Heidelberg 2015
H.M. Fardoun et al. (Eds.): REHAB 2014, CCIS 515, pp. 24–34, 2015.
DOI: 10.1007/978-3-662-48645-0_3

(PervasiveHealth '14) where proposal is described the without going into technical details [17].

2 State of the Art

Psychological therapies are based on the study related to human behavior as well as mental activity on human behavior. These therapies typically explore concepts such as perception, attention, motivation, emotion, brain function, intelligence, personality, relationships, consciousness and the unconscious.

Depending on the realized mode, the psychological therapies are distinguished among others, as in the following sections.

2.1 Physical Therapy

In the physical therapy, the psychologist sees his patients in his office; therefore, the patients are obliged to physical presence and are treated in the psychologist's office. During one session, the patient sees the psychologist or therapist in his office or therapy room, and the rest wait their turn in a waiting room.

This is the most traditional process of acquiring psychological support [4]. The psychologist and the patient are meeting face to face; they have personal discussion and review the discussion material together, so that the psychologist provides personalized instructions to the patient. Proximity and contact are the predominant features of this mode.

2.2 Online Therapy

In contrast to the traditional psychologist, the online one offers the same services from a distance [5]. Therapist and patient are not in the same location but they contact each other by electronic means; their communication is established via computer networks. Here, distance and borders do fall; however, this mode suggests that the patient's relationship with the psychologist is not as warm and close as with physical therapy.

Depending on the communication and technology used, this mode of therapy can be realized via synchronous or asynchronous communication tools such as Email/Chat/Teleconferencing (Skype) etc.

2.3 Virtual Reality

Simulation is a technique that creates experiences similar to reality [6]. Simulation functions are based upon predefined limits and have many advantages. For example, in "Technical Exposure", the therapy is more personalized and aids in coordinating and controlling situations that could not be done in the real world, improving the space-time relationship.

2.4   Mobile Application

Nowadays, applications are designed to provide basic information about anxiety and stress including meditation and breathing techniques as well as offline reading or graphic material that is accessible by the interested user [7]. In some applications, a user can find him/herself out of the suggested and normal stress level, based upon the results provided by an assistant. Here, there is no interactivity and no real and functional utilization, nor can we understand it as a process of rehabilitation, as it does not offer a professional therapy service.

3   mTherapy: 21st Century's Therapy

The research question in this research is the following: 'In what ways can we offer professional online service, that does not only get therapist and patient into contact, but also assists the patient on demand, even in cases the patient cannot contact the therapist?'.

The proposed solution is a mobile application that has several features (not available yet) taking advantage of the extensive technological utilization in the area of psychological rehabilitation. Its basic functionality is to assist people with stress or anxiety so that they can evaluate the degree of professional assistance acquisition using this application. In case they do not require professional assistance, the application would help them by suggesting appropriate ways to relax, providing them theoretical material and an available assistant for such purposes.

If professional help is needed, the application assists the user to search for a professional psychologist in order to acquire mobile therapy through web navigation from another device. This would help the patient in all stages of the rehabilitation process and would actively support a better diagnosis by monitoring the follow-ups throughout the rehabilitation process. Lastly, the mobile platform is easy and comfortable to use for both the patient and the therapist.

The next section describes the functions that distinguish, characterize and highlight the proposed mobile application as mTherapy, compared to other current applications. These functionalities are provided by the innate properties of the mobile device, as for example, portability and accessibility from any location the user finds himself, such as by GPS on specific geographic locations or the use of a camera as a means of visual contact in a live connection between patient and therapist. Also as a cloud-based application, mTherapy facilitates the complete and customized rehabilitation for the patient, as it is located and managed anchored in the flexibility and efficiency of the cloud computing technology.

mTherapy functions and related sections are described below.

3.1   Diagnosis

mTherapy features a section using a support assistant wizard to detect and identify stress and anxiety levels. Based upon specified and pre-programmed levels, that exceed the threshold of the normal levels, the software recommends the user several relaxation tools, including indications and techniques that reduce the levels of anxiety and stress.

Based on the wizard's results that reveal certain degrees of anxiety or stress levels, the application automatically shows the user the possibility to opt for a professional service therapy.

mTherapy does not only provide the user with the convenience of going to a therapist, but also facilitates practical and anonymous access to therapists so that the patient can contact the one s/he prefers.

Once the wizard completes the initial estimation, the patient can proceed to the basic registration of a series of concise data. After that step, the application suggests a number of therapists geographically nearby the user, accessing a professional network or use the mobile GPS function. These multiple choices provide the user with the flexibility and freedom to choose a face-to-face, blended (face to face and online) therapy or therapists offering their services exclusively online, regardless their geographic location. Such recommendations also accompany explanations on the benefits and convenience of an online therapy with respect to traditional therapy. For this purpose, the device accesses a therapists' database offering suggested services and simultaneously, stores the users' personal details in a database in order to choose a convenient and affordable way to access therapy.

The diagnostic wizard records observations and specific questions obtaining the maximum possible information regarding the type of anxiety disorder; this result is provided to the therapist for assessment when seeing the patient (Fig. 1).

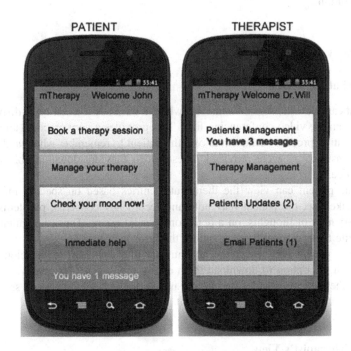

Fig. 1. Patient and therapist service access.

3.2 Therapy

Once the user has chosen the therapist using mTherapy and after agreeing to undergo a therapy for a short or medium term in order to solve his/her problems, sessions are scheduled via a mobile camcorder, also offering the option of using any other preferred device.

Once the patient initiates the session, the application provides him with the option to start the therapy session which has previously been booked through the appointment system. As such, the patient and the psychologist may have direct contact and establish a visual communication to provide the therapist and the patient with all possible information to support the therapy [8].

The therapy module offers the therapist as well as the patient with the following options for each scheduled session:

- Videoconferencing Section: establish direct communication between patient and therapist, with the possibility of the first to use a camera phone as an option for a video recording and to resources optimization available on the mobile device.
- Notes section: here, the therapeutic psychologist's advises and patient's concerns are collected.
- Files section: these are provided by the therapist, as for example, documentation, schedules or tasks, so to enhance the therapy process. They can be viewed and downloaded on the internal or external phone memory for later patient's review and consideration.

4 Therapy Management

4.1 The Patient's View

The patient can view the session's history, wherein each session can be re-displayed as extracted from the video conferencing files. This provides a very practical approach to the rehabilitation process because it allows the patient to remember where and how the therapist's instructions were provided. These video files are downloadable from the mobile device.

Also the patient can view the therapeutic entries based on specific information received. Likewise, the patient may note and record any concerns, problems, reflections, experiences or thoughts, on a draft for the next query. Thus, the patient has no need to write them manually or remember them for later use.

Also, the patient can access the attachments files uploaded to the cloud by the therapist with the option to download them at any time for a later review.

Lastly, the system provides an internal messaging system supporting specific and agreed communications between the patient and the therapist.

4.2 The Therapist's View

In addition to displaying the content (e.g. video, notes and attachments/documents/tasks) provided to the patient, the therapist may view the patient's history, as for example panic attacks or critical moments, both in frequency and intensity; these are collected by the assistant for primary patient care; the latter is used to assist the patient in situations in which the patient is not able to contact the therapist for any particular reason. This information serves to monitor the patient incidents, enquiries and steps during the rehabilitation process.

4.3   Monitoring

mTherapy provides access and use on demand at any moment so that the patient cannot only take advantage of the information received from the therapist at any time and place and revise it through his mobile, but in addition s/he can receive primary support and assistance in any situation as it occurs.

For this purpose, and for the patient's benefits, even if the patient does not have Internet connection at that moment, he can access an assistant (downloadable and updatable cache from the cloud), as for example, in critical intensive anxiety or panic attacks.

In occasions of emergency, the wizard provides the patient with interactive breathing patterns so to control the patient breathing using the screen and calm him/her. It also suggests distraction techniques or therapy reminders, which the therapist has already customized depending on the situation and knowledge on the patient. The patient can access and use these resources in order to overcome these critical situations. It is therefore a customized, and thus, not a general self-help information service.

Whenever the patient responds to the primary care assistant, the discomfort levels he has experienced are recorded. Thus, to be reported to the therapist along with the frequency of these unpleasant situations, the patient goes through it. This information is used by the system to provide the therapist with a visual graph of such incidents.

These notifications are sent to the therapist mobile platform as alerts, so to aid the therapist in knowing more about the patient's problems. Such information is critical for the therapist to decide on immediate or less immediate contact with the patient so as to supervise his condition enabling a progressive patient monitoring.

The therapist can also provide consultation to the patient about the usefulness of the advices to assist for the patient's primary care, and correct or modify any of these as necessary. Also, the patient can transmit the support service, or any other issues, derived from both the automated assistant and the therapist. This serves as feedback in order to improve the application and supporting services.

Any wizard assistant change and modification is updated from the cloud and is downloadable for offline use.

5   mTherapy: A Cloud Mobile App

mTherapy resources are constantly available to the user, regardless the user's time zone and location [9]. The documents are not physically stored on the user's mobile but are retrieved via the Internet. All that is needed is a mobile device or any other device connected to the Internet [10, 11].

Features and rehabilitation services are provided via cloud technology; therefore, they do not require the patient or the therapist being in a specific physical location, however, s/he may be at home, enjoying the convenience of the service incorporating an improved quality life (Fig. 2).

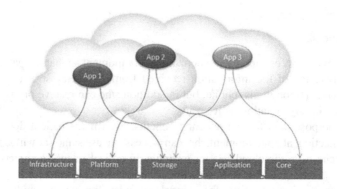

Fig. 2. Structure of the mTherapy cloud

Also, as for the interface and content customization of the patient module, these are easily achievable; furthermore, as the content location is on the cloud, both the therapist and the patient do not have to worry about the file management and the storage. This custom service takes place without the need for significant financial or technological effort [12].

Regardless the mTherapy introduction and the cloud-based mobile application, mTherapy may also be accessed via a computer through an enabled web browsing [13].

The technical details related to this cloud-based application refer to the following characteristics that support mTherapy to be an easy to use tool to support the rehabilitation purposes:

- The information (videos, database, users, and documents) is stored in a cloud.
- Data can be downloaded promptly (in this case, video of each session and material provided by the therapist) for offline access.
- Support for different user needs, as for example, application cloud data backup with different characteristics such as data compression, security, and backup schedule [14].
- Web browser access and use [15] and/or a mobile version via applications installed on Internet-connected devices, such as desktop computer and mobile phones.

Once the specific needs are determined for the patient, the next step is to carry out the system's conceptual design. The obtained design will describe the necessary for the patient services. Taking into account that the system is a cloud-based application, it is necessary to allow the user to work *offline*. With offline mode, the user can access to application information even when the mobile device isn't connected to the network. In this way, the system's connections are downloaded providing greater speed and safety.

The architecture is divided into four parts, the first is the *Kau Hospital cloud* [16]; this is where data related to patient's history is stored and also all clinical data management is performed.

Furthermore, the necessary services are grouped to support the EPT (Environments Personals Treatment), as illustrated in Fig. 3.B.2. These are divided into two main services. On the one hand, the methods that allow creating the patients' accounts, related to the medical information. On the other hand, therapies specifically generated for the patients' rehabilitation process. These are based on the data association provided by the therapist and patient history information.

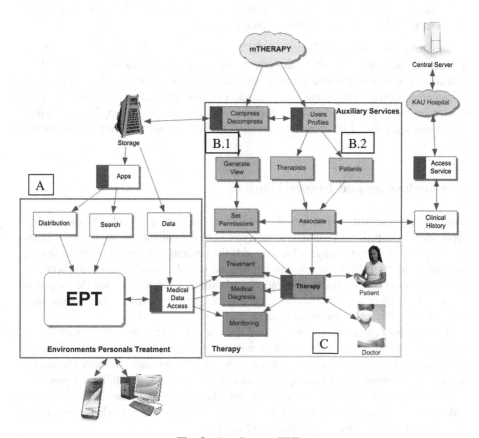

Fig. 3. Arquitectura EPT.

User profile component generates the therapy from the data of patient's history. The service *associate* obtains the necessary data setting permissions.

The architecture, as in the Fig. 3.B.1, supports the component-level security and information access. Users can access the information depending on their role in the system. Thus, they generate a view for each of the users participating in the system. These users are typically the medical experts/careers users in different specializations in therapy, doctors, nurses, physiotherapists, and even external ones supporting doctor's work. The therapy is divided into three components: *medical diagnosis, treatment, and monitoring* (See Fig. 3.C).

- Medical Diagnosis: with patient's medical diagnosis the doctor can analyze all medical data and test the patient.
- Treatment: In this section, the doctor can deal with the medical treatments prescribed to the patient. These treatments are medical data and are visible only to the doctor.
- Monitoring: In the follow-up therapy, there is a point when the doctor and the patient interact. The patient provides information about the improvements made through the rehabilitation. In this way the doctor can modify the treatment and achieve a rehabilitation process adapted to patient.

Environments Personals Treatment (EPT), as with Fig. 3.A, is a space that allows users to interact with each other and make the necessary queries to medical data. These data come from the user accounts; the association enables integration of the system and allows any medical system through a data access layer interaction EPT. In Fig. 3, the system provides medical data and applications. For the specific applications which obtain and send data, EPT must be connected to the Web Services responsible for the task.

6 Conclusions and Future Work

This chapter presented the concept of rehabilitation support using a cloud-based mobile application to improve the interconnectivity of both the patient and the therapist in the field of psychological therapy. mTherapy aids the communication, information sharing and maximum availability of a patient through the use of a mobile device. mTherapy is a prime support system for psychological and different scope therapies developed to support a comfort and continuous care for the patient so that s/he always feels accompanied during the recovery process.

Internet and cloud-computing technology are the mTherapy key elements, and unlike other existing applications, it is not a self-help option; however, mTherapy provides a full rehabilitation service using basic mobile functions. As such, the mobile device development opens new opportunities for the patients' rehabilitation process.

Mobility, user interface and services may be improved in the future; as such, additional resources may be needed to meet any arising needs towards the mTherapy access and utilization by both patients and therapists.

One architectural requirement is indeed anticipating such evolution so to provide data security. For this reason, a data layer was created in the environment allowing diverse applications access depending on the given security permissions level. Establishing information levels is controlled by setting security permissions. Furthermore, the compression level documents are determined by a compression service. There is a compression system standard file, decided to perform compression streams (compressed into the time) before shipping, and decompressed by the EPT.

There are two main components are highlighted in the system architecture. The first is the medical records, such as the user accounts. The second manages associations with user accounts, providing treatments, medical diagnostics and monitoring of patients. The system will support health related data evolution provided by future rehabilitation patients' therapy associated data.

References

1. Rojas, E.: La ansiedad, Debolsillo (2000). Ding, W., Marchionini, G.: A study on video browsing strategies. Technical report, University of Maryland at College Park (1997)
2. De Alda, Í.O., Espina, A., Ortego, M.A.: Un estudio sobre personalidad, ansiedad y depresión en padres de pacientes con un trastorno alimentario1 A study about personality, anxiety and depression in parents of patients with an eating disorder. Clínica y Salud **17**(2), 151–170 (2006)
3. Arenas, M.C., Puigcerver, A.: Diferencias entre hombres y mujeres en los trastornos de ansiedad: una aproximación psicobiológica. Escritos de Psicología **3**(1), 20–29 (2009)
4. Esparcia, A.J.: La psicología de internet y la psicología en internet. Regulación deontológica y ética de la intervención psicológica a través de internet. Psicología em. Revista **8**(12), 11–23 (2008)
5. Soto-Pérez, F., Franco, M., Monardes, C., Jiménez, F.: Internet y psicología clínica: Revision de las ciberterapias. Revista de psicopatología y psicología clínica **15**(1), 19–37 (2010)
6. Perpiñá, C., Baños, R.M., Botella, C., Marco, J.H.: La Realidad Virtual como herramienta terapéutica: Un estudio de caso en las alteraciones de la Imagen Corporal en los Trastornos Alimentarios. Rev. argent. clín. psicol **10**(3), 227–241 (2001)
7. PaulesCiprés, A., Fardoun, H.M., Alghazzawi, D.M., Oadah, M.: KAU e-health mobile system. In: Proceedings of the 13th International Conference on Interacción Persona-Ordenador, p. 29, ACM, October 2012
8. Pérez Villar, J.: El Análisis de la Comunicación en Psicoterapia (II Parte). Revista del Hospital Psiquiátrico de La Habana (1985)
9. Burdea, G.C.: Rubber ball to cloud rehabilitation musing on the future of therapy. In: Virtual Rehabilitation International Conference 2009, pp. 50–50, IEEE, June 2009
10. Fardoun, H.M., Altalhi, A.H., Cipres, A.P., Castillo, J.R., Albiol-Pérez, S.: CRehab: a cloud-based framework for the management of rehabilitation processes. In: 2013 7th International Conference on Pervasive Computing Technologies for Healthcare (PervasiveHealth), pp. 397–400, IEEE, May 2013
11. Fardoun, H.M., Cipres, A.P., Alghazzwi, D.M.: Distributed user interfaces in a cloud educational system. In: Lozano, M.D., Gallud, J.A., Tesoriero, R., Penichet, V.M.R. (eds.) Distributed User Interfaces: Usability and Collaboration, pp. 151–163. Springer, London (2013)
12. Ograph, B.T., Morgens, Y.R.: Cloud computing. Commun. ACM **51**(7) (2008)
13. Miller, M.: Cloud Computing: Web-Based Applications that Change the Way You Work and Collaborate Online. Que Publishing, Indianapolis (2008)
14. Kaufman, L.M.: Data security in the world of cloud computing. IEEE Secur. Priv. **7**(4), 61–64 (2009)
15. Wang, L., Tao, J., Kunze, M., Castellanos, A.C., Kramer, D., Karl, W.: Scientific cloud computing: early definition and experience. In: HPCC, vol. 8, pp. 825–830, September 2008

16. PaulesCiprés, A., Fardoun, H.M., Alghazzawi, D.M., Oadah, M.: KAU e-health mobile system. In: Proceedings of the 13th International Conference on Interacción Persona-Ordenador, p. 29, ACM, October 2012
17. Fardoun, H.M., Alghazzawi, D.M., Delgado, S.A.: mTherapy: a mobile based therapy. In: Proceedings of the 8th International Conference on Pervasive Computing Technologies for Healthcare (PervasiveHealth '14). ICST (Institute for Computer Sciences, Social-Informatics and Telecommunications Engineering), ICST, Brussels, Belgium, pp. 447–450 (2014). http://dx.doi.org/10.4108/icst.pervasivehealth.2014.255265,   doi:10.4108/icst.pervasivehealth.2014.255265

Assistive E-Health Platform
for Permanent Monitoring

Sebastian Fuicu$^{(\boxtimes)}$, Andrei Avramescu, Diana Lascu,
Roxana Padurariu, and Marius Marcu

Politehnica University of Timisoara, Timisoara, Romania
{sebastian.fuicu,marius.marcu}@cs.upt.ro,
{andrei.avramescu,diana.lascu,
roxana.padurariu}@student.upt.ro

Abstract. Chronic diseases, such as heart disease, stroke, chronic respiratory disease and diabetes are the major cause of death in the world. This paper aims at presenting a low cost, secure medical platform for mobile and desktop operating systems to monitor vital parameters, receive notifications when the pre-defined limits are out of range and foresee a patient's health status. This system processes medical data effectively by correlating the parameter trends with the patient's actual state to anticipate their health evolution. The purpose of the platform is to offer up-to-date information about chronic diseases in order to permanently ensure patients' safety and adequate treatment. In a systemic approach, this chapter is a complement to a publication presented in the workshop of the 8th International Conference on Pervasive Computing Technologies for Healthcare (PervasiveHealth '14) [1]. Taking into consideration the previous work, we present a concrete scenario of how the system works, describe the system components, and discuss some aspects regarding energy consumption and autonomy.

Keywords: Chronic diseases · E-health · Immediate response · Permanent watch · Future prediction · Complex rules · Cloud storage

1 Introduction

Taking into consideration the evolution of technology when it comes to the medical world, making life easier for patients is no longer only possible, but also compulsory. Nowadays, we can rely not only on monitoring a patient, but also taking action in the shortest time. Common diseases among the elderly include hypertension, diabetes, heart failure, and other chronic diseases. Patients with these diseases can live normal lives, but they must regularly monitor their conditions. Self-monitoring is a growing trend, and if medical professionals could analyze the supplied physiological information, they could more effectively prevent diseases and disease-related complications [2, 11].

Focusing only on people suffering of chronic diseases, thus on patients who should be permanently supervised, a history of the diseases evolution would be helpful not only for the particular patient, but also for those having similar symptoms. Recent advances in computing technologies including body sensors and wireless communications have revealed the possibility of providing remote health monitoring (RHM) to

© Springer-Verlag Berlin Heidelberg 2015
H.M. Fardoun et al. (Eds.): REHAB 2014, CCIS 515, pp. 35–44, 2015.
DOI: 10.1007/978-3-662-48645-0_4

patients at high risk of falls and with chronic diseases. The body sensors deployed in, on, or around the human body are able to measure the fundamental health parameters in a situation where large sized and standard medical examination equipment are not available; the pervasive use of mobile phones and the ubiquity of Wi-Fi connection enable medical informatics to overcome the time and location barriers [3].

In the WHO European Region report for 2008 is specified that 86 % of deaths are attributable to chronic diseases [4]. Most of the past health care system research efforts were focused on sensor networks design like routing, MAC design, and sensor nodes deployment. In those designs, sensor data are transmitted to remote server through access devices. Tasks like sensor data storage, patients' health states determination, and notifications are conducted by a central server while gateway only acts as an intermediate device. The response delay includes network delay and central server delay [5].

Cloud computing simplifies information sharing among various healthcare institutions involved in the care process, which is of utmost importance in healthcare. Healthcare cloud has a great market potential given the fact that less than 7 % of the US hospitals have a functional and integrated electronic medical record solution [6]. In our system, cloud storage and sharing information are relevant parts because there is no use of involving hospitals, to find out information that can be easily received by always collecting a patient's data, like medical tests before a surgery.

Although it may seem obvious, the continuous care a chronic disease sufferer needs is often overlooked. Helping them by taking action not only in case of an emergency, but whenever a treatment needs change or receiving information that can lead to something unexpected may turn out to be more important than focusing a doctor's entire energy only on a more severe point in somebody's disease.

This paper is structured as follows: Section 2 presents the description of the system including the data acquisition mechanism, the software components and the software architecture. Section 3 describes the data flow in the system and Sect. 4 provides a concrete example of how the system works.

2   System Description

An integrated healthcare system that enables health monitoring and disease management in the home environment has been a major research area for healthcare researchers [7]. Besides being watched over only at home, it is even better to be certain of your health any place and at any time. Moreover, changing the treatment according to the patient's needs, enables him to be aware of his health state and thus makes him more confident.

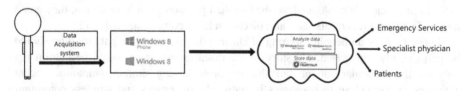

Fig. 1. Overview of the system

This section describes the complex e-health platform, beginning with the physical components, continuing with the software part and in the end the way the entire system works (see Fig. 1).

2.1 Data Acquisition System

The physical part of this complex system consists of:

E-health sensor shield used to monitor in real time the health parameters of a patient. This can be seen as the "center" of the hardware where all the sensors used into our prototype version of the system get engaged in collecting information.

Arduino Module used for programming the e-health sensors and also used for the power supply of the entire data acquisition system.

Sensors (for example: Pulse and oxygen in blood, airflow, body temperature, electrocardiogram, glucometer, galvanic skin response, blood pressure, patient position).

Bluetooth Module used to detect and connect to available devices available in the area (see Fig. 2).

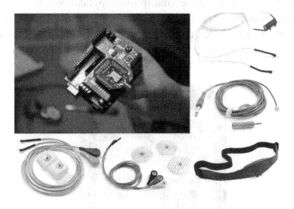

Fig. 2. Data acquisition system

According to the patient's diseases and the doctor's recommendations, a certain group of sensors can be used. The sensors shown above have been used only to prove the applicability of the system and a sufferer is able to choose his/her own set of sensors. This particular kit can be found at [8]. Because of high-technology used today in the medical field, there are sensors that can be worn without any discomfort. Moreover, the trend is to create ultra-wearable medical sensors or under skin sensors. There are also smartphones that have embedded sensors and that can be used for a medical purpose such as this system.

Modularity and flexibility are two of the relevant characteristics of this system. The first characteristic is proven by the possibility to use a large diversity of data acquisition systems. The platform is considered flexible because of the different types of diseases that can be kept under control by notifying the important actors when patient's health parameters are not found in the accepted limits for the patient's current state. It is important to have a clear image of the physical components and the way they are connected (see Fig. 3).

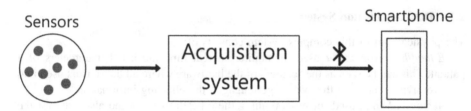

Fig. 3. Hardware communication

2.2 Software Components

To be able to keep a close connection between physicians and patients, the system offers applications for a variety of devices. These applications are mainly intended for the doctors. Patients can use a simple smartphone application.

Smartphone application – Patient - collects medical data from the sensors and sends them forward to be analyzed and stored in the cloud; localizes the person in case of an emergency situation; offers a brief preview of the patient's data (see Fig. 4).

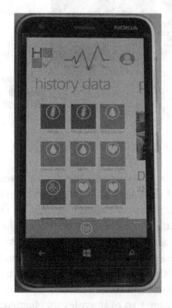

Fig. 4. Patient application - screenshot

Smartphone/tablet application – Physician – enables the doctor to always know the health parameters of any patient under his supervision and receives notifications according to his preset criteria/rules; provides a map to the patient in case of an emergency situation (see Fig. 5).

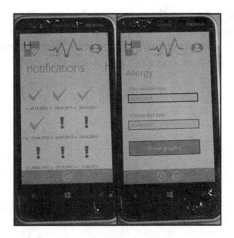

Fig. 5. Physician application - screenshot

Desktop application – Physician – this application creates the environment for the doctor to create complex criteria, individualized for each patient. These rules will trigger notifications if they are exceeded. The interface is user-friendly and the physician can visualize his rules by simply dragging and dropping blocks (see Fig. 6).

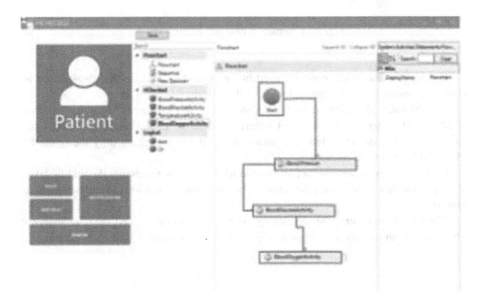

Fig. 6. Desktop application - screenshot

Website – offers a secure way for both patients and physicians to access the data from any public location; this represents a start point for creating a health community.

2.3   Software Architecture

For a better visualization for how the system works, we will use the next picture:

The medical data is acquired from the sensors worn by the patients via Bluetooth and transmitted to their smartphone, as describe below. From there, the information is forwarded into the cloud where it is analyzed in specific ways (see Fig. 7).

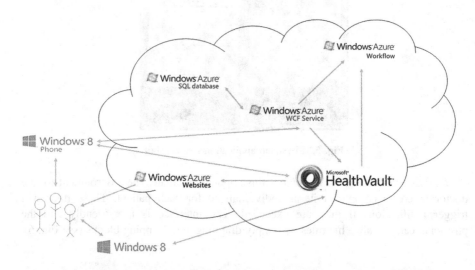

Fig. 7. Information flow and architecture

The main software technologies used in the current system are Microsoft based to assure the security and the performance of the solution:

HealthVault – all health information is stored into this safe medical database offered by Microsoft authorized in all E.U. Countries and in the U.S. This offers security for every connection in the system, the patient being the one granting only the rights he wishes to his personal doctors.

WCF (Windows Communication Foundation) Service – represents the middle layer of the system that assures the interaction between client applications, database and data analyzer.

Windows Workflows – the technology on top of which is created the data analyzer where physician can create complex rules that are individualized for each patient.

3 System Data Flow

The software system follows the idea of trading systems that are used on a regular basis by brokers all over the world. They offer efficient prediction with a high level of security. As brokers, the physicians are able to create complex rules in which they can correlate different health parameters.

These criteria set by the doctors can generate two types of notifications. First, there is the General Notification that announces the doctor that certain limits have been exceeded, but nothing urgent has happened. These kinds of notifications may lead to the change of the treatment or may require unplanned medical tests. Secondly, there are the Emergency Notifications that can announce both physicians from the community that are available in the vicinity and the ambulance. To know exactly to whom these notifications must be sent, it is necessary that the system localizes the doctors. In this purpose, the application uses its GPS feature, that also helps know the location of the patient in need. The two points given by the GPS system makes it easy to provide the physician with a map that show the way to the patient. While the GPS system works only in an outdoor environment, we also need a system for indoor positioning so that the location of the patient is accurately determined. Therefore, our system is able to use any indoor localization solution such as using Wi-Fi radio [12] or using the sensors embedded in smart phones such as accelerometers and magnetometers [9]. The Emergency Notifications come from any patient and that requires immediate care. When approaching a patient in a delicate situation, the doctor receives a small health profile to know what action to take.

Because the patient has to permanently wear the sensors and data is retrieved in real time, the amount of data that should be collected is huge. Knowing the normal limits of the health information for each category of supervised parameter, there is no use of collecting everything the sensors receive. The filtering of the data that is finally stored in cloud is done simultaneously with the continuous analysis performed to decide whether to announce medical actors.

Having the ability to analyze Big Data is of limited value if users cannot understand the analysis. Ultimately, a decision-maker, provided with the result of analysis, has to interpret these results. This interpretation cannot happen in a vacuum. Usually, it involves examining all the assumptions made and retracing the analysis [10]. This is why the physicians have only to supervise their patients and take the right decisions in case of any kind of notifications.

Furthermore, the system presented may help not only patients as individuals, but it can also come in handy for statistics and research projects. In this purpose, by collecting patient's health information with their approval and anonymizing them, they can then be transmitted to those institutions with interest in medical and pharmaceutical research and investigations.

Another direct advantage offered by big data analyzes is the reduction of energy consumption. The system discussed in this paper offers also a level of abstraction in terms of filtering on the smartphone. It is not only aimed for collecting information, but also to be a first step in the data processing flow. In practice, this means a decrease of data transmitted to cloud with an average of 30 % – 70 %, these percent being found in the energy consumption.

4 Scenario

Taking into consideration everything above, we will present a concrete example of how the system works.

HChecked implies a set of actors, for this example there will be two doctors, the patient's personal doctor, a volunteer doctor and one patient. The latter is suffering of multiple diseases: diabetes and a heart disease, which are linked and have symptoms that often fluctuate. This is why the generalist recommends that he is always aware of the modifications in the patient's (health) state. It is important to note that the doctor will treat each patient in an unique way, taking into consideration all particularities of each individual. This is why, patients that have the same diagnostic can be looked after in an individual manner, because the values that their prescribed parameters have are different. For this example, the situations that may occur in such circumstances are the following:

1. The specialist physician receives notifications that the parameters have been exceeded, but upon analysis he decides that no special measure has to be taken. In this situation the patient won't be announced and the prescribed treatment remains the same. Also, the volunteer doctor doesn't participate in this scene (Fig. 8).
2. The specialist physician receives notifications that the parameters have been exceeded, but he considers that he must take action and calls the patient for further investigations or just prescribes new medicine (Fig. 9).
3. The personal specialist physician receives a notification and observes an important difference in the patient's parameters. Because this case consists of an emergency situation, all of the doctors that are part of the HChecked community will also be announced. The first doctor that responds to the notification takes it upon himself to find the patient and to offer first aid to the person in need. This volunteer doctor is the firs who reaches the patient, receives his health profile on the smartphone and knows how to act. Simultaneously to reaching to all the doctors in the area, the ambulance service is also announced. Usually, the ambulance will reach the patient after he has received first aid. Although he has also received a notification, the personal doctor mostly doesn't intervene because he usually isn't in the vicinity. However, there are some situations when the personal doctor is also a volunteer that receives a notification from one of his patient and in this case he will also take action (Fig. 10).

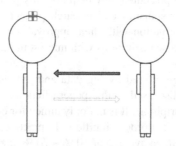

Fig. 8. The system notifies the personal physician

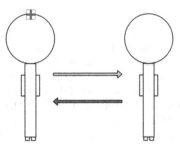

Fig. 9. The system notifies the personal physician who takes measures

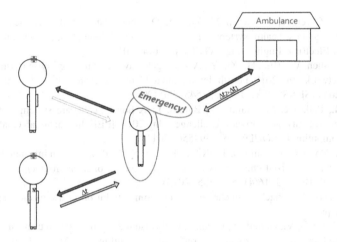

Fig. 10. Emergency situation

5 Conclusions

In this paper we have presented a health-platform aimed to improve the lives of chronic disease sufferers. Besides the improvement of the decision-making process based on the personal history of the patient, which is a common feature on monitoring systems, this medical platform assures that the decision is taken at the proper time by continuously analyzing data in real-time. The distinctive element in the current paper is the way in which the data is analyzed based on the complex criteria that the physicians can create.

Future work will be focused on creating and analyzing use cases to improve the system's functionalities.

Current research presented in this paper was focused on creating a viable, reliable and secure solution of analyzing patient's health data in real-time.

Acknowledgement. This work was partially supported by the research grant CHIST-ERA/1/01. 10.2012 – "GEMSCLAIM: GreenEr Mobile Systems by Cross LAyer Integrated energy Management".

References

1. Fuicu, S., Marcu, M., Avramescu, A., Lascu, D., Padurariu, R.: Real time e-health system for continuous care. In: Proceedings of the 8th International Conference on Pervasive Computing Technologies for Healthcare (PervasiveHealth '14). ICST (Institute for Computer Sciences, Social-Informatics and Telecommunications Engineering), ICST, Brussels, Belgium, pp. 436–439, Oldenburg, Germany, May 20–23 2014. doi:10.4108/icst.pervasivehealth.2014.255308
2. Lee, Y.-F.: Personal medical monitoring system: addressing interoperability. IT Prof. **15**(5), 31–37 (2013)
3. Liang, X., Barua, M., Chen, L., Lu, R., Shen, X., Li, X., Luo, H.Y.: Enabling pervasive healthcare through continuous remote health monitoring. IEEE Wirel. Commun. **19**(6), 10–18 (2012)
4. Ciorap, R., Corciova, C., Ciorap, M., Zaharia, D.: Optimization of the treatment for chronic disease using an e-health system. In: 2011 7th International Symposium on Advanced Topics in Electrical Engineering (ATEE), pp. 1–4 (2011)
5. Chen, Y., Shen, W., Huo, H., Xu, Y.: A smart gateway for health care system using wireless sensor network. In: 2010 Fourth International Conference on Sensor Technologies and Applications (SENSORCOMM), pp. 545–550 (2010)
6. Deng, M., Petkovic, M., Nalin, M., Baroni, I.: A home healthcare system in the cloud–addressing security and privacy challenges. In: 2011 IEEE International Conference on Cloud Computing (CLOUD), pp. 549–556 (2011)
7. Jeong, S., Youn, C.-H., Shim, E.B., Kim, M., Cho, Y.M., Peng, L.: An integrated healthcare system for personalized chronic disease care in home-hospital environments. IEEE Trans. Inf. Technol. Biomed. **16**(4), 572–585 (2012)
8. http://www.cooking-hacks.com/ehealth-sensors-complete-kit-biometric-medical-arduino-raspberry-pi
9. Martin, E., Oriol, V., Gerald, F., Ruzena, B.: Precise indoor localization using smart phones. In: Proceedings of the International Conference on Multimedia, MM 2010, pp. 787–790. ACM, New York, NY, USA (2010). doi:10.1145/1873951.1874078
10. http://www.cra.org/ccc/files/docs/init/bigdatawhitepaper.pdf
11. Fuicu, S., Marcu, M., Avramescu, A., Lascu, D., Padurariu, R.: Real time e-health system for continuous care. In: The Proceedings of 8th International Conference on Pervasive Computing Technologies for Healthcare, Oldenburg, Germany, 20–23 May 2014
12. Marcu, M., Fuicu, S., Girban, A., Popa, M.: Experimental test cases for wireless positioning systems. In: International Conference on Computer as a Tool, EUROCON 2007, pp. 900–907, Warsaw, POLAND (2007)

A New Quantitative Performance Parameter for Monitoring Robotics Rehabilitation Treatment: Technical Guidelines

Elisabetta Peri[1]([✉]), Emilia Biffi[2], Cristina Maghini[2],
Fernanda Servodio Iammarrone[2], Chiara Gagliardi[2], Chiara Germiniasi[2],
Alessandra Pedrocchi[1], Anna Carla Turconi[2], and Gianluigi Reni[2]

[1] Nearlab, Department of Electronic, Information and Bioengineering,
Politecnico di Milano, Milano, Italy
{elisabetta.peri,alessandra.pedrocchi}@polimi.it
[2] IRCCS E. Medea, Bosisio Parini, Lecco, Italy
{emilia.biffi,cristina.maghini,servodiofernanda.iammarone,
chiara.gagliardi,chiara.germiniasi,annacarla.turconi,
gianluigi.reni}@bp.lnf.it

Abstract. The great potential of robots in extracting quantitative and meaningful data is not always exploited. The aim of the present work is to propose a simple parameter that allows to follow the performance of subjects during upper limb robotic training with no additional effort for patients or clinicians.

The parameter has been computed using data automatically recorded by the robot during each session of training. In this chapter we give the technical guidelines to define the performance parameter and we use it to evaluate the training outcome in a group of 14 children affected by Cerebral Palsy.

Keywords: Robotics rehabilitation · Assessment · Upper limb · Armeo®Spring Pediatric · Cerebral palsy

1 Introduction

In clinical practice, it is substantial to identify among the multiple variables involved in rehabilitation treatments which ones might have a larger impact on outcomes and influence recovery. Moreover, such evaluations require the use of quantifiable, valid, and sensitive tools to guarantee reliable between-study comparisons and greatly improve the understanding of key treatment effects [1].

Unfortunately, many assessment methods commonly used today are based on subjective impressions and could depend on both the operators and the patients personality, attitude, and psychological state. All this makes it difficult to justify the effectiveness of therapy treatments [2]. Further, sophisticated 3D posture analysis systems, which allow assessing posture and movements in a quantitative fashion, are not always available [3,4].

© Springer-Verlag Berlin Heidelberg 2015
H.M. Fardoun et al. (Eds.): REHAB 2014, CCIS 515, pp. 45–54, 2015.
DOI: 10.1007/978-3-662-48645-0_5

During the past few years, robot-assisted rehabilitation has become a very active area of research not only because rehabilitation robots can provide controlled, intensive, task-specific training that is goal directed and cognitively engaging, but also because measures derived from robot data can contribute to the understanding of how different treatment variables (e.g., dosage, amount, and type of assistance provided) influence motor learning and recovery [5,6].

Previous studies have developed some ad-hoc assessment tools to extract outcome measures of patients performance, such as position of a hand effector, ability in following a trajectory and measures of forces exchanged [7]. This is the case of the i-match Project [8] that developed six assessment modules to quantitatively evaluate the upper limb performance. Often the main idea is to be inspired by functional test commonly used in clinical practice and to convert them in a virtual version that exploits all the advantages of the technology, i.e. accuracy and repeatability of the measures. An example developed in the i-match Project is the peg-in-hole test, inspired by the nine-hole peg test whose objective is remove a peg from a hole and insert it into another with normal speed and accuracy. It provides information about fine motor control.

Another possible approach is to exploit the built-in technology of the rehabilitation robots e.g. potentiometers that allow extracting trajectories and subjects kinematics during the robotic training. In this direction, Merlo and colleagues proposed normative values of 25 healthy subjects upper limb functionality [9] during an exercise of assessment with Armeo®Spring. The authors used the robot data to extract indexes of task precision, movement smoothness and velocity.

However, all the methods reported above require the development of ad-hoc technology and/or additional time for patients and clinicians to perform the rehabilitation assessments.

Furthermore, only few robotic assessment methods have been compared and validated with clinical and functional scales [7] thus their use in clinical practice is limited.

In this work we describe a simple parameter that can be easily derived from data automatically saved by the robot and that gives an indication of subjects performance. This assessment parameter combines information about time needed to finish an exercise, scores obtained during the exercise and level of difficulty. It can be used to follow the trend of a robot-aided treatment, to describe changes in performance before and after a rehabilitation and thus to investigate the effects of variations in the therapy on patients motor and functional recovery. Here we used Armeo®Spring (Hocoma, AG) and we evaluated 7 exercises. However, the core idea underpinning the presented parameter does not depend on the robot employed and on the exercise performed thus it could be extended to other devices.

2   Materials and Methods

Fourteen inpatients affected by cerebral palsy (CP) performed a training with the paediatric version of Armeo®Spring. Details about the subjects are reported in Table 1.

Table 1. Participants' details at baseline.

Etiology	CP (6 unilateral, 8 bilateral)
Age, years[a]	10.8 (2.9)
Gender, M/F	11/3
MACS[b], 1/2/3	2/7/5

[a]Median (interquartile range).
[b]Manual Ability Classification System.

All inpatients and their families gave voluntarily their consent to the clinical trial. The research protocol was approved on March 2010 by the ethics committee of IRCCS E. Medea.

2.1 Apparatus

Armeo®Spring Pediatric is an exoskeleton with five degrees of freedom (3 in the shoulder, 1 in the elbow and 1 in the forearm). It is not provided with robotic actuators but springs are used to guarantee passive arm weight support and guidance. The stiffness of the springs can be customized resulting in a different level of gravity support and patients muscular involvement. This enables patients to achieve a larger range of motion within a 3D workspace with their own residual functionality, promoting the rehabilitation process. A pressure-sensitive handgrip is also present providing grasp training.

The Armeo exoskeleton can be adapted to the patients morphology by changing the position and the length of the orthosis. The pediatric version is available to adapt the orthosis to children.

Through dedicated software, patients are engaged in exercises that aim at training functional and meaningful tasks (e.g. break eggs, clean a surface, etc.) involving different upper arm districts and joints.

2.2 Definition of P

Seven exercises among those commonly used by the therapists during rehabilitation sessions were selected to evaluate subjects performance over different joints and in different spaces (1D, 2D and 3D), accordingly to the indication of clinicians and physiotherapists. In particular, we evaluated a 1D exercise ("goalkeeper"), four exercises performed in a 2D space ("egg cracking", "fruit shopping", "stove cleaning" and "vertical catching") and two in a 3D space ("chase balloon"and"reveal panorama").

During each training session, information about the exercises (e.g. difficulty level, working area, arm weight support), the score obtained by the subject and the time required to perform the exercise were automatically recorded by the system, with no additional effort for the patients and the physiotherapists.

All these components have been taken into account in a comprehensive performance parameter (p_i) computed as in Eq. 1 for each ith exercise:

$$p(i) = \frac{S_i/S_{i,TOT}}{T_i/T_{i,TOT}} D_i \tag{1}$$

where S_i is the score obtained during the ith exercise, $S_{i,TOT}$ is the maximum score obtainable, T_i is the time required to complete the ith exercise, $T_{i,TOT}$ is the maximum time available. If the ith exercise was not time or score limited, $S_{i,TOT}$ or $T_{i,TOT}$ have been considered equal to 1. Finally D_i is the difficulty coefficient that considers level of the exercise (L_i in the following) and variation in autogrip and control threshold for each subject during the training.

Equation 2 summarizes the methods used to obtain the parameter of difficulty D_i.

$$D_i = L_i \pm AG \pm TH \tag{2}$$

where L_i is the difficulty level of the ith exercise, AG accounts for enabling or disabling the autogrip function and TH accounts for variation in control threshold.

Physiotherapists usually modify L_i, AG and TH to increase or decrease the difficulty of the exercises. In particular, if the grasping task was expected for the exercise, the autogrip (AG) could be enabled or disabled modifying D_i in terms of ± 0.5 points. Moreover if the autogrip is disabled, the precision required by the grasping could be modulated through thresholds (TH) that varied between 0 and 100. For each 10 points of variation, D_i was incremented or decremented of 0.05 points.

Other parameters such as the work-space and the arm weight support of each subject were not varied during our training thus they were not considered in D_i.

The value of L_i is strongly exercise-dependent and the methods used to compute it for each of the seven exercises are further detailed in the following paragraphs.

The first exercise considered was the "goalkeeper" where the patient is supposed to use the prono-supination of the wrist (1D movement) to save goals. As the difficulty level increases, more and quicker movements are required. The variation of difficulty due to this two factors have been taken into account evaluating the velocity of the balls (by the mean of a chronometer) and the number of shoot needed to complete the exercise over different levels. Thus two corresponding coefficients (C_V and C_N respectively) have been computed as in Eq. 3 in order to represent the amount of variation of difficulty with respect to the level "very easy".

$$C_X(i) = \frac{X_i^{levelj}}{X_i^{level\,"veryeasy"}} \tag{3}$$

where $C_X(i)$ is the coefficient related to the factor X of the ith exercise (i.e. in "goalkeeper" X corresponds to the velocity V and to the number of balls N) and level j is the level of difficulty considered ("very easy", "easy", "medium" and "difficult").

$L_{Goalkeeper}$ is the product of this two quantities ($L_{Goalkeeper}=C_V C_N$). All the mentioned values are reported in Table 2.

The "egg cracking" and "fruit shopping" exercises require to reach an object (apple or egg) with a cursor controlled by the end-point position of the exoskeleton in the 2D space, and to move it to a different portion of the space (cart or pot). They involves flex-extension/abduction-adduction of the shoulder, flex-extension of the elbow and the grip-release of the hand, when the autogrip function is disabled. The higher is the levels of difficulties, the higher is the number of object to be moved (coefficient C_N) and the smaller is their size (coefficient C_S). An estimation of the objects areas for each level of difficulties has been obtained by approximating the apples and the eggs using an ellipse. C_N and C_S are the coefficients computed as in Eq. 3 and the level coefficient L is obtained as the product between them. Results are detailed in Table 2.

"Reveal panorama" involves the same body districts but require exploring the 3D space with a sponge that becomes smaller as the difficulty level increases. An evaluation of the 3D surface of the parallelepiped that composes the sponge was used to compute the coefficient C_S (Eq. 3) that is the only term of $L_{RevealPanorama}$ (Table 2).

The "stove cleaning" exercise requires moving a sponge in 2D space and involves abduction-adduction of the shoulder, flex-extension of the elbow and the grip-release of the hand, when the autogrip function is disabled. The dimension of the sponge varies with the difficulty level. Similarly to "Reveal panorama" but in the 2D space, the sponge was modelled as a parallelogram and the coefficient C_S accounted for the variation of the sponge surface. $L_{StoveCleaning}$ is equal to C_S.

"Vertical catching" and "chase balloon" involve the same articular movement (flex-extension/abduction-adduction of the shoulder, flex-extension of the elbow) but are performed in the 2D and 3D space, respectively. Both exercises require reaching a target that appears on the screen.

Concerning the "vertical catching" exercise the increase of the difficulty level entails both higher number of target (C_N) to be reached and bigger area covered by this targets (C_S). For this exercise data concerning both the number of target and the area exploited were present in the Armeo manual and the correspondent coefficient are reported in Table 2. The value of $L_{VerticalCatching}$ is obtained by the product of C_N and C_S.

For the "chase balloon" exercise higher difficulty level means decreased dimension of the balloons. We modeled the balloons with ellipsoid and the correspondent reduction of the surface C_S was computed as described in Eq. 3 (values reported in Table 2). Also in this case $L_{ChaseBalloon}$ is equal to C_S.

Starting from the information described above it was possible to compute D_i.

The exercise "chase balloons" is an exception as it was possible to modulate the number of targets to be reached in order to obtain the maximum score independently from the difficulty level. The possible choice were "very few" (8 objects), "few" (12 objects), "many" (24 objects), "full many" (36 objects). Following Eq. 3 the correspondent coefficient C_N assumed the values 1.0, 1.5, 3.0, 4.5 respectively. Thus in this exercise the coefficient of difficulty $D_{ChaseBalloon}$ was computed starting from the product between $L_{ChaseBalloon}$ and C_N.

Table 2. Level coefficients (L) to take into account the variation of difficulty due to the variation of the level of the exercise.

		Very easy	Easy	Medium	Difficult
Goalkeeper	C_T	1.00	1.48	2.43	4.86
	C_N	1.00	1.54	2.00	2.86
	$L_{Goalkeeper}$	1.00	2.27	4.86	13.88
Egg cracking	C_N	1.00	1.50	2.00	2.67
	C_S	1.00	1.56	2.85	6.25
	$L_{EggCracking}$	1.00	2.34	5.70	16.69
Fruit shopping	C_N	1.00	1.55	2.18	3.45
	C_S	1.00	1.00	1.26	1.62
	$L_{FruitShopping}$	1.00	1.55	2.75	5.60
Reveal Panorama	C_S	1.00	1.84	6.70	6.45
	$L_{RevealPanorama}$	1.00	1.84	6.70	6.45
Stove Cleaning	C_S	1.00	1.99	5.94	73.07
	$L_{StoveCleaning}$	1.00	1.99	5.94	73.07
Chase Balloon	C_S	1.00	2.61	4.29	6.42
	$L_{ChaseBalloon}$	1.00	2.61	4.29	6.42
Vertical Catching	C_N	1.00	1.67	2.50	4.00
	C_S	1.00	1.35	1.87	2.57
	$L_{VerticalCatching}$	1.00	2.25	4.68	10.28

Afterwards, ones the parameter p_i was computed it has been divided on the maximum performance achieved over time by the group of subjects (p_i^{max}) obtaining P_i (Eq. 4) that was used to compare different exercises.

$$P_i = \frac{p_i}{p_i^{max}} \qquad (4)$$

For every session of each subject, the value of P_i corresponding to the ith exercise could range from 0 (if the subjects score is 0) to 1 (if the subject achieved the maximum p_i with respect to the overall group of patients).

Finally P was computed for every single session as the median value of P_i for all the exercises. P is considered as index of the overall motor performance.

In order to test and validate the parameter P, 14 subjects underwent 4 weeks of training of 20 sessions lasting 30 min. During each session, subjects performed a customized pull of exercises with the supervision of a physiotherapist. The exercises were chosen in order to provide an engaging and gradual training, increasing the difficulty level over time (very easy, easy, medium, difficult).

2.3   Data Analysis

In this work, we first used the performance parameter P to follow the training of each subject over time.

Then, for each subject the median value of P_i and of P within the first week (T_0), between the 12th and the 16th days ($T_{1/2}$) and within the fourth week (T_1) of training were computed obtaining their performance during 3 well-defined time points. The effect of time on the performance was assessed by using the non-parametric Friedman test for paired samples. If values of P_i and P in T_0, $T_{1/2}$ and T_1 were found significantly different ($p < 0.05$), a post-hoc analysis (Bonferroni-adjusted Wilcoxon test) was performed comparing pair of groups (T_0 vs $T_{1/2}$, T_0 vs T_1 and $T_{1/2}$ vs T_1).

3   Results

Figure 1 shows the values obtained session by session by all the subjects. Median and quartiles are shown as bold line and colored area.

The training tendency was highly variable but an overall improving trend can be observed (the regression line of the median value obtained correlation coefficient R equal to 0.95).

Table 3 summarizes the main results obtained for every exercise (P_i) and for the comprehensive parameter P. Medians and interquartile values computed for

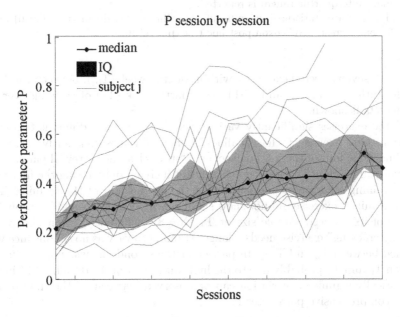

Fig. 1. Results of P obtained, session by session, during the eight exercises considered. Median and interquartile values of the population (bold and colored area respectively) and the values of P for each subjects are shown.

Table 3. P_i and P for the considered exercises over time (T_0, $T_{1/2}$ and T_1). N is the sample size on each time point of each exercise.

	T_0	$T_{1/2}$	T_1	p-value[b]		
				T_0 vs $T_{1/2}$	T_0 vs T_1	$T_{1/2}$ vs T_1
$P^a_{Goalkeeper}$	0.25 (0.09)	0.33 (0.31)	0.66 (0.18)	**0.002**	**0.005**	0.022
N	12	12	10			
$P^a_{StoveCleaning}$	0.25 (0.18)	0.53 (0.20)	0.54 (0.10)	**0.003**	0.018	0.889
N	12	12	8			
$P^a_{FruitShopping}$	0.45 (0.12)	0.43 (0.26)	0.62 (0.24)	0.248	**0.011**	**0.011**
N	11	11	9			
$P^a_{EggCracking}$	0.13 (0.19)	0.16 (0.14)	0.26 (0.12)	0.022	0.033	**0.003**
N	14	14	11			
$P^a_{RevealPanorama}$	0.10 (0.08)	0.17 (0.15)	0.30 (0.47)	**0.012**	**0.005**	0.066
N	13	12	10			
$P^a_{ChaseBalloon}$	0.26 (0.15)	0.47 (0.24)	0.68 (0.26)	**0.013**	**0.013**	**0.015**
N	13	12	10			
$P^a_{VerticalCatching}$	0.35 (0.11)	0.50 (0.15)	0.54 (0.14)	**0.002**	**0.005**	0.021
N	13	13	10			
P^a	0.27 (0.22)	0.43 (0.29)	0.54 (0.35)	**<0.001**	**<0.001**	**<0.001**
N	101	99	79			

[a]Median (interquartile range) is reported.
[b]Bold values are statistically significant according to Friedman (p < 0.050) and Bonferroni-corrected Wilcoxon post-hoc test (p < 0.0167).

each of the seven selected exercises, within the first week (T_0,), between the 12th and the 16th days ($T_{1/2}$) and within the fourth week (T_1) of training over all the subjects is shown.

All the exercises significantly varied over time but with different temporal evolution. One exercise ("chase balloon") showed values constantly increased over time while four of them ("goalkeeper", "stove cleaning", "reveal panorama" and "vertical catching") obtained a significant increase only during the first part of the training, showing a plateau during the second half of the training. The "stove cleaning" exercise did not show significance between T_0 and T_1 probably because of its reduced sample size at T_1 (N = 8). Differently, "fruit shopping" and "egg cracking" exercise needs a longer training to vary as no significance was obtained between T_0 and $T_{1/2}$. In particular the second one was not significant between T_0 and T_1 probably due to the high variability of the data in T_0. Finally a statistically significant variation can be observed between all the time points for the comprehensive parameter P.

4   Discussion

The need of reliable, quantitative and repeatable evaluations of training effectiveness is an up-to-date theme in the clinical practice. In fact, in some cases clinical scales are operator-dependent and not sensitive enough to highlight changes felt by patients and their parents [7]. Some quantitative evaluation could be obtained by the use of ad-hoc technology (e.g. optoelectronic analysis of the kinematics, sensorized robots) but these methods are time and money consuming.

Here we propose an innovative parameter P that takes into account the time needed to finish an exercise, the scores obtained during the exercise and the level of difficulty. This parameter is computed by mean of an excel macro in a simple and quick way from data automatically acquired by the robot during the training, and it does not require extra expensive devices.

The values obtained with P are patient-dependent and do not allowed classification of patients performances or disabilities. Indeed they can be used to compare the performance of each subject over time. In fact P allowed to follow each subject training session by session and to analyze performance variation between the beginning and the end of exercises.

All the exercises analyzed showed significant variation of P_i and P over the three time point analyzed. The different temporal trend give information about the time required to vary the performance, that is not the same for all the exercises. Anyway it seems to be not dependent from the dimension of the space used and from the body district trained. The specific behavior of "stove cleaning" may be due to the different size of the T_1 group ($N = 8$) with respect to T_0 and $T_{1/2}$ (both with $N = 12$).

As the parameter is built starting from data on the exercises trained, the variations observed could be due to a learning effect. Anyway the validation performed and described in a previous work [10], give some evidence that an increase in the values of P corresponds to a functional improvement in terms of Melbourne scale [11], thus the variation of the parameter may be due to the sum of the two effects: leaning effect and functional improvement.

To conclude, in this work we provide technical guidelines to compute a simple parameter aimed at evaluating robotic training. It seems to be a useful tool to follow the training and to give information about the performance on the exercises with no additional effort for patients and minimal additional effort for clinicians. The guidelines could be used by other researchers to reproduce the work or to apply the parameter to other exercises of Armeo®Spring and to other devices.

Further investigations are required to confirm these results and to validate the parameter with more clinical scales. Data of an age-matched healthy control group will be acquired in order to have a reference about the maximum performance achievable during the exercises. Moreover a validation with kinematics data would be important in order to compare the parameter with other quantitative and operator-independent data.

References

1. Lo, H.S., Xie, S.Q.: Exoskeleton robots for upper-limb rehabilitation: state of the art and future prospects. Med. Eng. Phys. **34**(3), 261–268 (2012)
2. Krebs, H.I., Volpe, B.T., Ferraro, M., Fasoli, S., et al.: Robot-aided Neurorehabilitation: from evidence-based to science-based rehabilitation. Top Stroke Rehabil. **8**(4), 54–70 (2002)
3. Granger, C.V., Hamilton, B.B., Keith, R.A., Zielezny, M., Sherwin, F.S.: Advances in functional assessment for medical rehabilitation. Topics Geriatr. Rehabil. **1**(3), 59–74 (1986)
4. Fortin, C., Ehrmann Feldman, D., Cheriet, F., Labelle, H.: Clinical Methods For Quantifying Body Segment Posture: A Literature Review. Disabil. Rehabil. **33**(5), 367–383 (2011)
5. Maciejasz, P., Eschweiler, J., Gerlach-Hahn, K., Jansen-Toy, A., Leonhardt, S.: A survey on robotic devices for upper limb rehabilitation. J. NeuroEng. Rehabil. **11**(1), 3 (2014)
6. Fasoli, S.E., Krebs, H.I., Stein, J., Frontera, W.R., et al.: Effects of robotic therapy on motor impairment and recovery in chronic stroke. Arch. Phys. Med. Rehabil. **84**(4), 477–482 (2003)
7. Brewer, B.R., McDowell, S.K., Worthen-Chaudhari, L.C.: Poststroke upper extremity rehabilitation: a review of robotic systems and clinical results. Top Stroke Rehabil. **14**(6), 22–44 (2007)
8. Amirabdollahian, F., Germano, T.G., Garth, R.J.: The peg-in-hole: a VR-based haptic assessment for quantifying upper limb performance and skills. In: 9th International Conference on Rehabilitation Robotics, ICORR 2005. IEEE (2005)
9. Merlo, A., Longhi, M., Giannotti, E., Prati, P., et al.: Upper limb evaluation with robotic exoskeleton. Normative values for indices of accuracy, speed and smoothness. NeuroRehabilitation **33**(4), 523–530 (2013)
10. Peri, E., Biffi, E., Maghini, C., Iammarrone Servodio, F., Gagliardi, C., et al.: A new quantitative performance parameter for monitoring robotics rehabilitation treatment. ACM Digital Library (2014)
11. Randall, M., Carlin, J.B., Chondros, P., Reddihough, D.: Reliability of the Melbourne assessment of unilateral upper limb function. Dev. Med. Child Neurol. **43**(11), 761–777 (2001)

An Exergame Concept for Improving Balance in Elderly People

Ather Nawaz[1(✉)], Mathilde Waerstad[2], Kine Omholt[2],
Jorunn L. Helbostad[1], Beatrix Vereijken[1], Nina Skjæret[1],
and Lill Kristiansen[2]

[1] Department of Neuroscience,
Norwegian University of Science and Technology (NTNU), Trondheim, Norway
{ather.nawaz,jorunn.helbostad,beatrix.vereijken,
nina.skjaret}@ntnu.no
[2] Department of Telematics,
Norwegian University of Science and Technology (NTNU), Trondheim, Norway
{mathildewaerstad,kine.omholt}@gmail.com,
lillk@item.ntnu.no

Abstract. Video exercise games (exergames) are becoming increasingly popular among elderly people. Many elderly experience reduced balance and muscle strength which make them at increased risk of falling. Muscle strength and balance training are the key components for preventing function decline and falls at old age. Exergames that are to be used among elderly users should be specifically designed for this group of people. This study aims to design and evaluate an exergame concept developed to fit the need and preferences of elderly users. First, seven elderly people tested three commercially available exergames. Feedback from focus group interviews revealed that the design of the existing exergames should be simplified and more closely related to activities that can be associated with older people's daily life. Based on the feedback a new exergame concept "in nature" was designed. The new exergame concept had a simple design, and included balance and muscle strengthening exercises related to real life activities. In the results of the workshop, the study provides eight design recommendations for exergame design for seniors.

Keywords: Exergames · Design · Seniors · Balance · Falls · Elderly

1 Introduction

The use of games for exercise is generally called exergames. The game industry mainly develops these games for a wider audience such as children and adolescents for the purpose of entertainment. The game industry is growing 9.1 % annually to $48.9 in 2011 and $66 billion in 2012, making it the fastest-growing component of the international media. Due to business goals, the game industry is mainly focusing on covering a large population without specific focus on the requirements of senior citizens.

However, the world's population is "greying", with the proportion of the world's population aged 60 and older set to double to more than 22 % of the overall population by 2050 [1]. The ageing process includes decline in visual and auditory systems,

© Springer-Verlag Berlin Heidelberg 2015
H.M. Fardoun et al. (Eds.): REHAB 2014, CCIS 515, pp. 55–67, 2015.
DOI: 10.1007/978-3-662-48645-0_6

as well as slowing down in movements [2]. Due to the increasing number of elderly people, movement impairments and the lack of physical activity among this age group will likely become one of the major societal challenges in the next decades.

One in three persons over the age of 65, and half of those over the age of 80, fall at least once per year. International guidelines on physical activity in older people highlight the need for balance and muscle strength training in order to prevent loss of physical function and falls [3].

Exergames have the potential to motivate senior citizens to be physically active. Exergames also have the potential to improve health-related issues among senior citizens, such as decreasing depression [4], and increasing physical function in general [5] and balance in particular [6]. However game technologies need to be designed and developed based on the older persons' needs and preferences. Furthermore, in order to prevent physical decline and falls, exergames developed for older people should also aim to work on balance control and muscle strength.

1.1 Relevant Work on Design of Exergames

A number of studies have focused on psychological effects of exergames [4, 7, 8]. However, not many studies have focused on designing senior-centered exergames for physical fitness in general and balance training in particular. To meet individual variability in level of physical function among older people, games should provide different difficulty levels so that seniors can adjust according to their comfort and needs. Gerling et al. [9] outlined four general points that are important for designing exergames for senior citizens: The possibility to (1) play both sitting and standing, (2) avoid too extensive and sudden movements, (3) adjust difficulty level and device sensitivity, and (4) simple interaction mechanisms and feedback in the gameplay. Furthermore, Jongman [10] expressed that design of an exergame for balance training should accommodate weight shifts during movements. A recent study [11] focused on the importance of assessing user experience of seniors when exergaming for balance training. The study finds that healthy seniors liked exergame that was specifically developed for seniors.

Seniors have different preferences, interests and taste of games that might not be the same as in a young population. Loneliness is a challenge among many older people, and reduced physical function makes it difficult to leave the house on their own. Therefore, exergames can offer an opportunity to exercise at home while socializing with others at distance through the gameplay [12]. A recent study [13] linked the movement elements in commercially available exergames with the game elements in each game and concluded that the interface should provide some kind of representation of the players' movements on the screen. However, a fully animated 3D representation is not necessary to achieve the required movements in the player's gaming behavior [13].

The current paper extends our work presented at rehab workshop2014 [17]. The current paper reported in evaluates existing off-the-shelf exergames and, based on feedback from the elderly players, presents a new exergame concept for elderly people for improving balance. The aim of this study is to design a simple concept of an exergame for elderly people using natural tasks that provide an opportunity to train aspects of balance and muscle strength. We conducted two workshops to evaluate previous off-the-shelf exergames and present a new exergame concept. On the basis of the results, this study highlights recommendations for designing exergames for seniors.

2   Method

In the context of exergames for seniors, the needs of seniors should be assessed through user-centered design process to make effective exergames for seniors [14]. We employed a user-centered design (UCD) method for designing the exergame [15].

We conducted two workshops with elderly users. The workshops were conducted at a seniors community centre that was familiar to the senior citizens. In the fist workshop the elderly users played three off-the-shelf exergames. After having played the off-the-shelf games they gave their feedback for these existing exergames and provided inputs for new game concepts. The requirements for a new game concept were made based on this feedback of elderly users and inputs for new game concept. Then, a prototype of a new game was designed. The same elderly users were invited to a second workshop aimed at evaluating the new exergame concept.

2.1   Participants

We recruited elderly people from a voluntary organization "Seniornett" or senior network. *Seniornett* is working with elderly citizens to become active users of ICT and internet. Seven elderly citizens participated in the first workshop and five elderly citizens participated in the second workshop. The average age of the participants was 70.6 (SD ± 7.9) years. All participants had their own computer and were familiar with using smartphones, but they had no prior experience with video game technologies.

Five out of seven participants used their computer several times a week. The senior citizens generally used computer for E-banking, email and news. Most of the senior citizens found social aspects of exercising important while four out of seven said that they would like to share information with family and friends through social media. Six out of seven participants said that they were physically active in everyday life and performed regular exercise in classes. Factors motivating them for performing exercise include: being in activity, socializing, achieving a good mood, and maintaining good health.

3   Workshop 1: Testing off-the-Shelf Exergames

The first workshop consisted of a gameplay section followed by a focus group where participants discussed their experience with the off-the-shelf exergames, their thoughts about the exergames and the technology, and their requirements for a new exergame.

The three off-the-shelf exergames used in the first workshop were "Kinect Sports: Season Two", "YourShape:Fitness Evolved", and "Fruit Ninja". Kinect Sports consists of six sports. We chose Tennis and Skiing because these games stimulate movement and balance activity in a fun and motivating way. YourShape is a fitness game that includes mini games. In the game pack YourShape, we chose "Aging with grace". We chose "aging with grace" because it was specifically designed for elderly.

Fruit Ninja is a game where players use their arms like a ninja to slice fruit that is thrown up into the air. This game was chosen on the basis of fun and balance requirements of the movements (Fig. 1) shows the interface of three games which were used in the study.

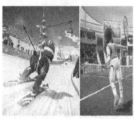 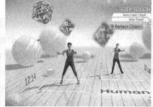 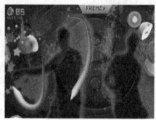

a) Skiing and tennis in   b) YourShape:Fitness   c) Fruit ninja
   Kinect sports   Evolved

Fig. 1. The three exergames in workshop 1

3.1   Procedure of Workshop 1

The first workshop was held over a period of two days. All seven seniors were present for introduction of the study on the first day of the workshop. However four seniors played exergames on the first day and provided their feedback. Three seniors played games on the second day of the workshop and provided their feedback. The workshop consisted of a gameplay section followed by a focus group. Before playing the three exergames, participants were introduced to the technology and how to interact with it. The participants in each group first played the games individually, and then competed against one another using a multi-players setting. Each participant played three games for a total of approximately 25 min. After gameplay, the participants provided feedback (Fig. 2) shows a screen-shot of two participants competing with each other in the skiing game in Kinect Sports on their experience with the gameplay and the technology for all three exergames in a focus group interview.

Two video cameras were used from different angles for recording. The first camera was placed in front of the TV and camera was used to capture facial expressions and movements with the game. The second camera was placed in a corner of the room to capture the overall environment of the room.

After playing game focus session was conducted with participants where participants discussed their experience with the off-the-shelf exergames, their thoughts about the exergames and the technology, and their requirements for a new exergame During the focus group, participants were asked about the challenges they faced while playing the exergames The feedback of the participants was transcribed and coded. A set of themes was derived from the feedback of participants in workshop.

3.2   Findings of Workshop 1

The participants expressed that they liked Tennis and Skiing because they could relate it to previous real life experiences with skiing and playing tennis. They also liked it

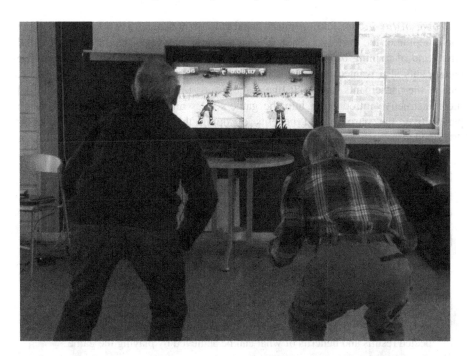

Fig. 2. Two participants compete in the skiing game in Kinect Sports

because these two games were physically more challenging, fun and entertaining than the other two games. Skiing was the game that engaged the players most while playing the game. Our interpretation is that seniors had higher level of engagement because Skiing is a popular sports in the area. Following are general points expressed by the seniors in the focus group discussion.

Information display: There was a general opinion among the seniors that too many things were presented at the screen during the game-plays of all games. For the Fruit Ninja game, one of the participants stated, "there are too many elements on the screen. Where should you look"? The participants stated that too many things were going on at the same time and that it was hard to do move hand simultaneously. The participants expressed that the interface was too complex in all games. One of the participants said: "the menu was extremely difficult", while another stated while trying to give input through hand gestures, "this is worse than working with the mouse on the computer". The participants wanted to see less information and elements on the screen at the same time.

> Recommendation1: The interface should be simple with minimal and relevant information only.

Outcome of the game: Participants wanted information regarding the specific effect and outcome of the exercises. They wanted to know why to do the different tasks and what kind of training benefits the games could give them beyond entertainment. The participants also wanted to know if they performed the movements correctly or not. One of the participants stated, "It [the game] needs to be softer and [there should be] more instructive introduction into the game's rules and objectives". From a design perspective, the purpose and benefits of doing the exercises should be clearly described.

Recommendation 2: The primary focus within game play experience should be on movement quality without too much distraction.

Recommendation 3: The exergame should provide a clear indication of expected results and benefits of what can be achieved by playing the game.

Progress and learning: The participants expressed that they wanted a simple way to display progress and learning in their game-play. One of the participants stated, "It is all about the experience of mastery, which is essential. The older you get, the more important it gets to progress". Another participant suggested different levels of tasks in the game and stated, eventually, "when you get better and manage to keep track of things, you can add more elements to the game. A lot of what happens in these games is not relevant". The other participant expressed that progress and learning in the exergame was not same as she experience in aerobic class, "we used to attend an aerobic class where they practiced exercises slowly before they could do it fast. I do not feel it [progress] the same way". Another participant stated that she did not want to get forced into something she did not want to do, and that she wanted to be able to choose which difficulty level to play in. "I am thinking that I do not want to get forced into something that is hard, that I do not master because then I get mad". One of the participant stated that she would like to see puzzle in the game.

Recommendation 4: The elderly users should be able to choose and add difficulty elements in the game for confidence and better progress.

Music: The participants did not like the music and background noise in the three game systems. Cheering, loud music, encouraging comments and fans were perceived as noisy and annoying by some of them. One of the participants stated, "I think everything about that [music] was too much". The participants rather wanted old music of their time, with less noise. Another participant stated, "You get sensitive to sound, you want to be active but without too much noise".

Recommendation 5: The game should provide age-appropriate music for elderly users, and the music should fit the aim of the game or the movements performed.

Game suggestions: In the feedback session in workshop 1, participants suggested that real-life activities for game design. These real-life activities includes wood chopping, sports, swimming, rowing, picking apples, biathlon, interval exercises, dance, puzzle games, and a walk in nature. In addition, it was mentioned that if the aim of the game was exercising, they wanted a full workout session including warm-up exercise, cool-down and stretching.

Recommendation 6: The game story should be close to real-life activities of seniors.

4   Prototyping the New Exergame

Based on the feedback from workshop 1, a horizontal prototype exergame concept was developed. A horizontal prototype provides a broad view of the system, focusing on user interaction more than on lower-level system functionality. A horizontal prototype reduces the level of functionality in prototype of the system. We made a horizontal prototype because it was a quick way of designing an interface and get feedback before moving to the next phase for development of an exergame. As shown in Fig. 3, the prototype focused on visual and sensory experiences of exergame design [16].

The two flow charts shown in Fig. 4 show how the game-story can be organized through two scenarios.

In Fig. 4(a), the player can choose to walk trail 1 without obstacles and hearts. This trail can be done just by walking. In trail 2, on the other hand, there are obstacles that need to be avoided, and hearts to gather. This trail will take some more time, but at the same time, exercises more of the body, which might result in a better score. In Fig. 4(b) the player can choose to walk the trail without obstacles and hearts, or choose to row a boat over to the other side of a lake. The second scenario provides the elements such as

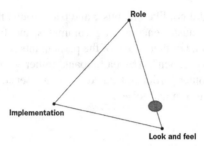

Fig. 3. Implementation of prototype in prototype triangle

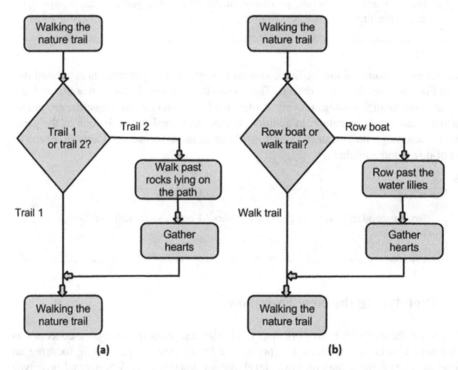

Fig. 4. Flow charts of two ways of "branching" in the game (a) The player can choose between two different trails and (b) The player can choose between walking the trail or rowing a boat over to the other side of a lake

water lilies that should be avoided, and hearts that are be gathered. After finishing the chosen trail, the player will end up on the same trail again. The new level can be added in the game by changing the tail and speed of the game.

4.1   Interface of New Exergame

Figure 5 provides an example of an exergame interface that was prototyped for seniors to fit their needs and preference. The exergame contains different levels of difficulties.

The player completes the easiest level first, and then proceeds to the next level. This is done for the player to be able to learn the game sufficiently before progressing to a more advanced level. The player could also play the game in collaboration with other players or compete against other players.

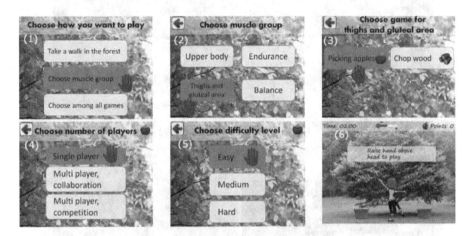

Fig. 5. The menu focuses on exercising different muscle groups

In the new concept, the seniors can choose exercises according to different body muscles and choose an exercise depending upon their own preference or the recommendation from a physiotherapist. This would provide elderly users with a clear objective and benefits of exercising. The design of the exergames reflects the goals of training muscle strength and/or balance For example, the goal of one of the exergames concepts is to pick as many ripe apples from a tree as possible within a given time. This activity requires players to stretch their body to reach for ripe apples (balance) and put them in a basket on the ground by performing deep squats (muscle strength). New, unripe apples appear on the tree and turn red when they are ripe. If the apple hangs on the tree too long, it rots and falls off the tree. The player gets points from picking red apples, and loses points both for picking unripe apples and from letting an apple rot.

As shown in Fig. 5, the prototype provides a simple interface with limited information, which is easy to understand for elderly users and helps them to focus more on the actual activity rather than confusing users with rich information displayed at different places on the screen.

Figure 6 presents the interface of different obstacles in the nature trail, which also challenges players' muscle strength and balance. A set of obstacles were added, necessitating the following actions: (a) jump from rock to rock to get over the river, (b) walk over the log lying across the path, (c) duck under the branch hanging over the path, (d) get over the lake by rowing the boat, (e) balance on the log to get over the river, (f) walk on the rocks lying on the path. As the seniors expressed the idea of doing a quiz in exercise, the design also included quizzes in the nature trail so participants could answer questions while maintaining their balance.

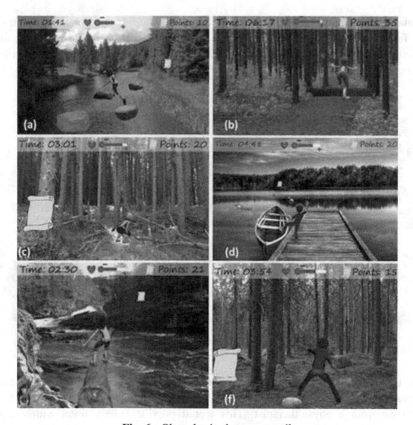

Fig. 6. Obstacles in the nature trail

5   Workshop 2: Presenting the New Exergame Concept

A second workshop was conducted at the same location as workshop 1 to get the feedback of senior citizens regarding the new exergame prototype. All participants from workshop 1 were invited to participate in the second workshop. The participants of the workshop were presented with the summary of the issues that were identified in the first workshop and the interface of the new game "Out in Nature". A computer and a projector were used to show the concept of the new game. The seniors were also provided with the paper prototypes of the interface.

5.1   Findings of Workshop 2

In the second workshop, the participants did not have many inputs and feedbacks. The participants of the second workshop generally liked that the exergame design of "out in nature" had a familiar environment. However, some of the seniors were concerned that including quizzes in the nature trail would take the focus away from the physical tasks to cognitive tasks. One senior stated, "Answering the questions in the quiz will become some kind of test on how good you are, and that is not how I have understood the point of these games".

Recommendation 7: The exergame concept must describe if the outcome of the game is a physical challenge, a cognitive challenge or both.

They liked that there were different difficulty levels in the game and another user stated, "I think that it is an advantage that everyone starts at the easy level, and the more confident you get the harder it gets. I think that is a good way to be controlled". However, the participants wished clearer description of what was required for different difficulty levels. Senior users liked the idea of having a nature trail to play an exergame, which would be entertaining and fruitful and at the same time increase their physical activity level. The users expressed that the design of the new game was simple to understand as it only showed limited information.

Recommendation 8: The exergame concept must make it clear what kinds of movements are required at different difficulty levels.

For music, the seniors were curious about what kind of music the games would get, "I am wondering, about the atmosphere and environment, when I am balancing there [on the log], will I hear the sound of water"?

Regarding methodological considerations of the study, it was challenging to present an interactive exergame with a paper prototype to such an inexperienced group, and the participants had little feedback and comments on the game design. This was one of the reasons that seniors did not provide many inputs on the new design. Future prototype should focus on developing more interactive prototypes to increase the users understanding of the game.

6   Conclusion

This study evaluates off-the-shelf exergame, designs new game concept, and evaluates exergame concept that fits the need and preferences of elderly users. The evaluation of three off-the-shelf exergames and presentation of a new exergame provided several important lessons for the design of exergames for senior citizens. First of all, it is important to show only limited information on the screen. Seniors prefer to focus on a single activity in the game rather than doing multiple activities such as physical activity and a quiz at the same time. Secondly, the exergame should provide the objective of the game at the start so that seniors are aware of the required activities and their potential effect. Thirdly, special focus should be given to progress and learning. Initial gameplay should be slower with subsequent progression in speed and difficulty as the senior advances. Lastly, age-appropriate music should be provided in accordance with seniors' choice. These are important aspects to take into consideration for exergames to be a relevant tool for senior citizens to train their physical function and prevent falls.

This study demonstrates the importance of designing exergames for seniors with simplified interfaces. The study provides a prototype that gives an example of how such a simple interface can be developed which can focus on different ways to train balance and strength in seniors. Designing the game with different exercises would allow seniors to train different muscle groups and enjoy the game at the same time.

Acknowledgements. The research leading to these results has received funding from the European Union Seventh Framework Programme (FP7/2007-2013) under grant agreement FARSEEING n° 288940. FARSEEING aims to promote better prediction, identification and prevention of falls with focus on ICT devices. We thank the older seniors from Seniornett for taking part in the project.

References

1. Factbox on video game industry. http://in.reuters.com/article/2013/06/10/gameshow-e-idINDEE9590DW20130610. Accessed 14 November 2013
2. Billis, A.S., Konstantinidis, E.I., Mouzakidis, C., Tsolaki, M.N., Pappas, C., Bamidis, P.D.: A game-like interface for training seniors' dynamic balance and coordination. In: Bamidis, P.D., Pallikarakis, N. (eds.) XII Mediterranean Conference on Medical and Biological Engineering and Computing 2010. Proceedings of IFMBE, vol. 29, pp. 691–694. Springer, Heidelberg (2010)
3. Gillespie, L.D., Robertson, MC., Gillespie, Sherrington, C., Gates, S., Clemson, L.M., Lamb, S.E.: Interventions for preventing falls in older people living in the community. Cochrane Database Syst. Rev. 2(CD007146) (2009)
4. Rosenberg, D., Depp, C.A., Vahia, I.V., Reichstadt, J., Palmer, B.W., Kerr, J., Jeste, D.V.: Exergames for subsyndromal depression in older adults: A pilot study of a novel intervention. Am. J. Geriatr. Psychiatry 18(3), 221–226 (2010)
5. Jung, Y., Li, K.J., Janissa, N.S., Gladys, W.L.C., Lee, K.M.: Games for a better life: effects of playing Wii games on the well-being of seniors in a long-term care facility. In: Proceedings of the Sixth Australasian Conference on Interactive Entertainment. ACM (2009)
6. Schoene, D., Lord, S.R., Delbaere, K., Severino, C., Davies, T.A., Smith, S.T.: A randomized controlled pilot study of home-based step training in older people using videogame technology. PLoS ONE 8(3), e57734 (2013)
7. Maillot, P., Perrot, A., Hartley, A.: Effects of interactive physical-activity video-game training on physical and cognitive function in older adults. Psychol. Aging 27(3), 589 (2012)
8. Anderson-Hanley, C., Arciero, P.J., Brickman, A.M., Nimon, J.P., Okuma, N., Westen, S.C., Zimmerman, E.A.: Exergaming and older adult cognition: a cluster randomized clinical trial. Am. J. Prev. Med. 42(2), 109–119 (2012)

9. Gerling, K.M., Schild, J., Masuch, M.: Exergame design for elderly users: the case study of silverbalance. In: Proceedings of the 7th International Conference on Advances in Computer Entertainment Technology, pp. 66–69. ACM, Taipei, Taiwan (2010)

10. Jongman, V., Lamoth, C.J.C., Van Keeken, H., Caljouw, S.R.: Postural control of elderly: moving to predictable and unpredictable targets. Stud. Health Technol. Inf. **181**, 93–97 (2012)

11. Nawaz, A., Skjaeret, N., Ystmark, K., Helbostad, J.L., Vereijken, B., Svanaes, D.: Assessing seniors' user experience (UX) of exergames for balance training. In: Proceedings of the 8th Nordic Conference on Human-Computer Interaction: Fun, Fast, Foundational, pp. 578–587. ACM, Helsinki, Finland (2014). doi:10.1145/2639189.2639235

12. Cornejo, R., Hernández, D., Favela, J., Tentori, M., Ochoa, S.: Persuading older adults to socialize and exercise through ambient games. In: 6th International Conference on Pervasive Computing Technologies for Healthcare (PervasiveHealth), pp. 215–218. IEEE, May 2012

13. Skjaeret, N., Nawaz, A., Ystmark, K., Dahl, Y., Helbostad, J.L., Svanaes, D., Vereijken, B.: Designing for movement quality in exergames: lessons learned from observing senior citizens playing stepping games. Gerontology **61**(2), 186–194 (2015)

14. Proffitt, R., Lange, B.: User centered design and development of a game for exercise in older adults. Int. J. Technol. Knowl. Soc. **8**(5), 95–112 (2012)

15. ISO 9241: Ergonomics of Human–System Interaction—Part 210: Human-Centred Design for Interactive Systems. International Organization for Standardization (ISO), Geneva, Switzerland (2010)

16. Houde, S., Hill, C.: What do prototypes prototype. In: Helander, M., Landauer, T., Prabhu, P. (eds.) Handbook of Human-Computer Interaction, vol. 2, pp. 367–381. Elsevier Science, Cambridge (1997)

17. Nawaz, A., Waerstad, M., Omholt, K., Helbostad, J.L., Vereijken, B., Skjaeret, Kristiansen, L.: Designing simplified exergame for muscle and balance training in seniors: a concept of 'out in nature'. In: Proceedings of the 8th International Conference on Pervasive Computing Technologies for Healthcare, pp. 309–312. Germany. ICST (Institute for Computer Sciences, Social-Informatics and Telecommunications Engineering), Oldenburg (2014). doi:10.4108/icst.pervasivehealth.2014.255269

Games-Based Therapy to Stimulate Speech in Children

Habib M. Fardoun[1(✉)], Iyad A. Katib[1], and Antonio Paules Cipres[2]

[1] Information Systems Department, King Abdulaziz University (KAU),
Jeddah, Saudi Arabia
{hfardoun, iakatib}@kau.edu.sa
[2] European University of Madrid, Madrid, Spain
apcipres@gmail.com

Abstract. There are speech troubles that can be a sign of speech disorders or speech sound disorders. Some causes include hearing loss, neurological disorders, brain injury, intellectual disabilities, and so on. It is therefore very important to include the speech therapy as part of the rehabilitation process for affected patients' phonation. This chapter presents a study on the ways sound creation develops, aiming at creating an application to aid the therapy session. The solution presented is used to improve speech problems through playing games.

1 Introduction

This is the first study of a series of studies on speech therapy. Here, the results show that this rehabilitation speciality was successful in primary schools as students with speech problems go to speech therapists for treatment.

According to the Royal Academy of the Spanish Language, speech therapy teaches phonation to those who experience pronunciation difficulties. It includes the diagnosis, rehabilitation, and prevention of problems related to communication skills and their associated functions. Following the Spanish ordination law of health professionals (Ley de Ordenación de las Profesiones Sanitarias L.O.P.S. Ley 44/2003, de 21 de Noviembre, de ordenación de las profesiones sanitarias), speech therapists graduate as health assistants. According to the associated legislation, "Graduated students in speech therapy develop the prevention, evaluation and restoring activities of audition, phonation and language problems utilising associated therapeutic techniques."

Speech problems may be divided into two categories: aphasias and dysarthria. Aphasias is produced as a consequence of a lesion or brain injury that leads to the loss of capacity to understand or produce language (either in adults or in children) [1]. Dysarthria is a language alteration produced by a brain lesion. It differs from aphasia in that alterations are not presented in the prolongation or in the language sequence but exist in associated difficulties with phonological components; in other words, by making language sounds [2].

This chapter is a complement to a publication presented in the workshop of the 8th International Conference on Pervasive Computing Technologies for Healthcare (Per-vasiveHealth '14) [11] taking into consideration the previous work, we describe in

© Springer-Verlag Berlin Heidelberg 2015
H.M. Fardoun et al. (Eds.): REHAB 2014, CCIS 515, pp. 68–77, 2015.
DOI: 10.1007/978-3-662-48645-0_7

detail the system functionality in order to help the reader to design similar systems focusing on speech rehabilitation.

2 State of the Art

Nowadays, most related exercises aiming at improving speech are created by therapists on hard copy paper format. The therapist prepares worksheets for children with these limitations; these exercises are found in specific topic books where there are patterns to perform the exercises. However, it is difficult to offer proper follow-up sessions with the children. Currently, there is no tool to prepare the exercises and carry out this follow-up for the children (Fig. 1).

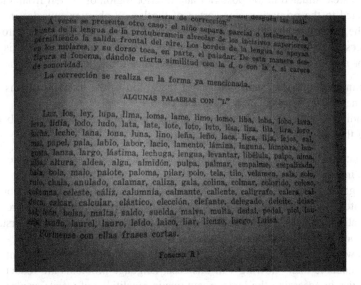

Fig. 1. Games and words to improve the pronunciation of specific words.

3 Objectives

In this paper, we aim to analyze, design and build a platform for specialists and also schools. The main goal is to support specific exercises so to improve the reading ability.

The procedure we have followed is as follows: First, we classify the problem for improvement. After the initial analysis, it is associated to the corresponding treatments. Then, the platform suggests personalized games for the child to perform rehabilitation activities from school or home. Both parents and teachers could also carry out the monitoring exercises, developed for mobile devices such as Smartphone, tablets, or other devices.

4 Classification and Treatment

A study was conducted based on the targeted diseases classification in relation to the language problems as well as the evaluation treatment. These details are presented next.

4.1 Classification

The areas in the brain responsible for language processing as well as the problematic areas in regards to language are [3]:

- Wernicke's area: situated in the posterior region of the left temporal lobe it decodes the language hearing information.
- Broca's area: situated in the posterior and inferior region of the left frontal lobe it is connected to the primary motor cortex of the larynx-pharynx muscles in order to code the patterns of the articular speech nerves. In written language, the information is processed to an occipital level (perception of graphical symbols) and is in relation, or not, to the hearing perception in reference to the left inferior parietal lobe.

The human phonetic system consists of the group of the different organs responsible for the language articulation [4].

Depending whether we talk about a neuropsychological alteration or bad functioning of the phonetic organs, the classification is [5]:

- Aphasia: it affects the spoken language (Broca's area) while receptive aphasia affects interpretation and language memory (Wernicke's area).
- Flowing: they are the aphasias that produce a lot of vocabulary without much articulatory effort; however, these may be responsible for many errors, little informative content, poor vocabulary and, definitely, a non understandable expression due to the presence of deform problems in the words.
- Not flowing: children make major articulatory effort, although the content is more understandable than "flowing". In this case, language problems are reductive with difficulties in accessing the lexicon, automatic repetitions of words or phrases, etc.
- Dysarthria: the articulatory alterations are manifested by omission, substitution, addition, or distortion of one or more phonemes, which affect the meaning of speech. In addition, children who suffer from dysarthria have difficulties in moving their phonetic-articulatory organs with difficulties on any activity. The following areas can be affected: articulation, speed, volume, prosody (intonation), and phonetic respiratory coordination. Dysarthria is the result of a lesion in the central or peripheral nervous system. The common causes include ictus, cranial accidents, neurodegenerative diseases (Parkinson, Multiple Sclerosis, etc.).

4.2 Treatment

Treatment associated to these anomalies is related to each of the organs taking part in the phonemes' creation [6, 7]:

- The respiratory system: articulating the phonemes is necessary so that several organs can work together. Oral language alterations are consequences of the unusual functionalities of these specific organs. In these cases, it is necessary that the correct process to breathe is demonstrated through respiratory exercises.
- The main phonation organ, the larynx: along with the tongue, phonation is created here. Treatment is usually related to respiratory, tongue, lips, and vocal exercises.
- The resonator system: formed by the inferior area of the supraglottal resonator system, the lips function as the articulator system. To deal with labial weakness, a child performs labial exercises in order to move the lips naturally.

5 Research Objective

The aim of this research is to bring these techniques closer to the ICTs rehabilitation so to be utilized by speech therapists in order to prepare appropriate exercises helping children performing their exercises from home. Nowadays, speech therapy is a forgotten area within TICS rehabilitation. Speech therapists are not located in educational centres; hence, this study offers an easy way for teachers to use these techniques with the assistance of a speech therapist.

6 Study Case

In this study, the speech therapist provides a set of exercises in an educational centre for young students, preparing them for their transition from childhood to puberty, this is when their voice changes (for when they leave aside their infantile voice). This is a very common physical problem for children at this age as their respiratory cavities are adapting and the deficiencies appear following a purely functional cause. These exercises can be classified as respiratory, labial, vocalization, and resonance.

- **Respiratory exercises:** Figure 2 shows the ways the children can improve their respiratory exercises and learn to breathe and increase their lung capacity through games. They are required to blow out the candle while breathing, in other words, providing a constant flow of air from the lungs to the iPad's sensors. A microphone detects the intensity and the airflow through the generated sound. The application offers different types of games for this treatment as seen on the right.
- **Labial exercises:** Using an iPad pressure sensor, designed and improved in later versions, the game consists of an activity of holding a ball in the air and requires more strength after each attempt. In this way, the child improves their labial strength. It is also aimed at increasing his/her capacity for pronunciation and phonation. As such, the child must blow through a mouthpiece connected to a rubber to guarantee that the lips are positioned correctly over the iPad pressure sensor. As in Fig. 3, the application shows a set of exercises including intensity and time factors.
- **Vocalization exercises:** In this case, the kids must vocalize, following a set of steps indicated by the application (Fig. 4).

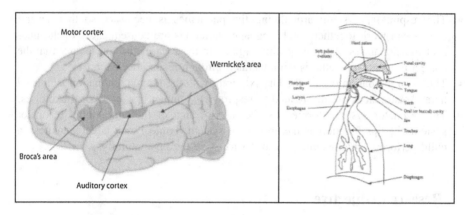

Fig. 2. Left: brain areas. Right: human phonetic system.

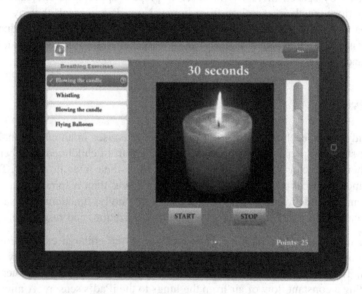

Fig. 3. Blowing the candle application.

As seen in Fig. 3, the child can perform the exercises by following the pronunciations shown in the application, for example, a karaoke. Thus, the student makes the interruptions and the phonemes' prolongations. Pre-visualization of the exercise content is available. Furthermore, exercise repetitions and examples are presented to show the student how to do the pronunciations.

These exercises can be performed at school or home with the parents' or teachers' help and support. The exercises are very simple to perform and do not require specific therapeutic knowledge. However, a specific period is required for the child to conduct the exercises in order to rehabilitate the voice's timbre.

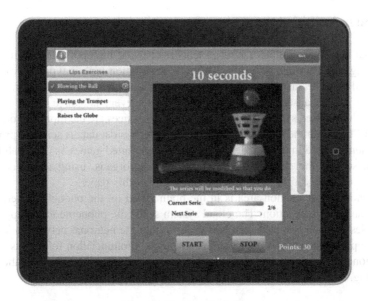

Fig. 4. Blowing the ball.

Nowadays, there are books related to speech therapy offering treatment guidelines. However, no specific platforms and applications exist to bring speech therapy closer to the educational centres and to the parents.

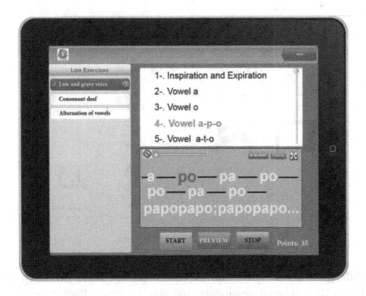

Fig. 5. Vocalization exercises (Color figure online).

7 System Architecture

During our study, an English language teacher checked the application utilisation in foreign language learning. She said that this rehabilitation type is typical for different languages. However, the option of using phonetic sounds was suggested as an essential application part because the phonetic is the same for every language.

In the cloud-based system architecture, the web services are the input and output for communication with the application as such. In other words, data is sent and processed in the system located in the cloud. The case study presented games as the rehabilitation exercises, so that the children could stimulate their organs, using vocalization and phonetic exercises, which were the research focus of this paper.

The phoneme generation area is in the brain based on the phonetic generation as with the language translation. The cloud system sends the phoneme to the application to processes it. Then complex activities occur within the neuronal network oriented to phonetics, phonetic symbols are created and sounds' pronunciation follows as a result. These phonetic languages and their combination in the brain area produce the vocalization (Fig. 6).

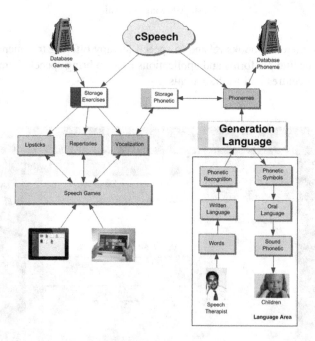

Fig. 6. Conceptual architecture.

Two different parts are presented in Fig. 5: on one hand (in blue), the game platform is classified in labial, respiratory, and phonetic types. Both the specialists and the teachers create these games. On the other hand (in green), the vocalization games is the locus where the phonetic exercises are responsible for the language generation.

The language treatment is emphasized in a light brown colour, where the speech therapist, using the introduced words into the platform, generates exercises. Therefore, the therapist generates vocalization exercises and the platform generates the sounds depending on the child's language. Thus, a layer in the cloud is consequently included for the phonetic function and the sound translation, in order to improve the vocalization for any language.

We have made a brief description of the system elements and its operation. Next, we will describe these features one by one, so to clarify the system functionality described in Fig. 5.

Exercises Storage: It provides an exercises collection and series to apply the treatment to the patients. The system offers several treatments depending on the associated disease. Then, in order to improve the related skill, different phonemes games are provided such as:

- Lipsticks: It contains lip exercises to position the lips correctly to improve pronunciation.
- Repertories: Breathing exercises aim to improve pulmonary capacity through the rehabilitation.
- Phonetic Storage: It provides a collection of phonemes needed to perform the exercises in the phonetic composition and stored phonemes pronunciation. This is to enable multilingual functionality, since the phonemes representation depends on the language as its composition is different for different languages.

Vocalization. Phoneme vocalization exercises. Based on the repetition of phonemes the patients can correct targeted defects in pronunciation. The phonetic exercises correspond to associated tables created by the therapist. In this case, only the phonemes are saved and then the composition of the specific exercise is performed.

The phonemes are performed by the language generation. It involves a process that the therapist and the child can carry out in the language area. It is a process the therapist must create for the child to follow.

The therapist generates concrete steps to improve the child's pronunciation such as:

- **Words**: The therapist creates a repetition of certain words addressing them in a concrete and precise order to generate exercises for the child; professional exercises produced here should be checked. If they are necessary for the word phonemes creation, and also, if not finalized, the system can make recommendations adapted to specific needs.
- **Writing Language**: Based on the words selected in the previous section, the specialist generates phrases and the necessary guidelines for the realization of phonemes phonetic exercises. At this point, the specialist acquires all the necessary phonemes and as such, guidelines for improving pronunciation child are easy to be created.
- **Phonetic Recognition**: Once the above steps, the system itself takes a phonetic recognition of the exercise. Therefore, the exercise is validated and the specialist can verify that everything is finalized, including suggested modifications. If

performance of phonemes is not correct in the database or not met, further validation is provided by the system to obtain validated phonemes existing in the system.

In this phonetic recognition process, the system must guarantee a number of steps between identification of phonemes, letters and words. This is necessary to establish a series of steps to be taken into account in the exercise, and the platform should contain to achieve the purpose:

- **Phonetic symbols**: the child must provide an acknowledgment of the phonetic symbols so to recognize the symbol and establish the relationship with the sound. In this section, the phonetic symbols are represented on the platform.
- **Oral:** The child's oral language should be enhanced by teaching the child; this is possible by the utilization of oral language phonetic symbols provided by the platform as banks of images and videos for the positioning of each phonetic symbol lips.
- **Phonetic Sound:** This is what the child hears and repeats, generated when following the guidelines. Upon recognition of the above steps, the child understands and associates the sound connected to the phonetic symbols.

Each of these steps takes an analysis of information concerning the composition and activities conducted by specialists; this data set should be verified by the system and stored for complete verification. These functions are generated separately in the system and should also be evaluated separately; hence the system should function in layers to analyze information from the various parties.

We will perform a root objects interrelationship between each of the parties, so that in this way the system will allow greater flexibility and maintenance. The object interaction is conducted by the layers i.e. each object operates independently supporting the top-level object; as such, the functionalities complement each other in order to provide a complete set.

Passing parameters between objects including objects creation can do this. The representation of an exercise object is a set of parameterized object, thus the object responsive to an interaction between them is coming from the user. Such functionality also facilitates objects monitoring towards data evaluation for each object to be associated with various sensors and devices that may arise as parts on the platform.

8 Conclusions and Future Work

Voice problems are essential to be treated early in the period between infancy and adolescence, delaying the teaching/learning process. However, using the suggested and performed exercises child with speech difficulties usually exhibits rehabilitation of the phonation system organs. Furthermore, this training also affects the brain where the sound is produced because the child associates those sounds with images, facilitating and accelerating training and rehabilitation.

This is the first research study on the speech therapy as a non-traumatic rehabilitation process produced and suggested by speech therapists.

In future work, we propose to create a system that allows the utilization of diverse rehabilitation devices (simulating real devices used by therapists). These devices were developed in the early twentieth century and they lack simple and intuitive graphics for contemporary user interfaces. A second research focus is on games performance connected to sensors to aid the necessary rehabilitation measures and evaluation.

References

1. Benson, F., Ardila, A.: What is Aphasia? In: Benson, D.F., Ardila, A. (eds.) Aphasia. A Clinical Perspective. Oxford University Press, New York (1996)
2. Aguado, G.: Trastorno específico del lenguaje. Retraso de lenguaje y disfasia. Ediciones Aljibe (1999)
3. Vázquez Sánchez, Juan, Mente y mundo: aproximación neurológica, AKAL (2007) ISBN 9788446025351
4. Hardcastle, W.J.: Physiology of Speech Production. Academic Press, London (1976)
5. Bases neurológicas y psicopedagógicas del tratamiento educativo de la diversidad. Gento Palacios Samuel, Sánchez Manzano Esteban. UNED (2010). ISBN:978-84-362-5987-2
6. Educación de la voz. María Purificación Veiga Liz, Ed. Ideaspropias editorial (2005). ISBN: 9788496578920
7. La voz. técnica vocal para la rehabilitación de la voz en las. disfonías funcionales.Tulon Arfelis, Carmen. Editorial Paidotribo (2000). ISBN:978-84-8019-491-4
8. Fardoun, H.M., Altalhi, A.H., Cipres, A.P., Castillo, J.R., Albiol-Pérez, S.: CRehab: a cloud-based framework for the management of rehabilitation processes. In: 7th International Conference on Pervasive Computing Technologies for Healthcare (PervasiveHealth), pp. 397–400 (2013). E-ISBN: 978-1-936968-80-0
9. Fardoun, H., Montero, F., Jaquero, V.L.: eLearniXML: towards a model-based approach for the development of e-Learning systems considering quality. Adv. Eng. Softw. **40**, 1297–1305 (2009). doi:http://dx.doi.org/10.1016/j.advengsoft.2009.01.019
10. Fardoun, H.M., Ciprés, A.P., Alghazzawi, D.M.: CSchool: DUI for educational system using clouds. In: Proceedings of the 2nd Workshop on Distributed User Interfaces: Collaboration and Usability, in conjunction with CHI 2012, pp. 684–695 (2012)
11. Fardoun, H.M., Katib, I.A., Ciprés, A.P.: Interactive speech therapy for children. In: Proceedings of the 8th International Conference on Pervasive Computing Technologies for Healthcare (PervasiveHealth '14). ICST (Institute for Computer Sciences, Social-Informatics and Telecommunications Engineering), ICST, Brussels, Belgium, pp. 377–380 (2014). doi: http://dx.doi.org/10.4108/icst.pervasivehealth.2014.255378

A Cost-Efficient Tele-rehabilitation Device for Training Distal Upper Limb Functions After Stroke

Patrick Weiss[1]($\boxtimes$), Alexander Gabrecht[1], Marcus Heldmann[2],
Achim Schweikard[3], and Erik Maehle[1]

[1] Institute of Computer Engineering, University of Lübeck, Lübeck, Germany
weiss@iti.uni-luebeck.de
[2] University Medical Center Schleswig-Holstein,
University of Lübeck, Lübeck, Germany
[3] Institute for Robotics and Cognitive Systems,
University of Lübeck, Lübeck, Germany

Abstract. Robotic rehabilitation devices offer prospects in improving the therapy outcome in stroke patients. In particular the combination with tele-rehabilitation functionality may be beneficial to reduce cost, which is especially required for home-based rehabilitation. In this paper a device is presented that allows for exercising supination/pronation, dorsiflexion, and finger training. Its communication architecture follows a modular design approach. The Qt-based graphical UI can be executed on different operating systems and devices including the cost-effective Rasperry Pi single-board computer. Tele-rehabilitation functionality is implemented based on SSL-encrypted RESTful web services following a three-tier architecture. Cost is reduced by omitting expensive sensors. A torque sensor is replaced with current-based torque sensing, used for progress measurement and interactive exercises. The evaluation shows accurate results after compensating the static friction, justifying the omission of an additional torque sensor. Torque measurements during passive exercises showed higher and more asymmetric ratings for a stroke patient than for a healthy subject indicating that this measurement may be used as an estimator of spasticity.

Keywords: Robotic rehabilitation · Tele-rehabilitation · Stroke · Home health care · Distal upper limb functions · Motor control

1 Introduction

In high-income countries, stroke is the third most common cause of death and the major cause of acquired adult disability [17]. Besides personal consequences, this means a high economical impact. The average lifetime cost for stroke rehabilitation per case in Germany is 43,129 € and projected 3.4 million new cases of ischemic stroke from 2006 to 2025 lead to estimated costs of 108.6 billion € [6].

© Springer-Verlag Berlin Heidelberg 2015
H.M. Fardoun et al. (Eds.): REHAB 2014, CCIS 515, pp. 78–90, 2015.
DOI: 10.1007/978-3-662-48645-0_8

Often, the upper limb is affected leading to significant problems in fine and gross motor skills. After three months, only 20 % to 56 % of all stroke survivors regain useful upper limb function [12]. In robotic therapy, training of the distal parts of the upper-limb appears to be a crucial factor in this recovery. A wrist extension for robotic upper-limb therapy device further increased the rehabilitation outcome in comparison to training of the shoulder and elbow alone [7]. Reaching and supination/pronation training is particularly important since it promotes progress towards more functional whole upper extremity movements [13].

Several robotic systems for upper limb rehabilitation have been presented [9]. While some studies show promising results in outcome [15], they are not consistently in favor of robotics in comparison to traditional therapy [8]. This underlines the necessity for a better understanding of motor learning which can be enhanced by means of robotic rehabilitation [14].

Seen from another perspective, these systems do not have to compete against traditional therapy, but may instead be complimentary, e.g. by deploying rehabilitation devices in the home environment. Home rehabilitation potentially reduces costs by increasing the amount of independent training time and relieving the load of therapists. Tele-rehabilitation gives them a means of control and surveillance over the training and the possibility of intervention if necessary.

However, most of the proposed devices are not suitable for home rehabilitation. Many systems are either too expensive, e.g. due to the use of force-torque sensors [11], do not offer modularity and virtual rehabilitation [5], or are fitted to other systems [1]. Nearly 75 % of the devices observed in a comprehensive review have not even undergone any sort of testing due to high complexity and poor usability [2].

Based on the aforementioned points, we propose a device called m·ReS^{R2} (second prototype of a modular Rehabilitation System for training of Rotational movements) for training forearm supination/pronation, dorsiflexion, and finger functions focusing on its application in the home environment. The system is required to be cost-effective and to provide an intuitive user interface. Essential to its function are an actuator and sensors for virtual rehabilitation or the study of rehabilitation paradigms, particularly visual feedback distortion [4], and the ability to give remote access to session data for tele-rehabilitation. The system has been described in [18]. This paper goes more into detail in the exercise modes and first experiences with a stroke patient training session.

2   System Implementation

2.1   Approach and Design

There are two basic approaches of training devices: End-effectors and exoskeletons. Rotational movements involve a high number of degrees of freedom (DOF) of the hand, which exoskeletons have to provide to allow fully unconstrained movements. Following a cost-effective approach, we chose an end-effector design

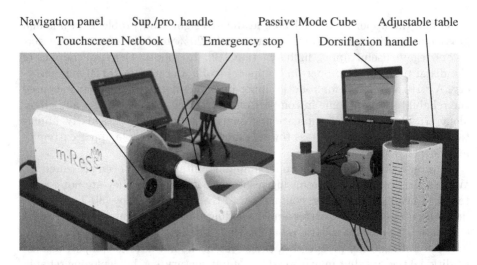

Fig. 1. Horizontal (l.) and vertical (r.) orientation of the training device

which allows tasks involving many DOF without the need for a high number of mechanical DOF.

The movements to be trained comprise supination/pronation, dorsiflexion, and fine finger exercises. These distal upper limb movements are strongly related to performing activities of daily living (ADLs) [5], such as drinking, eating, or knob manipulation. Moreover, these movements are important to orientate the hand before grasping an object [16]. Depending on the orientation of the device and the handle used, different movements can be trained. Supination and pronation exercises are performed in the horizontal position with the arm aligned to the motor axis. Dorsiflexion and fine finger exercises require the device to be orientated vertically (Fig. 1). To this effect the motor axis lies perpendicular to the arm such that the method of interaction changes and additional muscles are activated. This way, only one actuator is necessary reducing complexity and cost, while still allowing for different training methods. In contrast to the former prototype [19], not the motor is turned but the device can be either placed on the table-top or adapted in height and orientation using an adjustable table. The advantages are that the mechanical design is kept simpler, the height can be changed, and the table can be omitted, if a table-top device is sufficient. A chuck attached to the motor can fasten different handles giving more flexibility in training. Supination/pronation requires an additional handle other than dorsiflexion and by varying its size, the difficulty for fine manipulation training can be tuned. The modularity through these optional components helps to get closer to the patients' needs or to clinical demands.

The end-effector's main component is a motor that supports or impedes the patient in performing rotational movements. The motor is placed within a casing that also houses the power supply with a fused power switch, a microcontroller board, electronics, and a navigation panel. An emergency switch is included to

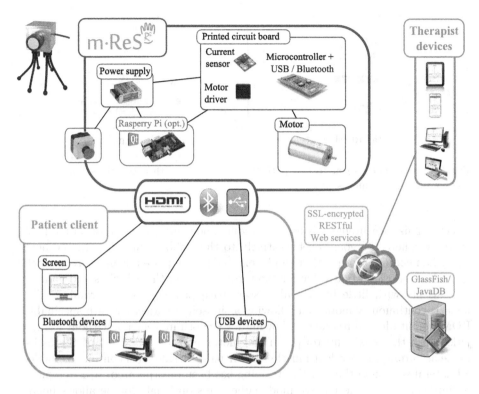

Fig. 2. Schematic of the system and possible interaction platforms

interrupt the power supply in case of a critical incident. Optionally, a single-board computer (Rasperry Pi) may be included to build an all in one device. Otherwise, a variety of devices such as common computers may be used to visualize sensor values and to allow for access to low-level functions over a graphical user interface (GUI). A system overview is depicted in Fig. 2.

2.2   Exercise Modes

Several training modes have been implemented. In the first step, the maximum range of motion (ROM) and torque are determined (GUI screens shown in Fig. 3). The ROM calibration consists of two steps. First, the anatomical range of motion (red area in ROM assessment screen) is determined which is a necessity to prevent the motor from turning beyond the joint's painless limit. Since the affected extremity is often not capable of performing this movement, the patient may be supported with stepwise motor-controlled angular position increments controlled via the user interface until the joint's maximum rotation is reached. This can only be performed by patients with sufficient sensory capabilities to feel the limit of the joint. Otherwise, a therapist has to lead through this step. The second step tests the ROM without the support by motor (green area in ROM assessment

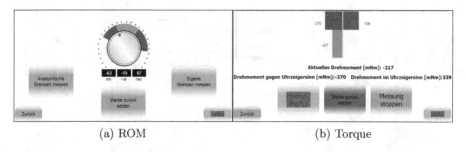

(a) ROM   (b) Torque

Fig. 3. Assessment screens to test patients' capabilities with range of motion (ROM) and torque measurements

screen). This measurement is used as a guideline value for the position mode of exercises where the goal is set relatively to this calibration value. In the next step, the maximum torque that can be exerted by the patient is measured, which is used as an orientation value for the torque-mode of the exercises and games.

Patients with little functionality start with passive/assisted training. The hand is continuously mobilized following a sinusoidal trajectory with specifiable ROM amplitude and frequency allowing for smooth movements without abrupt jerks. Also the maximum torque of the motor may be set to adapt the assistance according to prevalent muscle tone or pain. Besides this continuous mode, a bilateral version of the assistive training has been incorporated. It uses a piece of hardware called the passive mode cube. This optional module allows hemiparetic patients to control the motor's position by turning a knob with their healthy hand mobilizing the impaired hand [19]. Bi-manual exercises may positively influence the rehabilitation progress since it has a facilitatory effect on the affected extremity [5].

Depending on the progress of the patient, the support can be reduced or counter-torques can be applied. Moreover, torque profiles are provided. For instance, we implemented a virtual spring mode where the torque is linearly increased with the angle difference to a neutral position. The mapping between angle and torque may be freely adjusted or is set according to the initial calibration.

The calibration measurements of torque and range of motion over several sessions can serve as a means of progress evaluation. Furthermore, continuous samplings during the exercises with a frequency of up to 100 Hz can be taken. Other indicators may be extracted from this data.

Simple rehabilitation games have been implemented to make training more diverse. The game variable, for instance the range of a board in a breakout-style game, depends on the initial calibration.

The system may be used to study new rehabilitation paradigms. We focus on visual feedback distortion (VFD), which is subject to studies of the cooperating neurologists. It may help to overcome learned nonuse by exploiting the gap between visual and proprioceptive feedback. Thus, patients are encouraged to reach beyond their self-assessed abilities [3,4,10]. VFD has been included into several modes including the games where the mapping between the input torque or movement and the game variable is slightly changed.

2.3   Actuation, Sensing, and Electronics

A brushed motor and a gear with a reduction ratio of 7:1 were used achieving a maximum total torque of 1.7 Nm. The combination of a strong motor with a low reduction gear ratio results in low backdrivability while achieving a decent maximum torque. It may not be sufficient to work against strong spasms but safety concerns and backdrivability outweighed this possibility. An encoder with 1024 impulses per revolution delivers the relative angle in incremental steps of 0.05°. A motor driver amplifies the pulse-width modulated signals (PWM) from the microcontroller.

Torque measurements are an important factor in assessing the patient's capabilities. Force-torque sensors were not an option, since they cost many times more than the presented system. Therefore, the torque is measured by utilizing its linear relationship to the armature current. A Hall effect based current sensor IC, dimensioned for the Ampere range of the motor, converts the current to voltage measured by the microcontroller's 10-bit analog-to-digital converter (ADC). An operational amplifier circuit amplifies the sensor voltage to cover the whole range of the ADC. The torque is controlled with an integrative controller comparing the measured current to the setpoint and adjusting the PWM signal, accordingly. A serial connection between the microcontroller and a user interface device is established either tethered, using a USB to UART bridge, or wireless based on a Bluetooth module with Serial Port Profile (SPP). The printed circuit board (PCB) further comprises voltage smoothing components and a tilt switch that measures, whether the device is oriented horizontally or vertically.

2.4   Software and Communication

The software architecture is designed in a modular way. It consists of a client-server architecture to provide tele or home rehabilitation functionality. The client, located at the patient's side, connects to the microcontroller over a serial UART connection to gather data or set parameters like resistance or target position. For comparison of the training outcome, the patient's maximum range of motion and exerted torque are logged for every training or game session. Furthermore, the trajectory of each session is stored to provide data which can be useful to examine intrasession effects such as fatigue. The data of each session is transmitted to the clinic side server or cached locally while an internet connection is not available. With this implicit offline mode the training can be continued anywhere and anytime without losing track of the progress.

The server software consists of a three-tier architecture which supports the modularity concept. It uses a web front-end based on the JavaServer Faces Framework PrimeFaces and connects to a JavaDB database. It is hosted on a Glasfish application server implementing a SSL-encrypted RESTful web service which receives data from training sessions and sets configuration values to the client software (Fig. 2). The interface features administrative, therapist, and patient views with restricted rights. Patients can only monitor their training process whereas therapists can also set configuration parameters like VFD for their patients training sessions. The RESTful approach combined with the PrimeFaces UI ensures compatibility of the server with various clients and web-browsers. The communication architecture allows for a variety of platforms to access the functionality of the device and server.

To maximize the flexibility in client hardware, our prototype client software is a cross-platform implementation based on Qt4 which runs on standard PCs (Windows, Mac OS X, Linux) as well as on single-board computers like the Raspberry Pi. We ported and natively compiled our software on a Rasperry Pi Model-B running Raspbian Wheezy. This single-board computer is small enough to be put it into the casing providing an all-in-one client. The software includes a GUI for progress measurements, motivating rehabilitation games, and progress visualization. The interface can alternatively be controlled by the integrated navigational switch panel, touchscreen, or standard PC input devices (keyboard/mouse).

The screenshot in Fig. 4, taken in the therapist view of the servers web front end, shows a visualization of the torque measurements of a healthy subject's exercise data. Each entry in the table represents a calibration session with the measured extrema used for exercises or games. The therapists see the amount of visual feedback distortion, whereas this information is not visible in patient view. The upper chart in the server-side view visualizes the progress over several sessions to allow an estimation on the training outcome. Each session has the whole trajectory data available which can be visualized in a movable pop-up window by activating the magnifier symbol next to it. The trajectory shows the torque, or angular displacement in other exercises, as a function of the time. It is available for all calibrations, exercise modes and games. The session and trajectory data can be exported to a spreadsheet for external processing.

3   Performance Evaluation

3.1   Torque Estimation Based on Armature Current Measurements

The first experiment evaluates the accuracy of the torque estimation from the current measurement. For this, we use a force-torque sensor that is rigidly connected to the device. A current profile is applied on the end-effector and the estimated torque is compared to the measured one. The profile includes a step at the beginning and a drop at the end of the sampling period. These two points are used for synchronization and scaling of the two sensors that return samples with constant but different sample rates. The values after the initial step and before the increase of current define the baseline on which the force-torque sensor is calibrated. The results are plotted in Fig. 5.

The dotted line represents the initial setpoint current which is converted using the linear relation between torque and current. At the beginning of the slope, the increase of current does not result in higher torque. We blame unwanted

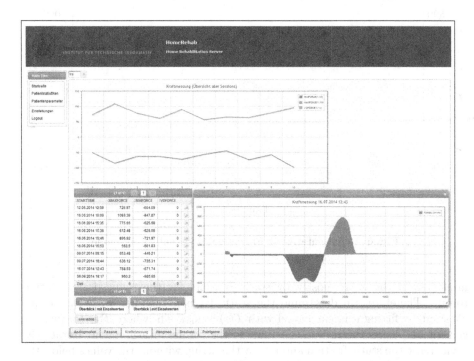

Fig. 4. Server-side visualization of a subject's training performance

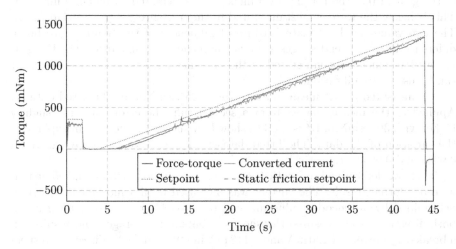

Fig. 5. Comparison of force-torque to current measurements including the setpoint trajectory with and without regarding the static friction. All currents are converted with the torque constant determined by the force-torque test

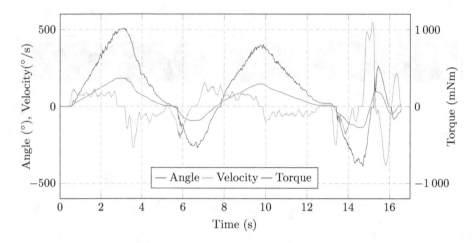

Fig. 6. Representative short session in virtual spring mode

influences of the gear, mostly by static friction, for the reduced transmitted torque. Therefore, we determine the static friction together with the torque constant by fitting a linear model with $T(i) = k_m i + b$, where T is torque, i is current and k_m is the torque constant, to the torque measurement. Iteratively, we increase the static friction and repeat the fitting without the values below the threshold until b is approximately zero. Thus, the static friction was determined to have a threshold current of 188 mA. The slope of the model represents the motor's torque constant. Regarding the reduction ratio of 7:1 and the efficiency of the gear of 0.9, the torque constant k_m was calculated to be 56.41 mNm/A. This is below the torque constant stated in the datasheet of $k_{m_d} = 64$ mNm/A. The two values might deviate because of influences of the temperature but a difference in this extend suggests further influences, for instance, that the gear has a lower efficiency than stated in the datasheet. Anyway, this measurement can be used for calibration.

We measured a root-mean-square error of 25.78 mNm for the fitted dataset. Applied to the measurements from a second run, the error was only slightly higher with 30.08 mNm. R^2 is used to show how successful the fit is in explaining the variation of the data. The fitted dataset and the second run have an R^2 of 0.9957 and 0.9943, respectively.

Then, we determined the static friction with a common method and compared it to our former result. The current was increased until a movement occurred, determined by an encoder value unequal to zero. After repeating 100 runs in both directions, the measured threshold currents were averaged and resulted in a breakaway current of 120 mA and −118 mA in CW and CCW direction, respectively. The lower value comes from the encoder's high sensitivity in conjunction with the gear's backlash. Since the application of the higher threshold current onto the motor does not lead to unwanted continuous movement, the higher

value is valid. It can now be utilized to decrease the initial user induced torque
and improve the accuracy of the torque estimation.

3.2   User Peformance in Different Exercises

The torque control can be applied in different training modes. First, a representative short session of the virtual spring mode, described in Sect. 2.2, is shown
in Fig. 6 with the angle, velocity, and torque plotted against the time.

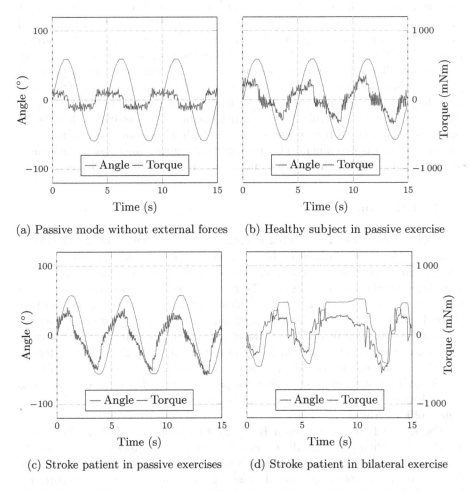

(a) Passive mode without external forces   (b) Healthy subject in passive exercise

(c) Stroke patient in passive exercises   (d) Stroke patient in bilateral exercise

Fig. 7. Automatic passive mode and bilateral exercise using the passive mode cube

Second, the passive mode is tested with a sinusoidal trajectory with a frequency of 0.2 Hz and an amplitude ranging from $-60°$ to $60°$ where $0°$ is the
semi-pronated position. This mode is tested without a user (no external force

on the handle), with a healthy subject whose hand is moved passively without working against the motor, and a stroke patient who tries to do the same. The trajectory is plotted together with torque that indicates the amount of resistance introduced by the user. Additionally, a session with the same stroke patient using the passive mode cube. The plots are grouped in Fig. 7.

The plots show that the controller achieves a smooth sinusoidal trajectory without abrupt movements. The curve follows the specified ROM and frequency. The measurement of the torque allows to draw conclusions about the resistance implied by the user. The first plot without external forces on the handle shows the lowest torque. The hand of a healthy subject imposes forces of the handle that the motor has to overcome in order to keep following the trajectory. Higher and asymmetric torques can be observed in the plot of the passive mode with a stroke patient. This can be explained with spasticity which is a common impairment after stroke. The increased muscle tone forces the hand towards a pronated position. Therefore, the motor has to overcome higher torques turning the hand into the supinated position which is reflected in the plots. The same can be observed for the same stroke patient using the bilateral passive mode cube. It can be seen that the torque peaks are not as high which can be explained with the lower angle displacements. The measurements during the passive modes may be used to observe spasticity and estimate the degree of the impairment.

4   Conclusion

A rehabilitation device for training forearm, wrist and finger functions has been proposed. The torque estimation based on current measurements and the angle sensing from the motor encoder readings permits virtual rehabilitation and studying rehabilitation paradigms. The performance evaluation revealed a relative root-mean-square error of 2.2 % which is reasonable especially considering the reduction in costs achieved by omitting a force-torque sensor. Therefore, expensive sensors can be omitted without relinquishing torque control and measurement. However, this method lacks the possibility of controlling the torque directly on the end-effector side, e.g., necessary for admittance devices. Still, the performance evaluation showed that torque profiles and passive exercises can be implemented and that the torque measurements allow conclusions about the degree of impairment.

The Qt GUI can be run on a Rasperry Pi which offers full capabilities of a PC for less than $35. The device can be accessed remotely and session data can be transmitted to therapists using web services. The cost-effective therapy device provides remote access capabilities which are important prerequisites for home rehabilitation. In future studies, we intend to validate the applicability, efficacy and reliability of the system with further stroke patients in the clinical and home environment.

References

1. Allington, J., Spencer, S. J., Klein, J., Buell, M., Reinkensmeyer, D. J., Bobrow, J.: Supinator extender (SUE): a pneumatically actuated robot for forearm/wrist rehabilitation after stroke. In: Annual International Conference of the IEEE Engineering in Medicine and Biology Society (EMBC), pp. 1579–1582. IEEE (2011)
2. Balasubramanian, S., Klein, J., Burdet, E.: Robot-assisted rehabilitation of hand function. Curr. Opin. Neurol. **23**(6), 661 (2010)
3. Brewer, B., Klatzky, R., Matsuoka, Y.: Feedback distortion to overcome learned nonuse: a system overview. In: Proceedings of the 25th Annual International Conference of the IEEE Engineering in Medicine and Biology Society, vol. 2, pp. 1613–1616. IEEE (2003)
4. Brewer, B., Klatzky, R., Matsuoka, Y.: Visual feedback distortion in a robotic environment for hand rehabilitation. Brain Res. Bull. **75**(6), 804–813 (2008)
5. Hesse, S., Schulte-Tigges, G., Konrad, M., Bardeleben, A., Werner, C.: Robot-assisted arm trainer for the passive and active practice of bilateral forearm and wrist movements in hemiparetic subjects. Arch. Phys. Med. Rehabil. **84**(6), 915–920 (2003)
6. Kolominsky-Rabas, P.L., Heuschmann, P.U., Marschall, D., Emmert, M., Baltzer, N., Neundörfer, B., Schöffski, O., Krobot, K.J., et al.: Lifetime cost of ischemic stroke in germany: results and national projections from a population-based stroke registry the erlangen stroke project. Stroke **37**(5), 1179–1183 (2006)
7. Krebs, H.I., Volpe, B.T., Williams, D., Celestino, J., Charles, S.K., Lynch, D., Hogan, N.: Robot-aided neurorehabilitation: a robot for wrist rehabilitation. IEEE Trans. Neural Syst. Rehabil. Eng. **15**(3), 327–335 (2007)
8. Kwakkel, G., Kollen, B.J., Krebs, H.I.: Effects of robot-assisted therapy on upper limb recovery after stroke: a systematic review. Neurorehabil. Neural Repair **22**(2), 111–121 (2008)
9. Maciejasz, P., Eschweiler, J., Gerlach-Hahn, K., Jansen-Toy, A., Leonhardt, S., et al.: A survey on robotic devices for upper limb rehabilitation. J. Neuroeng. Rehabil. **11**(1), 3 (2014)
10. Matsuoka, Y., Allin, S., Klatzky, R.: The tolerance for visual feedback distortions in a virtual environment. Physiol. Behav. **77**(4–5), 651–655 (2002)
11. Metzger, J.-C., Lambercy, O., Chapuis, D., Gassert, R.: Design and characterization of the ReHapticKnob, a robot for assessment and therapy of hand function. In: 2011 IEEE/RSJ International Conference on Intelligent Robots and Systems (IROS), pp. 3074–3080. IEEE (2011)
12. Nakayama, H., Jørgensen, H.S., Raaschou, H.O., Olsen, T.S.: Recovery of upper extremity function in stroke patients: the Copenhagen stroke study. Age (SD) **74**, 11–2 (1994)
13. Oblak, J., Cikajlo, I., Matjacic, Z.: Universal haptic drive: a robot for arm and wrist rehabilitation. IEEE Trans. Neural Syst. Rehabil. Eng. **18**(3), 293–302 (2010)
14. Reinkensmeyer, D.J., Emken, J.L., Cramer, S.C.: Robotics, motor learning, and neurologic recovery. Annu. Rev. Biomed. Eng. **6**, 497–525 (2004)
15. Takahashi, C.D., Der-Yeghiaian, L., Le, V., Motiwala, R.R., Cramer, S.C.: Robot-based hand motor therapy after stroke. Brain **131**(2), 425–437 (2008)
16. Van der Lee, J.H., de Groot, V., Beckerman, H., Wagenaar, R.C., Lankhorst, G.J., Bouter, L.M.: The intra-and interrater reliability of the action research arm test: a practical test of upper extremity function in patients with stroke. Arch. Phys. Med. Rehabil. **82**(1), 14–19 (2001)

17. Warlow, C., Van Gijn, J., Sandercock, P., Hankey, G., Dennis, M., Bamford, J., Wardlaw, J., Sudlow, C., Rinkel, G., Rothwell, P.: Stroke: practical management (2008)
18. Weiss, P., Heldmann, M. Gabrecht, A. Schweikard, A., Münte, T. M., Maehle, E.: A low cost tele-rehabilitation device for training of wrist and finger functions after stroke. In: Proceedings of the 8th International Conference on Pervasive Computing Technologies for Healthcare (PervasiveHealth 2014), pp. 422–425 (2014)
19. Weiss, P., Heldmann, M., Münte, T., Schweikard, A., Maehle, E.: A rehabilitation system for training based on visual feedback distortion. In: Pons, J.L., Torricelli, D., Pajaro, M. (eds.) Converging Clinical and Engineering Research on Neurorehabilitation, pp. 297–302. Springer, Heidelberg (2013)

Personalization of Assistance and Knowledge of Performance Feedback on a Hybrid Mobile and Myo-electric Robotic System for Motor Rehabilitation After Stroke

Davide Neves[✉], Athanasios Vourvopoulos, Mónica Cameirão,
and Sergi Bermúdez i Badia

Madeira-ITI, Universidade da Madeira, Funchal, Portugal
davideneves@gmail.com, {athanasios.vourvopoulos,
monica.cameirao,sergi.bermudez}@m-iti.org

Abstract. Upper limb motor deficits caused by stroke have a large impact on a person's daily activities and independence. The personalization of the rehabilitation tasks to the needs of the patient as well as the enhancement of the feedback provided to the patient are strategies for promoting motor relearning. In this paper we describe the development and pilot evaluation of a portable system that uses a robotic orthosis to deliver assistance and meaningful feedback during rehabilitative training. Two software modules are implemented, one that investigates an optimal calibration method for the personalization of the level of assistance, and another one that combines the orthosis with a mobile application running on a tablet that provides graphical knowledge of performance feedback to stroke patients while performing therapy. Here we present two preliminary studies and discuss the potential of this technology.

Keywords: Myo-electric orthosis · Personalization · Stroke · Motor rehabilitation · Knowledge of performance · Mobile devices

1 Introduction

Motor impairment of the upper limb, cognitive and emotional sequels are commonly observed in stroke survivors [1, 2]. These deficits have a huge impact on a person's activities of daily living (ADL), creating dependence on others in order to perform simple daily tasks. Rehabilitation is essential for motor learning and helping in the acquisition of skills that can improve independence in everyday tasks. Here, several elements can contribute to a more successful rehabilitation process for enhancing motor performance, from different occupational therapy approaches to the use of novel technology to stimulate the reorganization of the brain motor areas [2–4].

The benefits of the advances in technologies in the rehabilitation area are well known, and the applications range from brain computer interfaces [5] to robotic systems [6]. Technology provides novel ways to adapt the rehabilitation process to the patient's needs, which is essential to provide more personalized therapy training. In this area, several approaches have combined intelligent training personalization with

© Springer-Verlag Berlin Heidelberg 2015
H.M. Fardoun et al. (Eds.): REHAB 2014, CCIS 515, pp. 91–103, 2015.
DOI: 10.1007/978-3-662-48645-0_9

Virtual Reality (VR) or Games [7] and shown to have a positive effect on the rehabilitation [8]. Currently, it is known that training through passive movement exercising
is able to engage motor networks by means of proprioceptive feedback [9]. However, it
has been shown to be an ineffective way of engaging overt execution motor areas [10].
One way of restoring active movement is to use of an actuated upper extremity orthosis
that utilizes electromyography to support successful arm movements. For this reason,
novel approaches using robotic assistive devices have been developed to restore active
movement capabilities in order to engage patients in a physical training with meaningful goal oriented actions [11,12]. Thus, personalization and adaptation to each
patient can be achieved by adjusting the degree of assistance being provided by the
robotic orthosis according to the patient's muscular activity patterns [13]. Unfortunately, in most cases, the assistance settings of those devices are configured manually
through an interface or menu based on expert knowledge, making it difficult for
patients to be autonomous in their training. Ideally, these devices should be able to
personalize the assistance levels by self-adjusting the settings, thus minimizing the
need of expert knowledge.

As important as providing personalization through the use of novel assistive
technologies is to be able to provide meaningful and valuable feedback that supports
patients in their motor relearning tasks. Nowadays it is widely accepted that there are
two types of extrinsic feedback that play a crucial role in providing information about
motor task execution: *Knowledge of Results* (KR) and *Knowledge of Performance*
(KP) [14,15]. KR feedback is given after completing the desired task and relates to how
well the task has been performed, while KP provides information about what is being
done during the execution of the training task in order to aid the patient in achieving the
best outcome [15]. Current computer based approaches for motor rehabilitation are
very well suited to provide KR by embedding training in the form of games that
provide quantitative measurements of results [16,17]. However, KP has not been so
widely addressed, this type of feedback being generally provided verbally by trained
therapists during task execution. To be able to incorporate KP features in rehabilitation
systems requires specific sensing technology, such as wearable or remote sensing
devices, capable of measuring and assisting the rehabilitation process in a safe and
unobtrusive way. In this sense, the combination assistive technologies that can partially
restore active movement capabilities in patients with motor deficits - while allowing the
capture of important physiological and kinematic information such as
electro-myographic signals or arm position - with software applications that provide
appropriate KP have a large potential.

The goal of this project is to develop a fully portable system that uses an upper limb
myo-electric robotic orthosis to enable and enhance active movement therapy by means
of: an intelligent calibration module for personalizing the level of assistance to each
user; and a training module that provides KP based on multimodal information captured from the user in real-time during the execution of the task. Both, calibration
module and KP module, are implemented as an Android application that connects
wirelessly with the robotic orthosis. These modules allow the user to modify in
real-time the settings of the device by searching for the parameters that are more
suitable for his/her muscular performance, and are designed to provide real-time
feedback on KP during training from both physiological and kinematic data. In this

paper we present the development and results of two pilot evaluations to (1) identify the optimal calibration parameters concerning the assistance level of the myo-electric orthosis, and (2) assess the impact of KP feedback when physiologically based feedback or when kinematic based feedback are used.

2   Methods

We developed a portable system relying on a mobile device and a myo-electric limb orthosis that enables active movement training and provides KP. First, in order to identify the optimal settings for the robotic orthosis, we developed and evaluated a calibration module. Then, we created a feedback module to investigate which type of KP feedback (physiologically or kinematic based feedback) would provide the patient with more useful information during motor training. The software modules developed in this project were designed for mobile devices that run Android OS (Google Inc., Mountain View, California, U.S.), and were implemented using the Android SDK and Unity 3D (Unity Technologies, San Francisco, USA).

2.1   Myo-electric Limb Orthosis

We used the mPower 1000 (mPower 1000, Myomo Inc., Boston, USA), a robotic limb orthosis that is portable and has one actuated degree of freedom (elbow join). The orthosis uses two electrode sensors placed on the biceps and triceps of a user, thus reading his/her electromyography (EMG) plus the orthosis motor position (i.e. elbow flexion). By activating the biceps or triceps during the arm movement, the EMG readings enable the device to assist users with motor impairments of the upper limb in completing the desired movements. The mPower 1000 has several configurable parameters to determine the amount of assistance. Independent assistance levels can be set for extension and flexion movements. Each level of assistance can be set with values that range from 0 to 20 (where 20 provides the highest level of assistance) through a virtual serial port over Bluetooth communication channel. In addition, the device offers three control modes, allowing the user to control the orthosis using only biceps or triceps muscles individually or both of them simultaneously.

2.2   Data Collection

For further analysis, all software modules collect synchronously all kinematic and physiological data available from the mPower 1000. Recorded data include pre-processed normalized amplitude values of the envelope of EMG signals from biceps and triceps (0–14), position of the arm (degrees), time (ms), average speed (degrees/s), values of the assistance levels for both extension and flexion (0–20) and the number of arm flexions and extensions. Due the fact that the EMG signal is noisy, a finite impulse response filter was applied to smooth the EMG data. Data are logged directly on the mobile device, sampled every 100 ms and stored as a CSV text file.

2.3   Calibration Module

For the calibration module, we developed a native Android application implemented using Android SDK tools. It uses the built-in Bluetooth capability of a mobile device to connect to the mPower. This application allows the user to adjust the extension and flexion assistance levels, increasing or decreasing the assistance using the plus and minus buttons in the touch screen (see Fig. 1). Two additional functions were implemented for conducting experiments: 'Reset EMG' resets the baseline values of the EMG readings; and 'Reset' initializes the assistance levels with random values (0 to 20). Because the experimental task requires the participant to search for the optimal assistance settings, the calibration module does not provide information about the current assistance values. This way we prevent the participants from memorizing the settings and avoid biases in the search.

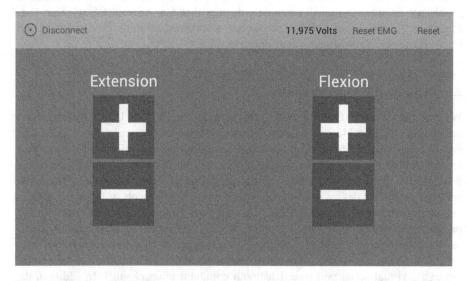

Fig. 1. Calibration module that controls the assistance levels of the mPower 1000. The module does not display the actual calibration values; it only has buttons to increase and decrease the assistance for extension and flexion movements.

2.4   Maximizing Movement Control Through Intelligent Adaptation

In order to identify the mPower 1000 settings that maximize performance for each user, we run a pilot study with 15 healthy volunteers with an average of 26.5 ± 4.3 years (see Table 1.). All participants were informed about the purpose of the study and gave their signed consent.

Before the experiment, participants had a training period to get familiarized with the robotic device and the mobile application. The experiment had duration of 20 min during which the participants wore the mPower 1000 and had to perform multiple elbow flexion/extension sequences. During that time they used the calibration module to change the levels of the assistance in flexion and extension movements with the goal

Table 1. Participant demographics

Participant	Age	Gender	Dominant arm
P1	28	Male	Right
P2	27	Male	Right
P3	22	Male	Right
P4	21	Male	Right
P5	28	Female	Right
P6	28	Male	Right
P7	39	Female	Right
P8	28	Female	Right
P9	23	Female	Right
P10	24	Female	Right
P11	24	Female	Right
P12	26	Male	Right
P13	24	Female	Right
P14	29	Male	Right
P15	27	Male	Right

of identifying the configuration that would give them more control over the orthosis device. After the user considered that he/she had found the best settings, the current assistance values were stored and replaced by random values, and the user had to repeat the process until new optimal settings were found. Each participant repeated the process several times during the 20 min experimental session. After the session, the user filled a questionnaire that consisted on 6 questions concerning the use of the mPower 1000, the level of control, comfort, fatigue, and also the perception of the participant about the "best calibration". To reduce the complexity of the task, in this study the assistance was determined using the biceps EMG information only. This means that users had to activate the bicep muscle to 'close' the device (flexion) and relax the biceps to 'open' de device (extension).

2.5   Feedback Module

This module leverages the information gathered from the myo-electric limb orthosis to provide stroke survivors with KP to assist and improve their rehabilitation exercises. This module has two main interfaces that are intended to deliver either physiologically or kinematic based KP feedback.

Physiologically Based Knowledge of Performance. In this KP mode, the mobile application presents feedback based on the physiological readings of the mPower 1000. Biceps and triceps EMG activation levels are represented in real-time as vertical bars accompanied by a numerical value (Fig. 2, top panel) under the label "flexion" and "extension". The bar values correspond to normalized EMG activation values, with 0 and 10 corresponding to the minimum and maximum muscular activation levels, respectively. This view enables the user to see their muscular activation patterns easily

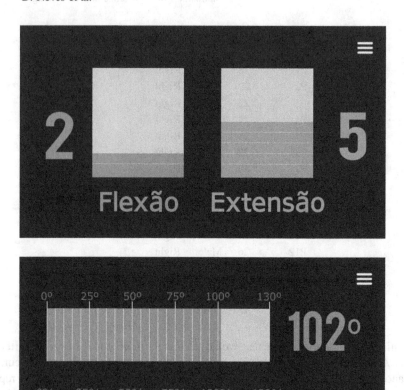

Fig. 2. Mobile assistance for knowledge of performance. The mobile application can provide a physiologically based feedback (top panel), and a kinematic based feedback (bottom panel) based on muscular activation or movement kinematic data respectively. 'Flexão' and 'Extensão' are Portuguese for 'Flexion' and 'Extension' respectively.

represented as bars, thus allowing the user to better understand how successful movement results from muscle activation.

Kinematic Based Knowledge of Performance. In this KP mode, the mobile application represents the real-time position and velocity of the arm movements in degrees/s (Fig. 2, bottom panel). Thus, this configuration relies on arm movement kinematic data and presents it, consistent with the physiologically based representation, as bars and their corresponding numerical value. Both kinematic and physiological data were chosen to be represented with the same amount of information channels (two bars) in a visually consistent manner. However, given the similarity of the two feedback representations and to avoid confusions, the kinematic based feedback is presented using horizontal bars.

2.6   Physiological vs. Kinematic Knowledge of Performance

In order to understand which feedback mode provides patients with a more useful and understandable information about their performance during the training, we ran a pilot study with stroke survivors. In this experiment we assessed how patients reacted to the two different types of feedback, i.e. physiological and kinematic (see Subsect. 2.5).

Three stroke survivors participated in this pilot evaluation (Table 2). The pilot took place at Hospital Dr. Nélio Mendonça and Hospital Dr. João de Almada, in Funchal. All the participants gave their informed consent and the study was approved by the ethics committee of the Madeira Health System (SESARAM).

Table 2. Patient demographics

Patient	Age	Stroke type	Side	Time post-stroke
1	74	Ischemic	Right	40 weeks
2	54	Ischemic	Left	5 weeks
3	78	–	Right	30 weeks

In this experiment, patients sat and wore the mPower 1000 robotic orthosis on their paretic arm (Fig. 3). Placed in front of them, a tablet ran the feedback training module (Fig. 2). Prior to the evaluation session, all patients had a training period to get familiarized with the mPower and the mobile application. After this period, the patients were presented with both KP feedback forms, that is, based on EMG activation and based on movement kinematics. The session consisted on the repetition of a simple arm movement (arm flexion and extension) during blocks of 4 min. Between blocks, patients had a few minutes to rest. After they completed the training, patients were asked about their opinion about each type of KP feedback.

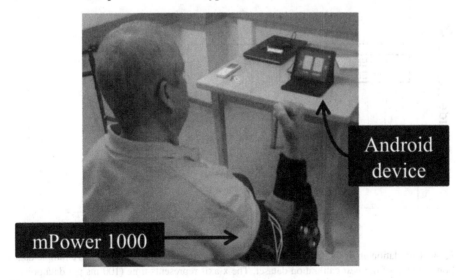

Fig. 3. Experimental setup. Stroke patient using the mobile knowledge of performance system for upper limb rehabilitation.

3   Results

3.1   Calibration Module: Maximizing Movement Control Through Intelligent Adaptation

This experiment involved healthy participants that had to find the optimal settings of the myo-electric robotic orthosis. For analyzing the data collected, all data collected were divided into two datasets: the first one containing all data related to flexion/extension exercising in which the optimal calibration settings were not found (*worst*), and the second one containing the data for the optimal calibration settings (*best*).

Figure 4a shows a best calibration data sample (EMG and elbow flexion) of a participant's session block. This particular data sample has a significant although very low Pearson correlation coefficient (r = -0.15, p < 0.001) between muscle activation (EMG) and actual movement (motor position). We computed the correlation coefficient for both datasets (Fig. 4b) and compared them with the non-parametric matched pairs Wilcoxon test. Although the correlation coefficient for the best configurations is statistically higher (p < 0.05), correlation values are low with a median below 0.4.

It can be observed that there is a large time lag between the muscle activation and the performance of the movement itself (Fig. 4a). Thus, in order to time correct the two time series (EMG and elbow flexion) a cross-correlation measure (Fig. 5a) was used. For the previous example in Fig. 4a we can observe that the maximum coefficient for the correlation (r = 0.81, p < 0.001) is found with a time lag of 10 time steps. Since each data point is collected at a rate of 100 ms, the 10 unit lag represents a second of delay between the muscle activation and the actual movement.

The analysis of all experimental sessions shows a higher time corrected correlation for the *best* settings dataset (r = 0.61) (see Fig. 5b), with an average time lag of

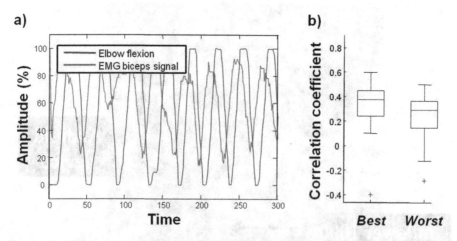

Fig. 4. Correlation analysis. (a) Normalized EMG vs. arm flexion (motor position) example data of one session of the *best* calibration dataset. The x axis represents time (100 ms per data point) and y axis normalized signal amplitude. (b) EMG vs. elbow position correlation analysis for all sessions of both datasets.

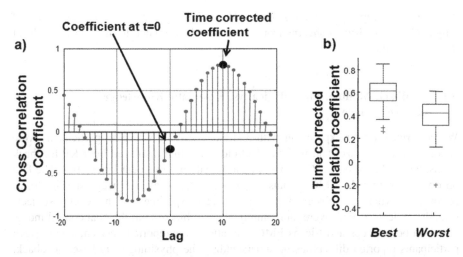

Fig. 5. Cross-correlation analysis. (a) Cross-correlation of the EMG vs. elbow flexion (motor position) of the example data in Fig. 4a. (b) EMG vs. elbow position time corrected correlation analysis for all sessions of both datasets.

12×100 ms. In this case, we find that the time corrected correlation is approximately 50 % better for the *best* dataset that when we consider all other settings in the *worst* dataset ($r = 0.4147$). A non-parametric matched pairs Wilcoxon test confirmed the differences to be significant ($p < 0.05$). Consequently, these data supports the idea that the best settings according to the user subjective reports are those that maximize the time corrected correlation between EMG activity and the movement performed by the myo-electric robotic orthosis. Further, an analysis of the parameter values used for the best calibrations for all sessions indicates that the median assistance levels for extension and flexion are $Mdn = 9$, $SD = 4.5$ and $Mdn = 16$, $SD = 4.6$ respectively, being the assistance in flexion about 40 % higher than in extension. These findings will lead to the implementation of an unsupervised algorithm that determines the mPower 1000 settings to maximize the time corrected correlation during motor movements (flexions and extensions).

Through the questionnaire (Table 3), participants reported a high level of control and comfort using Myomo ($M = 7.8$ and $M = 6.8$ respectively). In addition, users felt that the system was easy to use ($M = 8.1$) and understood well the calibration ($M = 7.9$).

Table 3. Responses to the user questionnaire (0-10).

Question	Responses
What was the level of control over Myomo?	7,8
What was the level of comfort when using Myomo?	6,8
What was the level of resistance that Myomo has provoked?	6,7
Level o fatigue after each block?	4,4
Do you think you managed to do calibration well?	7,9
Use of the myo-electric orthosis was easy?	8,1

Although users reported some resistance (*M = 6.7*), they did not report high levels of fatigue (*M = 4.4*). Most concerns from the users where related to the heavy weight of the robotic orthosis.

3.2 Feedback Module: Physiological vs. Kinematic Knowledge of Performance

We performed a pilot experiment with 3 stroke survivors where all participants were exposed to the mPower and with an Android tablet that displayed both KP feedback forms, that is, based on EMG activation and based on movement kinematics. The first observation is that the EMG signals of patients were weak and irregular (Fig. 6), as opposed to what was observed in the previous experiment with healthy subjects (Fig. 4a). Triceps signals were more unreliable than biceps; and the dual control mode, based on both biceps and triceps EMG activation, was reported very challenging. All participants reported difficulties in understanding the physiologically based feedback. We believe that the large oscillations on the EMG signals combined with the need of

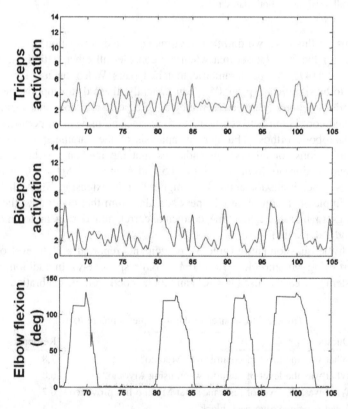

Fig. 6. Data sample for biceps and triceps EMG activation, and arm flexion for one patient performing repetitive arm flexion and extension training using the mPower 1000 myo-electric orthosis.

understanding the antagonistic nature of biceps and triceps EMG for the generation of the correct movement, made the physiologically based feedback less intuitive. When asked about which mode they preferred, all participants favored the more direct relation between kinematic feedback and movement execution, claiming that the kinematic feedback was easier to understand.

4 Discussion and Conclusions

In this project, we proposed a novel hybrid mobile rehabilitation approach by means of a myo-eletric driven orthosis in order to restore and enhance active movement training. To that end we developed a mobile system consisting of two software modules, a calibration and a feedback module, and evaluated them on healthy users and stroke patients. From the findings of the evaluation of calibration module, it is possible to conclude that a time corrected correlation on the muscular activation patterns (EMG) and actual movement can be used to assess the level of control by the user, and therefore to determine the best assistance settings. Hence, there is potential to build an intelligent system that is capable to self-calibrate only using actual user movements, without expert knowledge, and making myo-electric robotic assisted training more patient friendly. In addition, users reported high levels of acceptance of the technological solution.

On the feedback study, patients reported that the kinematic type of feedback was easier to understand. Unfortunately, we observed that also cognitive deficits derived from stroke interfered with the feedback comprehension, which resulted in a small sample of patients having criteria for participating in this evaluation. Despite these limitations, we believe that this tool has potential for supporting specific stroke survivors during their rehabilitation process. This mobile system does not only assist in action execution by virtue of the displayed feedback, contributing to generating knowledge of performance, it also serves to quantitatively assess and monitor changes in the muscular activation patterns of the biceps and triceps, making it also possible to quantify long term changes and improvements.

Overall, such a system can be valuable for supporting the execution of rehabilitation tasks in users with motor deficits of the upper extremities, offering personalized exercise assistance with enhanced feedback on performance. In the future we want to integrate both modules into a single application, providing both a self calibration method and enhanced feedback for the execution of motor tasks. We aim at conducting further experiments with a larger sample of stroke survivors to better understand both the effect of the nature of the feedback provided for knowledge of performance as well as its long term implications in the recovery of normal arm kinematics and muscle activation patterns.

Acknowledgements. This work is supported by the European Commission through the RehabNet project - Neuroscience Based Interactive Systems for Motor Rehabilitation - EC (303891 RehabNet FP7-PEOPLE-2011-CIG), and by the Fundação para a Ciência e Tecnologia (Portuguese Foundation for Science and Technology) through SFRH/BD/97117/2013, and Projeto Estratégico - LA 9 - 2013–2014.

References

1. Feigin, V.L., Barker-Collo, S., McNaughton, H., Brown, P., Kerse, N.: Long-term neuropsychological and functional outcomes in stroke survivors: current evidence and perspectives for new research. Int J. Stroke Off. J. Int. Stroke Soc. **3**(1), 33–40 (2008)
2. Legg, L.A., Drummond, A.E., Langhorne, P.: Occupational therapy for patients with problems in activities of daily living after stroke. Cochrane Database Syst. Rev. **4**, CD003585 (2006)
3. Dimyan, M.A., Cohen, L.G.: Neuroplasticity in the context of motor rehabilitation after stroke. Nat. Rev. Neurol. **7**(2), 76–85 (2011)
4. Bowden, M.G., Woodbury, M.L., Duncan, P.W.: Promoting neuroplasticity and recovery after stroke: future directions for rehabilitation clinical trials. Curr. Opin. Neurol. **26**(1), 37–42 (2013)
5. Bermúdez, S., García Morgade, A., Samaha, H., Verschure, P.F.M.J.: Using a hybrid brain computer interface and virtual reality system to monitor and promote cortical reorganization through motor activity and motor imagery training. IEEE Trans. Neural Syst. Rehabil. Eng. Publ. IEEE Eng. Med. Biol. Soc. **21**(2), 174–181 (2013)
6. Fasoli, S.E., Krebs, H.I., Stein, J., Frontera, W.R., Hughes, R., Hogan, N.: Robotic therapy for chronic motor impairments after stroke: follow-up results. Arch. Phys. Med. Rehabil. **85** (7), 1106–1111 (2004)
7. Nirme, J., Duff, A., Verschure, P.F.M.J.: Adaptive rehabilitation gaming system: on-line individualization of stroke rehabilitation. In: Conference Proceedings of Annual International Conference of the IEEE Engineering in Medicine and Biology Society, vol. 2011, pp. 6749–6752 (2011)
8. Cameirão, M.S., Bermúdez i Badia, S., Duarte, E., Verschure, P.F.M.J.: Virtual reality based rehabilitation speeds up functional recovery of the upper extremities after stroke: a randomized controlled pilot study in the acute phase of stroke using the Rehabilitation Gaming System. Restor. Neurol. Neurosci. **29**(5), 287–298 (2011)
9. Carel, C., Loubinoux, I., Boulanouar, K., Manelfe, C., Rascol, O., Celsis, P., Chollet, F.: Neural substrate for the effects of passive training on sensorimotor cortical representation: a study with functional magnetic resonance imaging in healthy subjects. J Cereb Blood Flow Metab **20**(3), 478–484 (2000). Off. J. Int. Soc. Cereb. Blood Flow Metab
10. Szameitat, A.J., Shen, S., Conforto, A., Sterr, A.: Cortical activation during executed, imagined, observed, and passive wrist movements in healthy volunteers and stroke patients. NeuroImage **62**(1), 266–280 (2012)
11. Bermúdez, iBS, Lewis, E., Bleakley, S.: Combining virtual reality and a myoelectric limb orthosis to restore active movement after stroke: a pilot study. Int. J. Disabil. Hum. Dev. **13** (3), 393–399 (2014)
12. Neves, D., Vourvopoulos, A., Cameirão, M., Bermudez i Badia, S.: An assistive mobile platform for delivering knowledge of performance feedback. In: Proceedings of the 8th International Conference on Pervasive Computing Technologies for Healthcare (PervasiveHealth '14). ICST (Institute for Computer Sciences, Social-Informatics and Telecommunications Engineering), ICST, Brussels, Belgium, pp. 440–442, May 2014. doi: http://dx.doi.org/10.4108/icst.pervasivehealth.2014.255278
13. Stein, J., Narendran, K., McBean, J., Krebs, K., Hughes, R.: Electromyography-controlled exoskeletal upper-limb-powered orthosis for exercise training after stroke. Am. J. Phys. Med. Rehabil. Assoc. Acad. Physiatr. **86**(4), 255–261 (2007)
14. Cirstea, C.M., Ptito, A., Levin, M.F.: Feedback and cognition in arm motor skill reacquisition after stroke. Stroke J. Cereb. Circ. **37**(5), 1237–1242 (2006)

15. Kilduski, N.C., Rice, M.S.: Qualitative and quantitative knowledge of results: effects on motor learning. Am. J. Occup. Ther. Off. Publ. Am. Occup. Ther. Assoc. **57**(3), 329–336 (2003)
16. Burke, J.W., McNeill, M.D.J., Charles, D.K., Morrow, P.J., Crosbie, J.H., McDonough, S. M.: Serious games for upper limb rehabilitation following stroke. In: VS-GAMES 200909. Conference in Games and Virtual Worlds for Serious Applications, pp. 103–110 (2009)
17. Cameirao, M.S., i Badia, B., Oller, E.D., Verschure, P.F.: Neurorehabilitation using the virtual reality based Rehabilitation Gaming System: methodology, design, psychometrics, usability and validation. J. NeuroEngineering Rehabil. **7**, 48 (2010)

Real-Time Feedback Towards Voluntary Pupil Control in Human-Computer Interaction: Enabling Continuous Pupillary Feedback

Juliane Georgi[1]([✉]), David Kowalski[2], Jan Ehlers[1], and Anke Huckauf[1]

[1] Department of General Psychology, Ulm University,
Institute of Psychology and Education,
Albert-Einstein-Allee 47, 89069 Ulm, Germany
{juliane.georgi,jan.ehlers,anke.huckauf}@uni-ulm.de
http://www.uni-ulm.de/in/psy-paed/allgemeine-psychologie.html
[2] Ulm University, Institute of Microelectronics,
Albert-Einstein-Allee 43, 89081 Ulm, Germany
david.kowalski@uni-ulm.de
http://www.uni-ulm.de/in/mikro.html

Abstract. Since the late 90's pupil size variations have been considered a possible input channel in Human-Computer Interaction [7]. [4,5] showed that it is possible to manipulate pupil size via self-induced regulation strategies. A training based on graphical real-time pupillary feedback supported the learning process towards voluntary pupil size control. For successful learning the feedback has to be reliable, stable and on time. Taking this into account, spontaneous blinking poses one important problem during real-time feedback. This paper presents the process and elaboration of real-time data filtering methods. The final implementation consists of a two-state process. Blink replacement is achieved with a data-driven threshold. The filter was programed and tested in the framework of a study by [3]. The testing results were promising.

Keywords: Real-time pupillary feedback · Voluntary pupil size control · HCI · Data filtering · Spontaneous eye blinks

1 Introduction

The success of Human-Computer Interaction (HCI) grounds on the necessity of providing a suitable link between human physical input actions and technical devices. [7] stated that "the fundamental task in computer input is to move information from the brain of the user to the computer" (p. 1). He stressed the importance of finding faster, more natural and more convenient means for information transmission. [7] was one of the first to mention eye pupil diameter as a future possible input channel.

Since then, various studies have shown that pupil size changes are related to cognitive and affective information processing, for example [6,11]. Yet, so far, the

© Springer-Verlag Berlin Heidelberg 2015
H.M. Fardoun et al. (Eds.): REHAB 2014, CCIS 515, pp. 104–114, 2015.
DOI: 10.1007/978-3-662-48645-0_10

majority of these studies have referred to pupil dynamics as merely passive, reactive information. Pupil size changes provide insight into affective experiences but seem to be defying any voluntary control, which is a crucial requirement in the case of feasible input channels. Ten years after [4,5,7] point to the possibility of intentional pupil size manipulations as a new way of transmitting information to a computer. They investigated the hypothesis that pupil variations can indirectly be controlled via several forms of physical and psychological self-regulation, for example positive thinking or changing the point of focus.

[4] provided real-time graphical feedback of the subjects' recorded pupillary behavior. This should allow the subjects to assess and learn to control their pupil variations, leading to voluntary pupil dilatations and constrictions. The authors see the quality and accuracy of the given feedback as essential to a successful learning process.

However, working with pupillary data raises two general problems. One is the sensitivity of the human pupil to changes in illumination, resulting in fluctuations of the recorded pupil size. This can be circumvented by providing constant lightning conditions, minimizing the possible influence of illumination on pupil size. The other one is the occurrence of spontaneous blinks. Blinking, characterized by a rapid closing and opening of the eyelid, causes the eye-tracker to record invalid values. During this process, the lid gradually occludes and uncovers the pupil leading to incorrect size measurements. The moment the eye is closed, the eye-tracker loses track of the pupil. For post hoc data analysis the method for removing the errors introduced by blinking does not have to meet any special requirements. Hence, with post hoc processing many methodical approaches are feasible.

However, in order to enable the control of a computer system by pupil size manipulations real-time eye tracking and feedback is required. Thus, handling blinks represents one important challenge. For providing real-time continuous feedback, the applied method has to be able to reliably detect and replace blinks by valid pupil size measurements without causing a too large delay and distortion in the data stream. Presentation of wrong or overly delayed values would disturb the feedback.

This paper presents the development and progress of an algorithm capable of fulfilling the above-mentioned specifications. In Sect. 2, the two filter approaches are presented, followed by their testing results and discussion. In Sect. 3 a conclusion is presented and implications for future work are elaborated.

2   Filtering Methods

The realization of real-time pupillary feedback needs to satisfy three premises, it has to be reliable, stable and on time. Reliability refers to the correctness and accuracy of the presented pupil size. Stability bears upon the ability to keep up reliable measurements when the pupil signal is disturbed which is particularly the case during blinking. The right timing assures that the depicted feedback values are related to the momentary pupil behavior at a specific time point.

Under these preconditions we developed and elaborated two filter algorithms for dealing with spontaneous eye blinks during real-time feedback.

Implementation and testing of the algorithms took place within the framework of a study by [3], evaluating the scopes and limits for training voluntary pupil control with real-time pupillary feedback. The subjects were instructed to try to control their pupil size as much as they can via self-induced imagination of positive or negative ideas, relaxation or by performing calculations. Figure 1 depicts the experimental setup and feedback schema presented to the participants. The basic feedback consisted of four circles. The use of graphical feedback instead of numeric values was considered to be more comprehensible. Likewise the presentation of circles was thought to be intuitive, since the shape of a circle is associated with the shape of the human pupil. The thicker black circle in the center represents the average pupil size of the subjects' baseline measurement. The two gray areas around the baseline circle depict the baseline average score plus/minus one standard deviation. These circles should serve the subjects as anchor points and remained constant during training. The dashed circle is the actual feedback. Its size varied according to the momentary pupil behavior. The fixation cross in the center should prevent the subjects' focus from drifting. For a more detailed description of the study refer to [3].

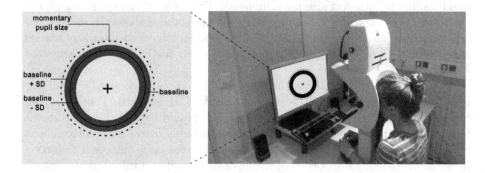

Fig. 1. Experimental setup and feedback schema as used in [3].

Pupil size was recorded with the SMI iView X™ Hi-Speed 1250 eye-tracker [13], featuring a sampling rate of 500 Hz. The experimental setup had a refresh rate of approximately 30 Hz, which implies one data point every 33.33 ms. The coding of the algorithms was done in PsychoPy v1.78 [12].

2.1 Value-to-Value Comparison Approach

Literature research of existing post hoc data analyzing methods indicates that one common rule to determine invalid data focuses on the comparison of consecutive measurement values. This approach is based on the assumption that the speed of pupil dilatation and constriction is physiologically limited. This proposes the definition of a criterion for the maximal allowed pupil diameter change during a fixed time interval. [9] have pointed out that applied criteria should best be derived from empirical data on actual physiological conditions. [10] investigated pupillary responses to emotionally provocative stimuli. They were recording pupil data with a 50 Hz eye-tracking system, hence the distance between two measurement points was 20 ms. They defined changes greater than 0.75 mm between two consecutive values as invalid measurements and removed them from the data set. In a subsequent study they halved their criterion to 0.375 mm [11]. Unfortunately, the authors did neither give a justification for their choice of criterion nor for its tightening in the second study.

Taken these considerations into account the first developed algorithm relies on a sample-to-sample comparison, as suggested by [10,11]. The filtering concept uses a criterion based on a study by [2]. This work provides a physiological foundation to the applied criterion. [2] investigated the amplitude and peak velocity of pupil constriction in the light reflex in 43 healthy subjects. The results yielded to an average peak velocity of 5.65 $\frac{mm}{s}$ ($SD = 1.17 \frac{mm}{s}$). Adaptation of the given peak velocity by [2] to our sampling rate of 30 Hz leads to a maximum sample-to-sample change of approximately 0.19 mm, as can be seen in the following equation:

$$5.65 \frac{mm}{s} = 0.0057 \frac{mm}{ms}$$
$$0.0057 \frac{mm}{ms} 33.33 \, ms = 0.19 \, mm. \tag{1}$$

The filtering process consists of the comparison of the absolute difference between each two measurement points to the criterion derived from equation (1). If a value is found to be exceeding this criterion, it is considered as invalid. The last valid measurement point is then taken as the comparison value for the following data points. Following the recommendation of [1], invalid values as well as zero values are replaced by the last valid value. Replacing ends once the last valid measurement and a following data point meet the criterion of 0.19 mm.

Testing Results and Discussion. Figure 2 depicts exemplary raw and filtered pupil diameter signals using the algorithm described in Sect. 2.1. The blinks are removed and replaced by the last valid measured value. However, the filtered data does not follow the raw data perfectly, especially between seconds 24 to 26. The lefthand side of Fig. 2 shows a close up of this time interval. A look at the raw data indicates a dilatation movement, consisting usually of two phases. The first one is a relatively steep and fast rising movement, whereas the second one is comparatively slower and continues until a certain base level is reached. This implies that the distance between two values, especially at the start of the upward movement could be somewhat bigger than 0.19 mm, as shown for the first two circled values. As a consequence the filter replaces the exceeding values by the last valid one and continues until one consecutive measurement meets the criterion, indicated for the third circled value.

These results point out one major drawback of this first filter implementation. They illustrate the trouble with keeping the comparison value fixed, once an

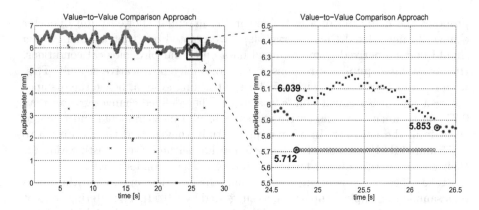

Fig. 2. Raw data signal (x) and filtered signal (o) after the Value-to-Value Comparison Approach. Close up of the time interval between 24 s to 26 s.

exceeding data point is found. Adherence of the comparison value leads to data replacements until a following measurement point matches the limit of 0.19 mm compared to the fixed value, potentially leading to massive data distortions.

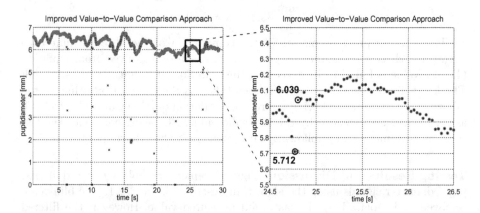

Fig. 3. Raw data signal (x) and filtered signal (o) after the Improved Value-to-Value Comparison Approach. Close up of the time interval between 24 s to 26 s.

In order to account for this issue, it is necessary to perform the value-to-value comparison independently of the last valid value. This requires buffering of two values and thereby introducing a delay. In the following explanation it is assumed that the first value is valid. The next incoming third measurement is then compared with the second. Two results are possible. If the comparison matches the criterion, then the second value becomes the next valid one and the following comparison is between the third and fourth value. If the criterion is not met, the first value is repeated, remains the valid value and the consecutive comparison is between the third and fourth value.

Figure 3 shows the same raw data and close up as in Fig. 2 with the modified filter. Studying the close up, it can be seen that the improvement leads to much less data distortions. However, correct data points are also replaced. This latter fact depicts two weak spots of a sample-to-sample change criterion.

The first problem is that the criterion is derived from a physiological characteristic. Therefore, it differs from person to person. This can be seen in the high standard deviation of the results by [2] (M=5.56 $\frac{mm}{s}$; SD=1.17 $\frac{mm}{s}$). These variations make it difficult to apply the same criterion to different persons. The second problem is that the applied criterion was based solely on average constriction speed and thus, disregarding the possibility that dilatation movements could be faster. A simple solution for both issues would be to enlarge the maximum allowed sample-to-sample change. However, the trade-off is that chances are increased to tolerate more invalid values.

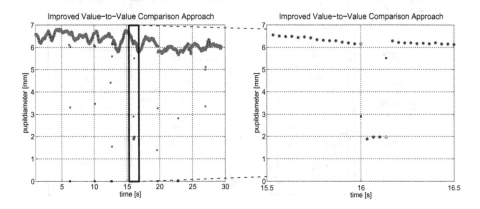

Fig. 4. Raw data signal (x) and filtered signal (o) after the Improved Value-to-Value Comparison Approach. Close up of the time interval between 15 s to 16 s.

Figure 4 illustrates another problem of the improved filter algorithm. Shortly after 16 s unusual small values are recorded. One reason for this might be, that the subject was blinking but did not close the eye completely. The close up on the left shows that the filter includes these values instead of replacing them, since the three adjacent values meet the criterion. This reveals a third weak spot of the applied criterion and filter. It does not check for unusual data.

As a consequence of these discussed problems of the first filtering concept an enhanced filtering algorithm was developed.

2.2 Enhanced Filter Approach (EFA)

The next proposed filter algorithm is built upon the improved value-to-value comparison approach and tries to overcome the implied problems. The implementation is based on a two-state-process and introduces the concept of a threshold. The threshold is a fixed value greater than zero, thereby indicating unusual small pupil diameter sizes, as well as blinks. This helps to detect blink movements at an earlier stage and to counteract the possibility of including unreasonable data. In this algorithm the value for the threshold is set to a maximal allowable pupil diameter of 3 mm. This choice is based on empirical experiences. Different than to the definition in the first algorithm, valid values are considered as three consecutive values which pairwise compared meet the allowable maximum deviation of 0.19 mm. This definition has proven to be more robust and reliable, than a simple value-to-value comparison. Figure 5 visualizes the basic working principle of the EFA algorithm, using a signal flowchart.

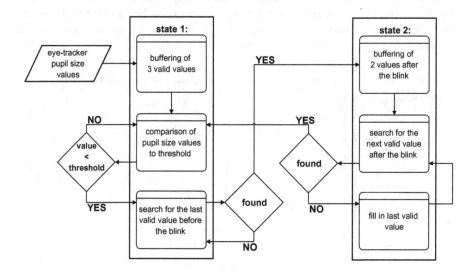

Fig. 5. Working principle of the EFA.

As shown in state one, each measurement starts with buffering three valid values. Three consecutive measurement points have to be greater than the threshold and meet the definition of valid values. This introduces a greater delay than in the previous filter where only two values need to be buffered. Nevertheless, these values constitute a save buffer, ensuring that a valid value is always given to replace invalid data. From then on, each incoming pupil size value is compared to the threshold. If it is greater, then it is considered valid and presented as feedback. If it is smaller, then a blink is detected and the actual filter process is activated. The EFA searches backwards in the preceding data for valid values, according to definition. The most recent valid value is taken as the replacement value and the filter switches to the second state. This state starts by buffering two values, thereby buying time to search for the next valid value in the prospective data. The two stored values are then again pairwise compared to the next incoming one, equivalent to the first process in state one. If they exceed the

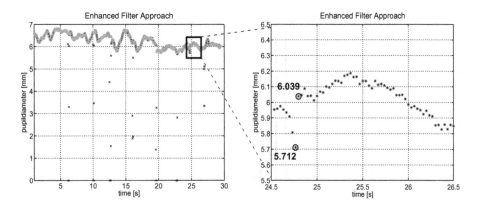

Fig. 6. Raw data signal (x) and filtered signal (o) after the EFA. Close up of the time interval between 24 s to 26 s.

threshold and are considered as valid, then the first one marks the endpoint of the blink and the filter switches back to state one. If they do not match both requirements, then the first value is replaced by the last valid value and the filter repeats the comparison process with the next incoming value.

Testing Results and Discussion. The EFA is compared to the previous filter concepts by using the same raw data signal and looking at the same time intervals.

Figure 6 depicts the time interval between 24 s and 26 s. The close up shows that the filter perfectly reproduces the raw signal course, in contrast to the previous approach (see Fig. 3).

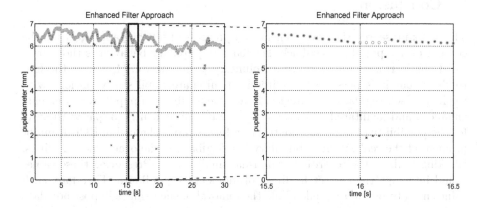

Fig. 7. Raw data signal (x) and filtered signal (o) after the EFA. Close up of the time interval between 15 s to 16 s.

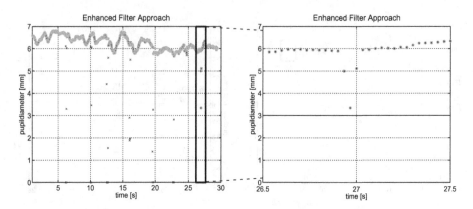

Fig. 8. Raw data signal (x) and filtered signal (o) after the EFA. Close up of the time interval between 26 s to 27 s.

The filter is also able to replace the unusual small pupil size recordings shortly around 16 s, as shown in Fig. 7. Both figures illustrate the benefits of the threshold. In contrast to a continuous comparison based on a fixed criterion, the threshold acts as a trigger to activate the search for valid values by pairwise comparison. This assures that valid values remain untouched by unusual large pupil size changes not associated to a blink.

Despite all of the mentioned aspects, introducing a constant threshold value does also create problems. The question to which value the threshold should be set is crucial. Figure 8 demonstrates this dilemma. The same data set but yet the invalid data around 26 s to 27 s, shown in the close up, are not intercepted. All three measurement points are greater than the threshold value.

3   Conclusion

This work presented the development and progress of filtering approaches in the context of live pupillary feedback. Feedback of pupillary behavior is thought to assist the learning process towards voluntary pupil control. [4,5] were the first to show that it is possible to indirectly manipulate pupil size variations with the help of self-regulation strategies. Real-time feedback of pupillary movements enhanced and facilitated this process. [4,5] and subsequently [3] paved the way for the possibility of pupil size control as a future input channel in HCI. A major problem of the realization of pupillary live feedback is the occurrence of blinks. Blinking leads to the recording of unusual small values. Presenting these values would interrupt the correct feedback of momentary pupil size. Therefore, such values need to be intercepted. While the removal of such values in post hoc data analysis does not need to meet any special requirements, the implementation of real-time filtering is a challenge. Real-time filters have to provide a reliable, stable and on time feedback. Feasible solutions for real-time filter concepts were elaborated. They were tested in the framework of a study by [3].

The first solution was a value-to-value comparison approach based on a maximal allowable sample-to-sample change criterion. The criterion was derived from average peak velocity of pupil constriction, given by [2]. This approach included a pairwise comparison of consecutive data points, with regard to the criterion. The implementation revealed the disadvantage of fixing the comparison value once two values were found to exceed the criterion. Potentially, this led to massive distortions in the filtered data, since the filter ceased to actually compare adjacent values.

In an improved version of this approach it was ensured that a continuous value-to-value comparison was maintained. However, the first results pointed out three major problems in applying a sample-to-sample change criterion. First, the derivation of the criterion from a physiological characteristic, introduces interindividual variations, thereby making it difficult to equally apply one fixed criterion. The second problem is the fact that the criterion based on average peak velocity of pupil constriction. Thus, this implementation did not respect that pupil dilatation movements could be faster. This led to replacement of correct data by the filter. A third weak spot is that this filter did not check for unusual data.

The EFA concept was based on the improved first approach and resolved its issues. The biggest advantage of this filter implementation, when compared with the first approach, is the use of a threshold. The threshold served as a trigger to activate the actual filtering, if there were values recorded which were smaller than the threshold. This helped to detect blinks and unusual data and, at the same time, ensuring that valid values remained untouched by unusual large pupil size changes not associated to a blink.

The results of the filter testings encouraged the implementation of the EFA. It could be proved that the EFA leads to better results as the first approach and overcomes its problems. Nevertheless, testing also revealed that the value of the threshold is crucial for successful filtering.

For a future development it is proposed to implement an adaptive threshold which is associated with actual pupil behavior. This should make it possible to identify unusual values dependent on the momentary signal trend, leading to more robust and reliable results. Furthermore, it is suggested to individualize the sample-to-sample change criterion, making it less susceptible to interindividual variations. Therefore, at the beginning of the data collection, the criterion could be adjusted by measuring a subjects peak velocity of constriction. Moreover, it might be possible to use linear interpolation to approach the actual signal course during the replacing of invalid values, as it was proposed by [8].

The current filter implementation and the proposed improvements still need to be investigated. It is important to further examine them in the context of real-time pupillary feedback, working towards a continuous, stable and direct feedback, which ensures a successful training on voluntary pupil size manipulation. This is a critical step towards the examination of how useful pupil size variations can be as one further input channel in HCI.

114   J. Georgi et al.

References

1. Bernhardt, P.C., Dabbs, J.M., Riad, J.K.: Pupillometry system for use in social psychology. Behav. Res. Methods. Instrum. Comput. **28**, 61–66 (1996)
2. Bremner, F.D.: Pupillometric evaluation of the dynamics of the pupillary response to a brief light stimulus in healthy subjects. Invest. Ophthalmol. Vis. Sci. **53**, 7343–7347 (2012)
3. Ehlers, J., Bubalo, N., Loose, M.C.A., Huckauf, A.: Towards voluntary pupil control - Training affective strategies?. Manuscript submitted for publication (2014)
4. Ekman, I., Poikola, A., Mäkäräinen, M., Takal, T., Hämäläinen, P.: Voluntary pupil size change as control in eyes only interaction. In: Proceedings of the 2008 Symposium on Eye Tracking Research & Applications, pp. 115–118. ACM, New York (2008)
5. Ekman, I., Poikola, A., Mäkäräinen, M.: Invisible eni: using gaze and pupil size to control a game. In: CHI 2008 Extended Abstracts on Human Factors in Computing Systems, pp. 3135–3140. ACM, New York (2008)
6. Hyönä, J., Tommola, J., Alaja, A.M.: Pupil dilation as a measure of processing load in simultaneous interpretation and other language tasks. Q. J. Exp. Psychol. A **48**, 598–612 (1995)
7. Jacob, R.J.K.: The future of input devices. ACM Comput. Surv. **28**, 177–179 (1996)
8. Marshall, S.P.: Method and Apparatus for Eye Tracking and Monitoring Pupil Dilation to Evaluate Cognitive Activity. US Patent No. 6,090,051 (2000)
9. Merritt, S.L., Keegan, A.P., Mercer, P.W.: Artifact management in pupillometry. Nurs. Res. **43**, 56–59 (1994)
10. Partala, T., Jokiniemi, M., Surakka, V.: Pupillary responses to emotionally provocative stimuli. In: Proceedings of the 2000 Symposium on Eye Tracking Research & Applications, pp. 123–129. ACM, New York (2000)
11. Partala, T., Surakka, V.: Pupil size variation as an indication of affective processing. Int. J. Hum-Comput. St. **59**, 185–198 (2003)
12. Peirce, J.W.: PsychoPy - psychophysics software in python. J. Neurosci. Methods. **162**, 8–13 (2007)
13. SensoMotoric Instruments, iView X™ Hi-Speed 1250. http://www.smivision.com/en/gaze-and-eye-tracking-systems/

Applying 3D Graphics to Computerized Cognitive Rehabilitation

Anna Alloni[1(✉)], Dani Tost[2], Silvia Panzarasa[1], Chiara Zucchella[3], and Silvana Quaglini[1]

[1] Department of Electrical, Computer and Biomedical Engineering,
University of Pavia, Pavia, Italy
{anna.alloni, silvia.panzarasa,
silvana.quaglini}@unipv.it
[2] Computer Graphics Division, CREB, UPC, Barcelona, Spain
dani@lsi.upc.edu
[3] IRCCS C. Mondino National Institute of Neurology Foundation, Pavia, Italy
chiara.zucchella@gmail.com

Abstract. Cognitive rehabilitation is usually administered in form of paper-based exercises the patient is required to solve. With the availability of new and advanced technologies, computer science is gaining more and more importance in the treatment routine. In this paper a software system for the rehabilitation of cognitively impaired subjects will be presented. Its features guarantee many advantages, both for patients and therapists, but to prevent the risk of reduced compliance, which, considering the intended target of the system- typically elderly people with low computer skills- cannot be ignored, 3D technology has been introduced. The project choices made and implementation strategies applied to increase immersion and entertainment and prevent boredom and drops in compliance will be described. Open issues and future works will also be illustrated.

Keywords: Computer-aided therapy · Cognitive rehabilitation · 3D graphics · Serious games

1 Introduction

Cognitive rehabilitation is usually administered in form of exercises, which the patients are expected to execute with pen and paper. In the latest years computer science applications have been developed to support this kind of treatment [1–7]. While these applications are in general well-accepted by young people or children, that need rehabilitation for example after a trauma or for learning and behavioural problems, the older patients (e.g. post-stroke or with degenerative diseases) may have some problems with them, since third age is a part of the population which normally doesn't show much familiarity with modern technology [8–10]. Such lack of comfort with PCs and informatics tools often entails negative consequences when it comes to trying to integrate such technology into the therapy routine: feeling this kind of innovation-something new and very likely never seen before, for which they are completely unprepared- "forced" upon them often leads to a decrease in the willingness of the

© Springer-Verlag Berlin Heidelberg 2015
H.M. Fardoun et al. (Eds.): REHAB 2014, CCIS 515, pp. 115–128, 2015.
DOI: 10.1007/978-3-662-48645-0_11

patients to actively participate in the process, to the point of developing some sort of "hostility" towards a tool they are not able to handle with ease.

Beside the matter of old age, also the particular condition of subjects suffering cognitive impairments could make them even more reluctant when confronted with a new type of therapy. All of this could even lead to a decrease of the patient's compliance.

On the other side, the "pen and paper" style in the mid-long term can make the therapy boring for the patients and time-consuming for the psychologists. As a matter of fact, the range of different stimuli (images and texts) available is limited by the (usually small) number of existing variants of the printed exercise sheets, and the therapist must be careful to not repeat the same stimuli within a short time. Moreover, the lack of an automated way of recording the results of the sessions prevents the therapists from monitoring the evolution of the patients' clinical condition with ease.

For this reason, being able to integrate computer science into the rehabilitation path in a way that reduces the potentially negative impact to the patient as much as possible is extremely important.

This paper, which is an extension of [11], describes how the developed system tries to achieve this goal.

2   Methods

The collaboration between the "Mario Stefanelli" Laboratory for Biomedical Informatics of the University of Pavia and the IRCCS Fondazione C. Mondino led to the creation of a software tool for computerized cognitive rehabilitation. The system, named CoRe (from **Co**gnitive **Re**habilitation), allows the user (the psychologist) to easily generate a computerized version of exercises aimed at restoring logical and executive brain functions, usually undergone with pen and paper during face to face rehabilitation sessions; besides, since the system keeps track of several performance parameters during the execution of the session, it can provide therapists a great help: by analyzing those parameters, CoRe is able to automatically assess the patient and thus to adjust each exercise's difficulty accordingly. As stated before, patient-tailoring of the exercises plays a vital role in preventing fatigue and boredom, since perceiving the rehabilitation as a stressful situation could very likely reduce the subject's compliance.

2.1   System Characteristics

CoRe features four main components:

- a graphical user interface allowing the therapist creating the treatment plans to set the parameters needed to start an exercise (difficulty level, number and maximum duration of the stimuli to be shown etc.);
- two databases, used to store the patients' personal information and performance parameters, as well as all the stimuli (texts, sounds and images) needed for the execution of the sessions;
- a software engine to generate the customized exercises based on both the options set by the therapist and the patient's performance;

- the exercises, which have been created with E-Prime, a commercial tool whose main advantage is the extreme flexibility, that allows a user to easily implement all the types of rehabilitation exercises needed.

The structure of CoRe is shown in Fig. 1. Just after setting the parameters, the therapist can start the exercises; the databases are accessed for Create Read Update Delete (CRUD) operations and three main purposes:

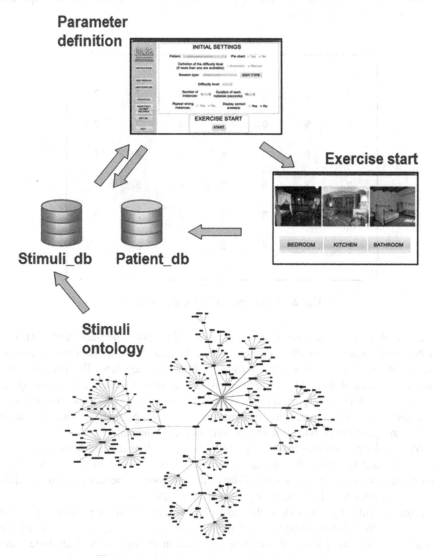

Fig. 1. Functional architecture of the CoRe system.

- when the database must be updated, and new stimuli inserted;
- when these stimuli need to be extracted in order to generate a new session;
- when the system needs to read/write the patient's performances and personal information.

The exercises featured in the system require the completion of several types of tasks based on the patient correctly recognizing the stimuli proposed. For example, Fig. 2 shows an instance of "Pick the element": the patient is shown a matrix of textual stimuli (the numbers visualized in each slot), among which he must choose the one requested by the system (here, the number 0).

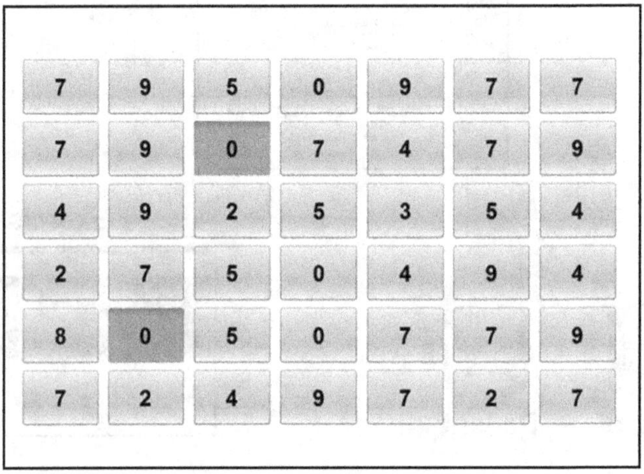

Fig. 2. An instance of "Pick the element"

To be able to generate the sessions correctly, the system interacts with a stimuli database containing about 6000 entries- words, images and sounds. This, of course, makes it possible to create exercises dynamically, thus exponentially increasing the number of variants available for execution: it's almost impossible that during an exercise the patient undergoes more instances based on the very same stimuli. This implementation choice- generation of dynamic sessions- represents the first step taken to solve the problem of boredom and prevent non-compliance.

Some tasks also require the user to identify relationships defined between stimuli. This is the case for "Find the intruder", shown in Fig. 3: five buttons are shown on screen, each one labeled with a word. Four of them belong to the same category, while one of them does not. The patient's goal is to select the intruder.

From a technical point of view, the most effective way of building such system- that is, one able to generate relation-based exercises correctly- is by organizing all the stimuli in an ontology, which describes every element through a set of attributes, and its relations with other entities. For example, the attribute "difficulty level" ("low", "medium", "high") associated to every single concept of the structure and related to the meaning of the concept itself, may be considered initially to retrieve stimuli according

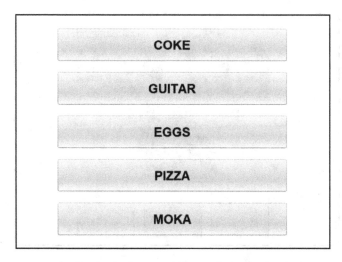

Fig. 3. An instance of "Find the intruder"

to the patient's scholarship (even if exercises will then be adjusted according to the patient's performance). "Is-a" relations among stimuli can instead be used to generate exercises for classification tasks, as in Fig. 3. A detailed description of the ontology is beyond the scope of this paper and can be found in [12].

3 Test Phase and Issues

The system as described above was first tested by volunteers who underwent simulated rehabilitation sessions in presence of a therapist and then were asked to comment the system: during this phase some issues emerged, that lead us to look for new strategies and solutions to make CoRe as compliant to the patients' needs as possible. Later the system has been tested on 9 Parkinson patients, who were supposed to undergo 12 sessions in a 1-month time range (6 patients performed all the sessions, while 3 were discharged before the end of the trial and dropped out after respectively 9, 10 and 11 sessions). While the general opinion about the system was positive, it was not hard to notice that certain types of tasks were generally preferred to others. In particular, the subjects appeared more entertained and involved when they were asked to solve exercises that featured visual stimuli- for example "Unscramble the images", shown in Fig. 4, in which the user has to put a scrambled series of cartoons in the right order to tell a short story.

This is confirmed by the fact that once the session was over and the volunteers were asked to solve a "text-only" exercise, it was not infrequent to hear them ask "Can't we do some more scene unscrambling instead of this?", even if the new exercise was based on the exact same task, as is the case with "Unscramble the sentence", that requires the user to select words in the right order to form a phrase (Fig. 5).

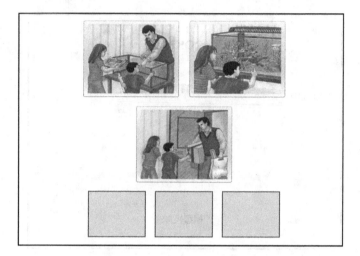

Fig. 4. An instance of "Unscramble the images"

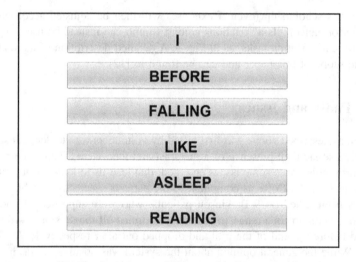

Fig. 5. An instance of "Unscramble the sentence"

Among the "text-only" tasks, CoRe features the previously described exercise called "Find the intruder" (Fig. 3) that exploits the relations between the concepts represented in the ontology.

Despite being a very simple exercise that requires only one click to be solved, the volunteers didn't seem to enjoy this task very much- for the reason explained above.

The strategy we chose to solve this problem consisted in transforming "Find the intruder" in a visual exercise: contrary to "Unscramble the sentence", in which grammar and syntax play a vital role, this exercise is based on recognition of concepts and thus better suited for re-engineering, that can be both 2D or 3D based. In the following section we focus on the latter solution.

4   3D Graphics

4.1   Reasons of the Choice of 3D

In the latest years, with serious games gaining public attention and becoming an object of interest for researchers, 3D graphics have been introduced in many fields of the medical practice, among which psychological rehabilitation [13–17].

We chose to develop the visual version of "Find the intruder" as a 3D-based exercise for one main reason: for a human subject a direct interaction with actual, material objects is perceived as more natural than its "abstract" counterpart, that is interacting with bare text (the words that "represent" said objects).

Being the use of (hundreds of) physical items during rehabilitation sessions a clearly non-viable option, the best alternative is setting up an interaction between the user and a visual representation of every object.

This, of course, could be achieved using simple.jpg images easily available online, but the advantages entailed by the use of 3D models are clear: first of all, it allows a more complex interaction, giving users the chance to have a 360° view of the solids and, in general, to manipulate them at pleasure: secondly, the programmer has complete control over the looks of a model- every single vertex, edge and face of a solid is editable in any moment- something that does not happen with 2D images.

4.2   Implementation Strategy: Interactivity and Simplicity

In the implementation phase, carried out in collaboration with the Computer Graphics Division of the Polytechnical University of Catalonia (UPC), some important matters had to be taken into consideration. First and most important, during the creation of object models a compromise had to be reached between detail and complexity: the more the vertices composing the solid, the bigger the resulting object file and the computational power needed to render the scene. This will be even more important when the time comes to use CoRe and the re-engineered 3D exercises for telereha-bilitation sessions: our typical cognitively impaired patients, that is mostly elderly people with very limited familiarity with modern technologies, very likely do not own powerful PCs. Thus it was necessary to keep the system requirements of our software as low as possible. As a thumb rule, we chose to set the maximum number of vertices-per-object to about 10.000.

Secondly, the 3D version of the exercise features a scenario (a room with 3 bare walls and a floor, with a big table as the only piece of furniture, see Fig. 6) that, though very simple and limited in space, the user is allowed to navigate freely, to get as close to the objects as possible.

This, together with the possibility to have a 360° view of the single objects, implies the need of a "complex" control system: it is clear how the combination of mouse buttons and direction arrows cannot be able to guarantee the needed degree of inter-action, and introducing more keyboard keys to the control system may well be considered way too complicated for our target users. For this reason another compromise is needed, this time between the degrees of freedom allowed to the user and the complexity of the controls.

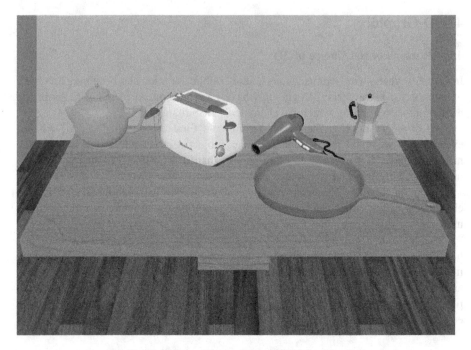

Fig. 6. The 3D implementation of "Find the intruder"

This is the main reason why different versions of the same 3D task have been implemented, to meet the needs of patients with different degrees of impairment.

Beside the previously described "basic" version, with the five objects randomly scattered on the table, another, apparently more complex one was implemented. Here, the elements are not immediately visible, but hidden into five closed boxes lined up on the table; in order to successfully complete the task, the user needs to open every box first, and see what's inside.

Since the introduction of the boxes increased the difficulty level of the exercise (and, consequently, the complexity of the control system required), the need to simplify some aspects of the execution emerged. This was done in order to avoid the introduction of unwanted complications that could interfere with the achievement of the main task.

The very idea of introducing boxes in the exercise made it necessary to choose the right approach to one particular issue. As mentioned above, our stimuli database is very wide and made up of elements belonging to diverse domains; it is clear that the difference between the objects' orders of magnitude can be substantial, and this can represent a problem. Let's say, for example, that the two categories are 'means of transport' (a car, a bike, a motorbike and a truck) and 'sports equipment' (a soccer ball): of course, simply "wrapping" rectangular boxes around the objects would render the exercise useless, because the size difference itself would basically give away the solution to the task: for this reason, boxes with fixed size and shape are used, and a scaling algorithm has been created to fit all the objects in.

A choice needed to be made between maintaining a constant scale for all the objects (that is, keeping the size difference realistic in order to contextualize the exercise and help the patient identifying the categories at the price of a potentially significant loss in objects' visibility- see the example of truck/car etc. vs. soccer ball) and scaling every object down/up to fit the box size (losing the information about the size difference, but guaranteeing the recognisability at a glance of all the objects).

The second solution was chosen (Fig. 7c–d), based on the fact that the main acceptability criterion for any 2D image is the visibility of the subject and no size difference information are ever available in picture-based exercises.

At that point, the only apparently trivial problem of the interaction with the boxes had to be tackled; while the initial intention was to develop a mouse-based drag-and-drop type of command, that would have required the user to simulate the gesture of lifting the lid in order to open the box, the simplification led to the choice of a much simpler approach: a click on a box triggers a default animation of its lid lifting and moving out of sight.

To pursue the simplification mentioned above, the free roaming feature, available in the "no-box version" of the task, has been disabled here: at the start of the game the camera is placed in front of the table, so that all the boxes are within the field of view at the same time, and all the patient is required to do to see what's inside a box is click on it.

This selection, as already mentioned, triggers a default animation (Fig. 7): while the lid lifts, the camera zooms to the selected box and tilts down to show the content. After a few seconds of wait, the camera zooms out and back to the starting position. The player is allowed to look into the boxes multiple times to re-examine objects already seen (a counter will keep track of the total number of views for each box). After that, he can complete the task by selecting the solution with the press of one of five aptly assigned keys within the keyboard.

A very important issue was brought to light by the therapists during the analysis of this implementation schema: some of the patients could be afflicted with visual-spatial processing deficits, and the camera motions featured in the exercise could cause confusion and disorientation. This is why an alternative version of the task was implemented: here, when the player clicks on the box, the camera moves parallel to the table until it stops in front of the selected box. The lid still opens automatically, but there is neither forward motion nor tilt of the camera. Instead, the object flies out of the box and then towards the player; It hovers in front of the camera, slowly spinning on its vertical axis for a few seconds to allow a better view, and then goes back into the box (Fig. 8).

5   Discussion

5.1   3D Models

The advantages implied by the 3D approach to the implementation of rehabilitation exercises have already been mentioned: pseudo-natural interaction with the objects, increased entertainment and involvement of the patient into the rehabilitation process, possibility to introduce new elements into the therapy (like training of spatial perception/processing through virtual navigation, when allowed by the health condition

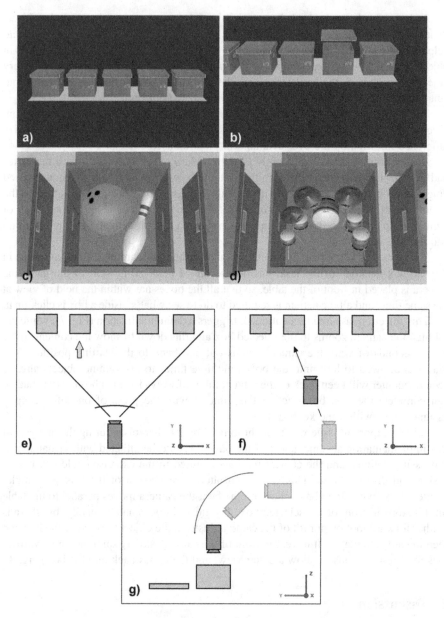

Fig. 7. Camera motion during the automated animation in the "box version" of "Find the Intruder": once a box is selected (a), the lid opens (b) and the camera zooms in and tilts down over the box (c). Besides, (c) vs. (d) show how all the objects are scaled to fit the dimensions of the boxes. The camera positions and movements during the animation are schematised in (e), (f) and (g).

of the patient). To achieve this, care has to be put in the modeling phase of the implementation: recognizability is fundamental, for, unlike what happens with photos,

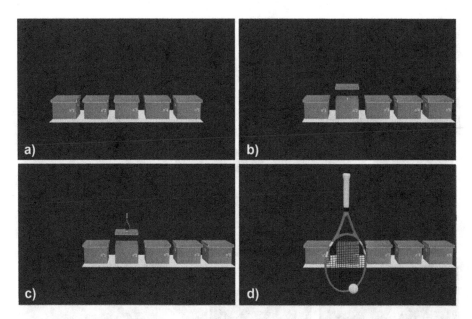

Fig. 8. Camera motion during the automated animation in the alternative "box version" of "Find the Intruder": once a box is selected (a), the lid opens (b) and the object flies towards the camera (c) and rotates on its vertical axis for a few seconds (d) before flying back into the box.

3D models are not (and cannot be) 100 % accurate representations of the original object. To date, about 50 models have been created, belonging to 7 different categories; the work is not over, others will be generated to enrich the archive as much as possible: this way 3D-based tasks will be allowed the same variability that text/image/sound-based exercises already show (Fig. 9).

5.2   Controls

To solve the still open question regarding the creation of a control system simple enough to be handled by patients, and at the same time able to provide the navigability and interactivity needed for the execution of the exercises, the introduction of particular hardware solutions must be also taken into consideration: being the manipulation of objects an essential feature for some tasks, the use of a touch screen (maybe even a multi-touch for zooming purposes) and adaptive push-button panels could represent an interesting option. As soon as a stable version of the exercises is ready to be integrated into the software system, usability tests will be undergone to assess which type of control is better accepted by the users.

5.3   Aids, Complexity and Difficulty Levels

As previously stated, the walls in the game scenario are left blank by default, in order to avoid possible distractions that would interfere with the achievement of the main goal

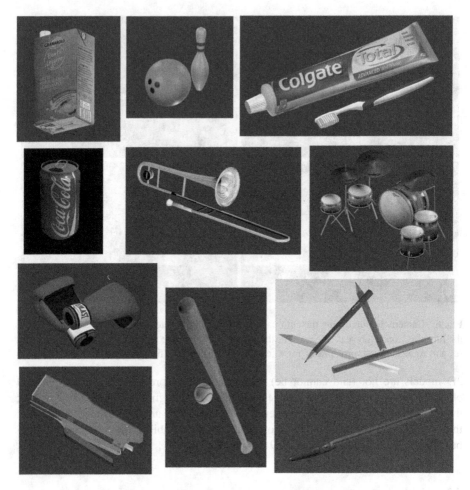

Fig. 9. Some of the models created for the 3D exercises

of the exercise. But if needed, an optional feature can be introduced, allowing a texture to be dynamically applied to them in order to create a meaningful context and help the patient solve the task. For example, if the main category is "kitchen supplies", the texture could show a kitchen, complete with cupboards and appliances (Fig. 10): this way it could be easier for the player to identify the intruder. If provided by the patient himself or his caregivers, the picture of the actual patient's kitchen could even be shown, to personalized the exercise and make the scene more familiar.

This is only one of the several aids that can be optionally introduced during the execution of an exercise (navigation ON/OFF, manipulation ON/OFF, manual actions vs. automatic animations etc.). Thus, the complexity of each session depends on many variables; for this reason the assessment of the overall difficulty level of an exercise is way more complex for 3D exercises than it is for text/picture/sound based ones and must be performed in close collaboration with the medical staff.

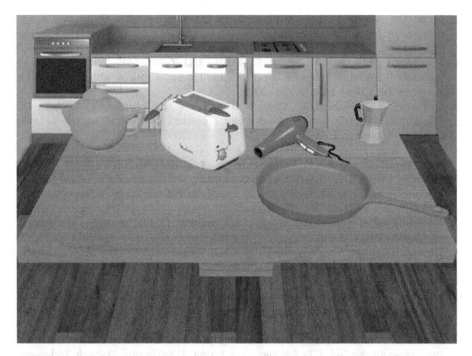

Fig. 10. The "Find the Intruder" task featuring the help texture

5.4   Acceptance

Also, it is not possible to assess which approach (text-only vs. 2D vs. 3D) will be preferred by every patient. Our goal is to offer, within one tool, the widest possible range of approaches from which to choose from. This way the therapist will be able to test different options in the early phase of the treatment and decide which one represents the most suitable solution for the specific subject.

Elderly patients (or, in general, people with little familiarity with modern technology) might refuse the 3D approach in the beginning, and switch to it later, after acquiring familiarity with the computerized therapy, while younger individuals, accustomed to playing videogames, will very likely prefer undergoing 3D exercises from the beginning.

Acknowledgments. Our thanks to Prof. Giorgio Sandrini and Dr. Elena Sinforiani, from IRCCS C. Mondino Foundation, who collaborated on the development of the system and agreed to test it.

References

1. Schuhfried. CogniPlus - I programmi di training (1995). http://www.schuhfried.it/cogniplus-cps/i-programmi-di-training/

2. Giunti, O.S.: ERICA - Esercizi di RIabilitazione Cognitiva per Adulti (2010). http://www.riabilitazione.giuntios.it/it. Accessed 25 Feb 2014
3. Anastasis. COG.I.T.O (2007). http://cogito.integrazioni.it/. Accessed 25 Feb 2014
4. Fernández, E., Bringas, M.L., Salazar, S., Rodríguez, D., García, M.E., Torres, M.: Clinical impact of RehaCom software for cognitive rehabilitation of patients with acquired brain injury. MEDICC Rev. **14**(4), 32–35 (2012)
5. Dwolatzky, T., Whitehead, V., Doniger, G.M., Simon, E.S., Schweiger, A., Jaffe, D., Chertkow, H.: Validity of the Mindstreams computerized cognitive battery for mild cognitive impairment. J. Mol. Neurosc. **24**(1), 33–44 (2004)
6. Kueider, A.M., Parisi, J.M., Gross, A.L., Rebok, G.W.: Computerized cognitive training with older adults: a systematic review. PLoS One **7**, e40588 (2012)
7. Tornatore, J.B., Hill, E., Laboff, J.A., McGann, M.E.: Self-administered screening for mild cognitive impairment: initial validation of a computerized test battery. J Neuropsychiatry Clin. Neurosci. **17**(1), 98–105 (2005)
8. Eurostat. Computer use in individuals in EU countries (2014). http://appsso.eurostat.ec.europa.eu/nui/show.do?dataset=isoc_ci_cfp_cu&lang=en. Accessed 4 Apr 2014
9. Eurostat. Individuals' level of computer skill in EU countries (2014). http://epp.eurostat.ec.europa.eu/tgm/refreshTableAction.do?tab=table&plugin=1&pcode=tsdsc460&language=en. Accessed 4 Apr 2014
10. Richardson, M., Zorn, T. E., Weaver, K.: Seniors' perspectives on the barriers, benefits and negative consequences of learning and using computers (2002). http://www.academia.edu/download/31048190/resource1.pdf
11. Alloni, A., et al.: Enhancing computerized cognitive rehabilitation with 3D solutions. In: Proceedings of the 2nd ICTs for Improving Patient Rehabilitation Research Techniques Workshop - REHAB 2014 (2014). doi:10.4108/icst.pervasivehealth.2014.255358
12. Leonardi, G., Panzarasa, S., Quaglini, S.: Ontology-based automatic generation of computerized cognitive exercises. Stud. Health Technol. Inform. **2011**(169), 779–783 (2011)
13. Abreu, P.F., Werneck, V.M.B., Costa, R.M.E., Carvalho, L.A.V.: Employing multi-agents in 3-D game for cognitive stimulation. In: Symposium on Virtual Reality (SVR), 2011, 23–26 May 2011, vol. XIII, pp. 73–78. IEEE (2011)
14. Grau, S., Tost, D., Campeny, R., Moya, S., Ruiz, M.: Design of 3D virtual neuropsychological rehabilitation activities. In: Second International Conference on Games and Virtual Worlds for Serious Applications (VS-GAMES), 25–26 March 2010, pp. 109–116 (2010)
15. Rego, P.: Serious games for rehabilitation: a survey and a classification towards a taxonomy. In: 5th Iberian Conference on Information Systems and Technologies (CISTI), 16–19 June 2010, pp. 1–6 (2010)
16. Tost, D., Grau, S., Ferre, M., Garcia, P., Tormos, J.M., Garcia, A., Roig, T.: PREVIRNEC: a cognitive telerehabilitation system based on virtual environments. In: Virtual Rehabilitation International Conference, 2009, June 29–July 2 2009, pp. 87–93 (2009)
17. Rizzo, A.S., Wiederhold, B.K.: Virtual reality technology for psychological/neuropsychological/motor assessment and rehabilitation: applications and issues. In: IEEE Virtual Reality Conference, 2006, 25–29 March 2006, p. 308 (2006)

Systems-of-Systems Framework for Providing Real-Time Patient Monitoring and Care: Challenges and Solutions

Roman Obermaisser[1]([⊠]), Mohammed Abuteir[1],
Ala Khalifeh[2], and Dhiah el Diehn I. Abou-Tair[2]

[1] University of Siegen, Siegen, Germany
{roman.obermaisser,mohammed.abuteir}@uni-siegen.de
[2] German Jordanian University, Amman, Jordan
{ala.khalifeh,dhiah.aboutair}@gju.edu.jo

Abstract. Systems-of-Systems (SoS) enable new emerging services in many application domains such as healthcare systems, transportation systems and the smart grid. However, satisfying real-time and reliability requirements is a prerequisite for the deployment of SoS in safety-relevant applications with stringent timing constraints. This book chapter describes a SoS framework for patient monitoring services, which supports the openness, dynamic nature and lack of global control in a SoS. The framework enables rehabilitation and recovery from illness by introducing sensing services, data analysis and real-time alert messages via monitoring centers. We address the temporal constraints by online scheduling of communication activities. In addition, data protection as well as security and privacy challenges are solved in the healthcare monitoring process.

Keywords: System-of-systems · E-health · Healthcare monitoring · Real-time communication · Scheduling · Reliability · Time triggered ethernet · Wireless communication

1 Introduction

In recent years, the number of people suffering from multiple chronic conditions is growing. An important demographic fact is the increase in percentage of people with chronic conditions that depend on the healthcare system and require costly long-term care, especially with elderly people. In order to provide an integrated system that can monitor and report the conditions of people as they travel through their everyday life, and then to make informed decisions on their care, based on this information, an integrated healthcare system supported with robustness, security assurance, reliability and real-time capabilities is needed to ensure smooth patients' rehabilitation and recovery.

The potential benefits of Systems-of-Systems (SoS) in healthcare applications are already clearly recognized, and societal trends indicate that they will be

© Springer-Verlag Berlin Heidelberg 2015
H.M. Fardoun et al. (Eds.): REHAB 2014, CCIS 515, pp. 129–142, 2015.
DOI: 10.1007/978-3-662-48645-0_12

attractive to a large and increasing number of people. As a part of the medical SoS, the elderly people environment will be equipped with sensors to obtain a range of normal and abnormal medical data (e.g., cardiac sensors, pulse oximetry sensors). If the analysis of the sensor data indicates that anything abnormal is happening, an alert will be generated to enable a safe, timely and efficient handling of the patient. Building such a medical SoS is challenging due to the fact that the system monitors patient in different ambient assisted living spaces (homes, and care centers for elderly) as well as the development of distributed embedded system architecture for constantly evolving and dynamic SoS with support for verifiable real-time, reliability and safety properties.

This book chapter provides a SoS framework for patients' healthcare monitoring and reporting, that takes into account several design and implementation challenges and proposes potential solutions. This framework extends previous work [1] patient monitoring and care for focusing on the following challenges:

- Providing a realistic model for the healthcare SoS based on upcoming IEEE standards with particular emphasis on QoS properties and architectural models specifying the building blocks, services and interfaces in healthcare SoS.
- Reliable and predictable communication services using heterogeneous in-home networking technologies. The framework provide solutions based on upcoming IEEE standards with support for time-triggered communication, wire-bound and wireless communication networks that are integrated into a reliable and temporally predictable communication infrastructure that supports healthcare components with different criticality-levels, QoS requirements (e.g., bandwidth, latency, reliability) and communication modes (e.g., streaming, cyclic control messages, events).
- Distributed algorithms for runtime coordination of constituting systems: Algorithms for coordinating the constituent systems are required based on distributed algorithms for the discovery and peering of components, dynamic resource allocation with guarantees concerning real-time behaviour and reliability.
- Security: The runtime coordination will be secured preventing attacks on the mechanisms for dynamic configuration in the healthcare SoS. In addition, privacy for exchanged medical data will be ensured.

The book chapter is organized as follows: Sect. 2 reviews the related literature work. Section 3, describes the components of the proposed framework. Section 4 describes the design challenges and proposed potential solutions. Section 5 demonstrates a case study for a realistic healthcare SoS. Finally, Sect. 6 concludes the book chapter and provides a road-map towards future research directions.

2   Related Work

The SoS paradigm is getting increasing attention in the design of large systems such as healthcare systems. In what follows, a literature review of the most related work is provided with an emphasis on the challenges and proposed solutions related to healthcare monitoring systems.

The authors in [2] provided a comprehensive literature review of some solutions that aim at building platforms for real-time health monitoring that use wearable wireless sensors to monitor the patients' health information. Examples of these platforms are: Mobihealth [3], Telemedicare[1], Osiris-SE[2] and PhMon[3]. The clinical safety and effectiveness for a medical application platform is addressed in [4]. Modelling and tooling was addressed in the VAALID[4] project.

SoS security is a relatively new area of research that attracted attention over the past few years. In the literature Kennedy et al. [5] surveyed security research related to SoS and pointed out some security concerns related to SoS. The authors also highlighted the fact that security issues in SoS environments are complicated and incur many challenges. Agrawal et al. [6] inspected SoS security and offered a security schema that considers dynamic uncertain environments. The proposed schema allows to keep the SoS environment under monitoring and feeds its security observations to adapt and alter its security status. Trivellato et al. [7] emphasize on protecting information in SoS and proposed a security framework for SoS. The framework aims at protecting information in SoS by combining context-aware access control with trust management and ontology-based services. Zhou et al. [8] examined the data flow within the SoS network, and showed that there are security risks due to data flow forwarding between different systems within the SoS networks. Earlier research efforts in the field of WSNs has pointed out the importance, sensitivity, and challenges of using WSNs within the eHealth sector. For example, Alemdar and Ersoy [9] provided a comprehensive survey about the state-of-the-art of WSNs for healthcare. The authors considered privacy as well as security issues by presenting an overview about known threats and solutions. Another example is [10], in which the authors are concerned with (technical) challenges regarding trustworthiness as well as security and privacy in WSNs for healthcare. Al Ameen et al. [11] recently discussed security and privacy of WSNs in healthcare applications. Related to security they differ between information security and system security and define possible attacks for each domain and also various practicable countermeasures to reduce the risk.

There are, however, critical challenges that must be tackled in order to leverage the results from these initiatives; system robustness, reliability and real-time capability are not extensively addressed in the state-of-the-art architectures, Furthermore, most of the published works consider some of these challenges

---

[1] Telemedicare project.

[2] OSIRIS-SE project, "Runtime Environment for Data Stream Management in Healthcare".

[3] PhMon project, "Personal Health Monitoring System with Microsystem Sensor Technology".

[4] Accessibility and Usability Validation Framework for Ambient Assisted Living (AAL) Interaction Design Process, FP7.

separately and not jointly. As such, there is a real need for proposing a scalable, reliable and secure framework that gives comprehensive solutions to all the afore-mentioned challenges. In this book chapter, the system architecture is introduced to support reliable closed loop control with stringent real-time requirements for applications such as medical monitoring and therapeutic support.

3   Framework Architecture

In this section, a general description of the SoS framework will be given, then it will be customized to the context of patients' monitoring and healthcare. As depicted in Fig. 1, the SoS framework comprises Constituent Systems (CSes), each of which consists of a set of the medical devices and actuators connected to each other through wire-bound or wireless communication networks. We distin-guish between the behaviour within CSes and the coordination between them. To support this interaction, it is planned to deploy in each CS a Constituent System Manager (CSM) and an Inter-Domain Gateway (IDG). In fact, this architecture is inspired from the Internet network hierarchical architecture where there are two levels of networking and communications, the intra-domain level where nodes communicate within the same domain specified by the Autonomous System (AS) using specific communication protocols such as the Open Shortest Path First (OSPF) intra-domain routing protocols for example, while inter-domain com-munication process takes place between different AS domains and run another suit of communication protocols such as the inter-domain Border Gateway Rout-ing Protocols (BGP). Such a hierarchical architecture proved to be both efficient in reducing the communication overhead and reducing the end-to-end delay, and extremely scalable in the Internet context, which is quite applicable to our SoS framework that requires both efficient communication processes and scalable, flexible and extensible capabilities. Further, an IDG is used to manage the com-munication process between different CSes, especially when each CS may have different communication media and protocols, such as the case of having a wire-less communication media and protocols within the CS and wired media and protocols between the CSes or vice versa.

In what follows, a description of the proposed SoS in the context of health-care monitoring is provided. As depicted by Fig. 1, the CSs can be represented as patients' who need healthcare monitoring and follow-up. Notice that each CS has a group of medical sensors and actuators connected to processing units that report their measurements and communicate with the Analysis and Notifi-cation Unit (ANU) using an intra-domain communication protocol. A detailed description of the CS components is provided in the next subsection.

3.1   Constituent System Components

This subsection presents a description of the CS components and functionalities, starting from acquisition sensors and actuators, the analysis and notification unit, and ending with the inter-domain communication protocol.

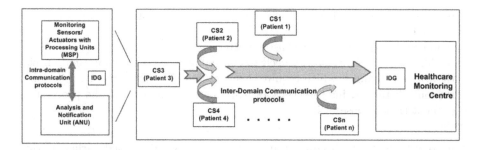

Fig. 1. Healthcare monitoring SoS

Monitoring Sensors and Actuators: The main purpose of these components is to provide timely and accurate information about the monitored events. In our case, the patients' health information. For example, blood pressure, skin temperature, heart monitoring, oximeter, glucose level, etc. Each sensor is attached to a processing element. This Monitoring Sensors Processing unit (MSP) could be a microcontroller for example[5], with a wireless transceiver that enables the sensor to send its information over the wireless channel to the ANU for further analysis and processing.

Notice that in some scenarios, where sensors' physical locations are close to each other, several sensors can be directly connected to a single microcontroller. For example, a skin temperature sensor and a blood pressure sensor are normally close to each other and can be both connected to a single processing element, while a video monitoring sensor, which is normally placed far away from the patient, will be connected directly to another processing element. In this configuration, the processing element has several crucial roles in managing the sensors' communication and data dissemination process, which in turns will result in a better usage of the wireless spectrum, less communication overhead, less interference, and fast transmission. These roles can be summarized as follows:

– Early data analysis and recording
  The processing element can analyse the sensed information values and if it is below or above certain thresholds, then it will send it to the ANU. This is much more efficient compared with the other schemes where the sensors continuously access the wireless channel and always send their information to the ANU, which may cause interference and collision especially in cases where there are large numbers of sensors and monitored patients.
– More efficient media access mechanisms and scheduling
  Access to the wireless media channel is very crucial in providing real-time data transmission and dissemination. With the existence of distributed scheduling algorithms (discussed later), different sensors can access the wireless channel more effectively without loading the wireless channel with collided and resent

---

[5] With the extensive spread of smartphones, the processing element can be also a smartphone with the proposer applications designed for that purpose.

packets. Further, each sensor can have a different priority for accessing the channel.

- Power and energy saving in sensors batteries
  In this design, sensors do not need to continuously send their information via the wireless channel, which requires a significant amount of energy, especially for long distances, instead, sensors will convey their data to the processing element that is close to it.

The Analysis and Notification Unit: The ANU described earlier as the Constituent System Manager is the brain of the CS where critical data sent from various sensors via their processing elements is analysed and a decision is made and sent to the healthcare monitoring center, where emergency doctors look at the alert messages and take appropriate actions. In addition, this unit also receives the sensors' log data and sends it to the healthcare center for archiving and later viewing and analysis.

The Inter-Domain Communication Protocols: In order to send the captured and analysed data to the ANU, a communication protocol is provided that is responsible for providing the appropriate communication media and access among all sensors' processing elements. In this proposed system, this communication protocol has the major role of delivering the patients' data in real-time to the ANU.

3.2   Healthcare Center Unit

After describing the CS components and communication requirements, it is important to complete the cycle and describe the Healthcare Center Unit (HCU) and its role in communicating with the CSs.

As can be seen in Fig. 1, each CS represented by its ANU needs to send its information to the HCU Inter-Domain Gateway for further processing and decision making. The IDG is simply a processing node that accepts the sent information from the ANU which may be from a different communication network such as the wireless media, and relays it to the HCU network, which is normally a wired network. Normally, physicians and healthcare personnel monitor these notifications and may take actions for their patients. To achieve that, an inter-domain communication protocol is used which has similar functionalities to the intra-domain protocol in terms of scheduling, real-time data assurance, and data protection and correction. However, here the scheduling will be among different CSes utilizing the TTEthernet technology.

4   Design Challenges and Solutions

This section focuses on the design challenges of the aforementioned healthcare monitoring system and proposes potential solutions. Mainly, two major challenges are discussed, real-time delivery assurance for the critical patients' data, and providing security mechanisms while sending, processing and storing these data.

4.1 Real-Time Assurance

Real-time assurance on delivering the patients' information, especially when an emergency case happens, is extremely important and it is a lifesaving process. In the proposed framework, the sensors' processing elements have to send their information to the ANU in a timely manner, which in turn will be sent to the healthcare center for further processing and response. As such, several mechanisms have to be deployed to assure real-time delivery for this information. In the following subsections, two mechanisms that are still under development are described to achieve that purpose: scheduling , data protection and prioritization.

1. **Scheduling**
   The goal of the scheduling mechanism is to develop distributed algorithms for online scheduling in a healthcare SoS consisting of multiple CSes each with a time-triggered communication network.

   It is important to mention that the scheduling mechanism will be managed within each CS (with different sensors belonging to one patient) and between different CSes (between different patients). The static control structure of present-day systems with time-triggered protocols is not suited for SoS. While several protocols improve flexibility with additional event-triggered communication primitives (e.g., rate-constrained and best-effort communication in TTEthernet), the time-triggered schedule is built off-line and remains fixed at run-time. Off-line scheduling and schedulability analysis of time-triggered systems have been intensively studied during the past years (e.g., OSIRIS-SE and PhMon projects). There are several approaches to tackle the scheduling problem in time triggered systems. The static scheduling and partitioning of processes, and allocation of system components is introduced in [12,13] based on a Mixed Integer Linear Programming (MILP) problem. The drawback of this approach, the complexity of solving the (MILP) model grows quickly with the number of the processes or services. Therefore heuristic approaches have been used for scheduling such as list scheduling heuristics using different priority criteria (e.g. [14,15]), branch-and-bound algorithms [16,17] and heuristics based on neighbor-hood search (e.g. [18–20]). Popular meta-heuristics in the neighbor-hood search are Simulated Annealing, Tabu Search and Genetic Algorithms. The authors of [21] present a scheduling algorithm for time-triggered and rate-constrained traffic based on neighbourhood search to minimize transmission delays and execution times, while also supporting service dependencies. An algorithm to handle event-triggered sporadic tasks based on offline schedules is introduced in [22]. The use of a plug-in approach to add functionality to existing scheduling schemes is proposed in [23]. However, online scheduling and reconfiguration in time-triggered communication networks based on real-time and reliability requirements is an open research problem. Furthermore, the heterogeneous nature of the SoS is another challenging aspect that should be taken into account, when designing the scheduling algorithms. Within the CS, some sensors may have time-triggered capabilities, especially the one with wired connection, while other sensors may not have such capabilities (wireless sensors for example). The latter sensors may require a gateway device that interfaces the wireless devices with the time-triggered network.

The conventional scheduling problem involves the definition of an input model that describes the scheduling problem, followed by the search for a feasible schedule using a scheduling algorithm and the adoption of the feasible schedule [24]. During the search, the input model remains fixed. In a SoS, this assumption of a strictly sequential process is unrealistic. Rather, further change requests for the input model must be incorporated while the scheduling is ongoing. The concurrent processing of change requests with consistent scheduling results is a novel research problem. For example, when adopting a new schedule for a given set of change requests in one CS, the other CSes should adopt corresponding schedules to satisfy the dependencies between CSes. Also, when new change requests arrive, intermediate schedule results must be mapped to new input models in order to prevent the invalidation of prior search results.

To achieve that, we extend previous scheduling algorithms for time-triggered systems [24] to support distributed scheduling with constrained knowledge about other CSes, as well as concurrent change requests to the scheduling problem. The scheduling results include the configuration parameters for the CS as well as the configuration parameters for the interaction between them. We plan to support standard Internet and Ethernet protocols (e.g., IEEE 802.1 standards) where scheduling results include parameters for traffic shaping, priority assignment and clock synchronization (e.g., 802.1Q, 802.1AS). A candidate for a wire-bound protocol within constituent systems is Time-Triggered Ethernet (SAE AS6802) [25], for which the computation of a time-triggered communication schedule will be performed. Candidates for wireless protocols are WiFi, Bluetooth and Zigbee. However, with the existence of different communication media, one should take into account that the overall communication architecture needs to be heterogeneous.

2. **Data Protection and Prioritization**

In the proposed framework, the most important part of the CSes is the medical sensors and actuators that capture the patients data and send them to the CSM for further processing and analysis. In order to have a flexible system, these sensors communicate with the CSM using the wireless channel. Consequently, these sensors can be viewed as a Wireless Sensor Network (WSN). In order to provide the sensors with access control to the wireless media channel, a proper scheduling mechanism should be implemented that takes into account the time constraints for each sensor and reliability issues. QoS assurance and reliability are very important in wireless media due to the fact that data is prone to both packet loss and bit errors. Delivering data without any errors and in a real-time manner is of high importance in the proposed

SoS framework, especially in the case of wireless media channels. In order to provide the sensors with access control to the media channel, as described above, a scheduling mechanism is required that takes into account the time constraints for each sensor. This scheduling mechanism must be designed while also considering reliability issues. QoS assurance and reliability are very important in wired and wireless media, and it is more urgent in wireless media due to the fact that data is prone to both packet loss due to congested links and bit errors caused by channel fading and interference. The framework will be designed in conjunction with the scheduling algorithm to assure delay constraints of the sensors, to minimize interference, and to support suitable error protection and correction mechanisms that reduces packet re-transmission. In the literature, there are many data transmission frameworks proposed to protect data from transmission errors using different mechanisms such as error correction and detection code, the prime example of such code is the Reed Solomon Forward Error Correction codes [26]. However, QoS for different data streams should be taken into account such that more important data sources (like the data coming from the blood pressure monitoring devices for example) are given more channel time and stronger correction capabilities than the less important ones (the measurement of body temperature for example) which can be achieved using proper scheduling mechanisms. Consequently, an unequal error correction codes that are applied on the stream level is proposed, such that different streams can be protected differently according to their importance and real-time requirements. In other words, more important data streams can be given higher priority in terms of protection than lower important data streams. In the proposed framework, the CSM is responsible for assigning unequal channel coding budget for different data streams according to their importance. Further, the CSM estimates the wireless channel connection conditions of the sensors, such that more channel coding is assigned for sensors that suffers from high interference and bad wireless channel condition. In conclusion, the CSM will take into account both factors (stream importance and wireless channel condition) while assigning the channel coding budget.

4.2   Security

The security framework aims to provide a secure infrastructure that enables the integration of patients' data (i.e. health records) from various and distributed data sources of involved parties in a secure and legal compliant way. Further, the security framework encompasses common requirements (i.e., technical, legal and economical), related security and privacy technologies (i.e., cryptographic mechanisms, privacy enhancing technologies, identity and access management), interoperability and compliance mechanisms. The patients should be aware of the complications caused by their illnesses; they should also have secure access to any pertinent data concerning these. Moreover, this information should not be misused by third parties. A secure and reliable communication and configuration service will support the interaction between the different entities following event-based triggering and execution of emergency processes.

Providing security in the context of SoS is a challenging task since SoSs are composed of heterogeneous systems. These systems may be secure as a stand-alone application but might not be when they are integrated within the SoS framework. The security framework should consider the dynamic nature of SoS and address the following aspects: access control, systems' integration interfaces, network security and data protection. In the proposed framework, a Security Configuration Manager (SCM) is proposed as part of the security framework to be implemented within both the MSP and CSM unites. The responsibility of SCM is to automatically and dynamically manage the security of the SoS depending on context information of the integrated systems. The SCM will support key management, device configuration, context-aware access control policies and generate alarms when anomalous behaviour is detected. Further, SCM will provide the security assurance for both frontend users and backend servers to defend against potential threats. To illustrates that, a walk through the data flow security is provided. First, patients' data captured by the sensors are sent through the MSP over a secure channel to the ANU where data is analyzed and processed. In fact, all MSPs and the ANU creates a virtual security boundary where link layer encryption on wireless LAN with WAP2 is used. Furthermore, the communication channel between the ANU and the Healthcare Monitoring Center is secured over a network layer encryption through an IPsec IDG.

Further, the security framework provides privacy-enhancing, and trust-leveraging infrastructure that enables the integration of patients' data (i.e. health records) from various and distributed data repositories of involved parties in secure and legal compliant way. The framework enforces data access policies, data anonymizing, adherence to privacy laws when creating privacy policies, and data encryption requirements for storage and transmission. In addition, the framework alerts the end-users to risk situations, employs trust-based metrics to warn patients; monitors and audits of information use, and withdraws of rights.

5   Medical Use Case

A medical case study is provided to demonstrate the usefulness of the proposed framework. In this section, three medical case studies are presented: (1) a real-time alert case study, (2) an ambulance case-study and (3) a surgery case-study (Fig. 2).

The real-time alert case study uses sensors to obtain a range of normal and abnormal medical data from a patient (e.g., cardiac sensors, pulse oximetry sensors). At the hospital, observed parameters and medication for a patient are recorded in health records. After the emergency treatment at the hospital, sensors continue to obtain medical data at the patient's home. All departments at the hospital get the real-time information from the patient. If the analysis of the sensor data at the hospital indicates that something abnormal is happening to the patient, an alert is generated for dispatching an emergency doctor to

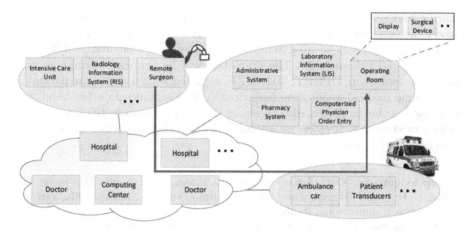

Fig. 2. Medical case use

the patient. The alert system enables a safe, timely and efficient handling of many patients with limited personnel of emergency teams and existing medical infrastructures. Security is essential to ensure privacy and prevent denial-of-service attacks. The SoS is dynamic and requires frequent reconfigurations, e.g. upon new patients, changes in emergency teams (e.g., new doctor) and changes in medical devices. Also, the open-world assumption is required in order to manage hospitals, medical teams and their capacities (e.g., carry-over to another hospital in case of overload).

The ambulance case study models a scenario, where emergency treatment starts before arriving at the hospital. Medical data is obtained (e.g., using ECG) and sent to emergency doctors at the hospital, who can give advice to ambulance teams as well as take actions remotely (i.e., telemedicine). For example, the emergency doctor can remotely administer drugs to increase blood oxygen concentration. The case study involves wireless communication links (e.g., patient monitoring using medical sensors) as well as wire-bound communication links (e.g., in-vehicle network of ambulance car, hospital networks). This case study involves stringent real-time and reliability requirements to realize control loops for emergency treatment encompassing patients, ambulance teams, emergency doctors and hospitals. The targeted scenarios are highly dynamic SoS scenarios where component interactions have to be established within predictable time.

The surgery case study includes emergency room equipment as well as remote analysis, computing and store services. For example, cameras and surgical robots are modelled to enable the participation of remote senior surgeons (e.g., surgeon from Europe supporting a surgery in the Middle East). The case study includes stringent real-time, reliability and security requirements for medical SoS.

6 Conclusion and Future Work

We present a SoS framework for healthcare monitoring service, with particular focus on the design challenges such as real-time data assurance, reliability and security, and suggests how they can be solved. As this is an ongoing research project, we are currently implementing the simulation environment of the SOS framework, which will be an extension of the simulation environment for the Time Triggered Ethernet [27]. The simulation will be performed using network simulation tools (e.g., OPNET, OMNET) integrated with tools for simulation of the dynamic medical application behaviour (e.g., Simulink). In other hand, we are designing the proper scheduling algorithms and data protection and prioritization mechanisms. Besides, we are investigating other important factors such as security and privacy.

Acknowledgement. Our thanks to Dr. Ala'aldeen Al-Halhouli, Dr. Samil Al Muhtasib, Dr. Yaser Mowafi, Dr. Mahmoud Sitohy, and Dr Mohamed Shaheen for their valuable comments and feedback.

This work has been supported in part by the European project DREAMS (No. 610640).

References

1. Khalifeh, A., Obermaisser, R., Abou-Tair, D.e.D.I., Abuteir, M.: Systems-of-systems framework for providing real-time patient monitoring and care. In: Proceedings of the 8th International Conference on Pervasive Computing Technologies for Healthcare. PervasiveHealth 2014, ICST, Brussels, Belgium, Belgium, ICST (Institute for Computer Sciences, Social-Informatics and Telecommunications Engineering), pp. 426–429 (2014)
2. Gay, V., Leijdekkers, P.: A health monitoring system using smart phones and wearable sensors. Int. J. ARM **8**(2), 29–36 (2007)
3. Jones, V., Halteren, A., Widya, I., Dokovsky, N., Koprinkov, G., Bults, R., Konstantas, D., Herzog, R.: Mobihealth: mobile health services based on body area networks. In: Istepanian, R., Laxminarayan, S., Pattichis, C. (eds.) M-Health. Topics in Biomedical Engineering. Springer, US (2006)
4. Hatcliff, J., King, A., Lee, I., Macdonald, A., Fernando, A., Robkin, M., Vasserman, E., Weininger, S., Goldman, J.M.: Rationale and architecture principles for medical application platforms. In: Proceedings of the 2012 IEEE/ACM Third International Conference on Cyber-Physical Systems. ICCPS 2012, pp. 3–12. IEEE Computer Society, Washington, DC (2012)
5. Michael, K., Llewellyn-Jones, D.Q.S.M.M.: System-of-systems security: a survey. In: The 11th Annual Conference on the Convergence of Telecommunications, Networking & Broadcasting. Liverpool, UK (2010)
6. Agrawal, D.: A new schema for security in dynamic uncertain environments. In: Sarnoff Symposium, SARNOFF 2009, pp. 1–5. IEEE (2009)
7. Trivellato, D., Zannone, N., Etalle, S.: Poster: protecting information in systems of systems. In: ACM Conference on Computer and Communications Security 2011 (2011)
8. Zhou, B., Arabo, A., Drew, O., Llewellyn-Jones, D., Merabti, M., Shi, Q., Waller, A., Craddock, R., Jones, G., Yau, A.: Data flow security analysis for system-of-systems in a public security incident in a public security incident. In: 3rd Conference on Advances in Computer Security and Forensics (2008)

9. Alemdar, H., Ersoy, C.: Wireless sensor networks for healthcare: a survey. Comput. Netw. **54**(15), 2688–2710 (2010)
10. Ko, J., Lu, C., Srivastava, M., Stankovic, J., Terzis, A., Welsh, M.: Wireless sensor networks for healthcare. Proc. IEEE **98**(11), 1947–1960 (2010)
11. Ameen, M., Liu, J., Kwak, K.: Security and privacy issues in wireless sensor networks for healthcare applications. J. Med. Syst. **36**(1), 93–101 (2012)
12. Bender, A.: Design of an optimal loosely coupled heterogeneous multiprocessor system. In: Proceedings European Design and Test Conference, ED TC 96, pp. 275–281 (1996)
13. Prakash, S., Parker, A.C.: Sos: synthesis of application-specific heterogeneous multiprocessor systems. J. Parallel Distrib. Syst. **16**(4), 338–351 (1992)
14. Sinnen, O., Sousa, L.: Comparison of contention aware list scheduling heuristics for cluster computing. In: International Conference on Parallel Processing Workshops (2001)
15. Kwok, Y.K., Ahmad, I.: Dynamic critical-path scheduling: an effective technique for allocating task graphs to multiprocessors. IEEE Trans. Parallel Distrib. Syst. **7**(5), 506–521 (1996)
16. Nessah, R., Yalaoui, F., Chu, C.: A branch and bound algorithm to minimize total weighted completion time on identical parallel machines with job release dates. In: 2006 International Conference on Service Systems and Service Management, Vol. 2 (2006)
17. Eles, P., Kuchcinski, K., Peng, Z., Doboli, A., Pop, P.: Process scheduling for performance estimation and synthesis of hardware/software systems. In: Proceedings 24th Euromicro Conference, vol. 1, pp. 168–175 (1998)
18. Tian, Y., Sannomiya, N., Xu, Y.: A tabu search with a new neighborhood search technique applied to flow shop scheduling problems. In: Proceedings of the 39th IEEE Conference on Decision and Control, vol. 5 (2000)
19. César Rego, A., Renato Duarte, B.: A filter and fan approach to the job shop scheduling problem (2006)
20. Eswaramurthy, V., Tamilarasi, A.: Hybridizing tabu search with ant colony optimization for solving job shop scheduling problems. Int. J. Adv. Manuf. Technol. **40**(9/10), 1004 (2009)
21. Abuteir, M., Obermaisser, R.: Scheduling of rate-constrained and time-triggered traffic in multi-cluster ttethernet systems. In: 2015 13th IEEE International Conference on Industrial Informatics (INDIN) (2015)
22. Isovic, D., Fohler, G.: Handling sporadic tasks in off-line scheduled distributed real-time systems. In: Proceedings of the 11th Euromicro Conference on Real-Time Systems, pp. 60–67 (1999)
23. Lennvall, T., Fohler, G., Lindberg, B.: Handling aperiodic tasks in diverse real-time systems via plug-ins. In: Proceedings Fifth IEEE International Symposium on Object-Oriented Real-Time Distributed Computing (ISORC 2002), pp. 137–144 (2002)
24. Obermaisser, R.: Time-Triggered Communication, 1st edn. CRC Press Inc., Boca Raton (2011)
25. Tamas-Selicean, D., Pop, P., Steiner, W.: Synthesis of communication schedules for ttethernet-based mixed-criticality systems. In: Proceedings of the Eighth IEEE/ACM/IFIP International Conference on Hardware/Software Codesign and System Synthesis. CODES+ISSS 2012. ACM, New York, NY (2012)

26. Khalifeh, A., Yousefi'zadeh, H.: Optimal audio transmission over error-prone wireless links. IEEE Trans. Multimedia **12**(3), 204–214 (2010)
27. Abuteir, M., Obermaisser, R.: Simulation environment for time-triggered ethernet. In: 2013 11th IEEE International Conference on Industrial Informatics (INDIN), pp. 642–648 (2013)

A Virtual Rehabilitation Solution
Using Multiple Sensors

Nuno Matos, António Santos$^{(\boxtimes)}$, and Ana Vasconcelos

Fraunhofer AICOS, Rua Alfredo Allen 455, 4200-135 Porto, Portugal
{nuno.matos,antonio.santos,ana.vasconcelos}@fraunhofer.pt
http://www.fraunhofer.pt

Abstract. Stroke is the major cause of long-term motor impairments
that are affecting millions of people. The process of physical rehabilitation is sometimes not available to some patients and is also usually slow
and demotivating. In this paper we introduce a new solution that uses
the concept of interactive games using motion sensors to improve the
rehabilitation results. It features a motion sensor server that supports
a growing array of sensors (currently Microsoft Kinect, Leap Motion,
Orbotix Sphero and Smartphones) and merge their data into a single
protocol that can be used for any purpose. The use of different sensors, even simultaneously, allows the rehabilitation of specific parts of
the body. This data can be stored in a server for physicians to analyse
and can clearly reveal the evolution of the patient in the rehabilitation
process.

Keywords: Physical rehabilitation · Stroke · Virtual reality · Natural
User Interfaces · Kinect · Leap Motion · Sphero · Smartphone

1 Introduction

According to the World Health Organization [1], 15 million people suffer a stroke
worldwide each year. Of these, 5 million die and another 5 million are permanently disabled. About 80 % of people who survive a stroke experience motor
impairments. One such impairment is hemiparesis: a partial paralysis of one
side of the body [9]. Hemiparesis usually causes chronic disability in the upper
extremities (arms) more than the lower extremities (legs). People with hemiparesis experience limitations in fine motor control, strength, and range of motion [2].

Repetitive exercises can provide the brain with sufficient stimuli to remodel
itself and provide better motor control [8]. However, only 31 % of stroke patients
perform these exercises as recommended [16], which can lead to an incomplete
recovery [10]. Therefore, finding motivating and effective ways to encourage people with hemiparesis to perform therapeutic exercises is crucial in helping them
achieve a more complete recovery.

Video games with motion-based input devices may provide a motivating way
to help people with hemiparesis complete therapeutic exercises and regain lost

© Springer-Verlag Berlin Heidelberg 2015
H.M. Fardoun et al. (Eds.): REHAB 2014, CCIS 515, pp. 143–154, 2015.
DOI: 10.1007/978-3-662-48645-0_13

motor control. Some research has already demonstrated that potential in game-based therapy [3,5]. In addition, game systems should monitor and measure users motion abilities and detect when improvements occur in both supervised and unsupervised settings.

Due to the ever growing set of affordable and commercially available motion sensing devices, it is now being perceived by therapists that they may be used for physical rehabilitation purposes. With this work, the authors introduce a novel physical rehabilitation solution [12] comprised of several games that can use different motion sensors (even simultaneously), being their data provided by a sensor server and using a common protocol.

2   State of the Art

The use of IT in physical rehabilitation programs is not new and is making huge improvements in terms of effective results.

VirtualRehab [17] is a VirtualWare product developed for PC that uses Microsoft Kinect to track and capture the movements of the patients and to allow them to play the provided games. These games are particularly focused on the balance, coordination and posture of the patients and use customized rehabilitation programs to help treat these physical symptoms. Thanks to a cloud based platform, there is also the possibility of registering the results obtained each time a patient plays one of the games so the therapist can be always supervising his patients' evolution whether they are having their sessions at a clinic center or at home. Kinerehab [4] is also a Kinect-based system used for rehabilitation purposes but instead of being used in healthcare centers, it is used by therapists in public schools. The main goal of this project is to give students the opportunity of having a different and less monotonous recovering process and to give the therapist a useful tool to monitor the students' information and progress. REMOVIEM [11] is a very recent project that is being used in the rehabilitation of patients from the Association of Multiple Sclerosis of Castellon and also promotes body movements, tracked by the Kinect sensor, through three motor rehabilitation games that try to improve the gait, the balance and weight transfer of the patient. Kitsunezaki et al. [7] implemented a solution that uses the Kinect sensor in a quite different way. This solution is based on an exercise that requires two sensors and two PCs, connected via an Ethernet hub, and where the user must cross the radius of action of both motion sensor devices by starting in front of one sensor and walking about ten meters until he reaches the other one. This exercise will allow the measurement of the step frequency, step length and velocity of the patient when doing the route, three essential gait parameters [14], with the help of the system's PCs that record the time spent on the exercise. Another different usage for this device was proposed by Saini et al. [15] and consists in a home-based platform that gathers an online biofeedback component to the movement tracking and exercises, which allows the system to store the patient's movements and knowledge result and display them to both patient and therapist. This type of solution is convenient for the patient because he can have his sessions at home without the need of his therapist.

3   Architecture

When this project started to take shape, it was decided that one of the requirements was to have the ability to provide motion sensor data to any application that implements Natural User Interfaces. Therefore, it was decided to split the solution in two main components: a motion sensor server, providing sensor data using a single protocol and through a common communication mechanism, and the client, in this case the application that runs the rehabilitation games and which processes the incoming sensor data. As such, this model allows the server to be expanded without affecting the client applications or be reused in different contexts.

3.1   Server

The development of the motion sensor server started to be just a mean to provide motion sensor data to a platform that does not support motion sensors (p. ex. Android). However, soon it became clear that the idea just makes sense, namely if there is the need to add support for such a sensor in applications that implement Natural User Interfaces. Instead of having to dig deep in the SDK of a specific motion sensor and limit the support to just that sensor, application developers can instead use this server and support the used protocol, no matter which sensor is being used. And if at the beginning the server only supported Microsoft Kinect, now it currently supports other completely different sensors like the Leap Motion, Orbotix Sphero and even Smartphones. Furthermore, the applications can use more than one sensor simultaneously using the same protocol (Fig. 1).

Supported Sensors. As mentioned previously, the development of the server started by providing support to the well-known Microsoft Kinect sensor. This sensor, apart from the video stream provided by the included RGB camera, provides a depth map that is obtained through the use of a IR light emitter and receiver. This allows software frameworks to be able to detect bodies in the field-of-view and track their skeleton through the detection of 20 joints. Through the use of a common SDK (OpenNI/NiTE), the support was expanded to other similar sensors like the Asus Xtion Pro.

Later, with the release of the Leap Motion, it was inevitable to add support to this sensor due to its characteristics. Leap Motion allows a real-time tracking of the hands and pointables (it may be fingers or other tools like pens) (Fig. 2). The sensor provides precise values regarding the position and orientation of the hands and pointables, allowing not only the tracking of these objects but also the detection of gestures. The main drawback is the limited field of view, which only allows the detection of hands up to 60 cm from the sensor. However, it brings clear advantages for the rehabilitation of the hand.

The *Kinteract* server was also added with the support to another sensor, the Orbotix Sphero (Fig. 3). This device is mostly well known as being a "robotic ball", with nearly the size of a tennis ball and featuring Bluetooth communication

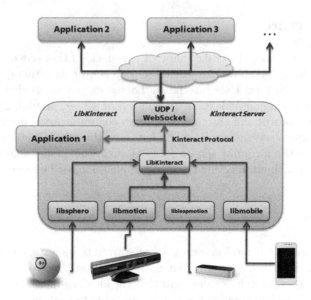

Fig. 1. *Kinteract* server architecture

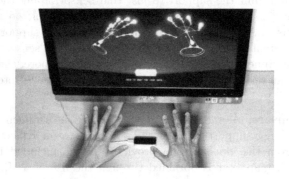

Fig. 2. Leap Motion

and being able to be controlled by a mobile device, but it can also be used as a controller due to the powerful IMU it has integrated. Therefore, it can also be used as a motion sensor and may be applied in monitoring some hand movements like rotation.

Finally, recently also smartphones were supported, due the fact that almost anyone available features accelerometer, gyroscope and magnetometer, and therefore can be used as a motion sensor, streaming their data using Bluetooth.

Architecture. The *Kinteract* server was designed to fit in every context, being provided as shared library that can be easily integrated into an application under

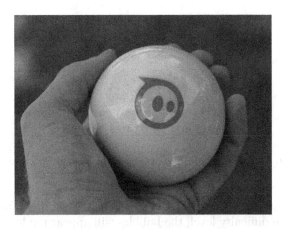

Fig. 3. Orbotix Sphero

development or providing a server-client model, opening an UDP/Web socket to receive connections from clients and providing a stream of motion sensor data. Although this is an unlikely scenario, the server supports several clients at the same time. Developed in C++, it currently runs on Windows, Linux and Android and the support to the different sensors is provided through individual shared libraries/DLLs, which are dynamically loaded on demand. The server is highly configurable and may easily be adapted to the clients needs. Apart from normal hand tracking, the server is able to detect common gestures performed with some sensors and, of course, retrieve and stream data from the sensors to the clients. The server is also able to perform open/closed hand detection with 3D motion sensor by applying Computer Vision algorithms implemented using OpenCV, although the accuracy is still not optimal.

3.2   Client

The client component of this solution is an Android application running on Google TV providing a platform for physical rehabilitation games. The application features a background service that is in charge of processing the sensor data sent using the *Kinteract* protocol. The user can either use Google TV's remote control or one of the available sensors to navigate the menus and may play the games as a guest or as a registered player if an external Personal Health Record is being used to manage patient profiles and store measurements. When playing as a guest, there will be no player profile and the results will not be saved. Several difficulty levels are available, each one with different combinations of available time and goal, which allow keeping up with the evolution of the patient and keep challenging him.

Chasing Bubbles. This game is played with the 3D motion sensor (Xtion Pro/Kinect) and its goal is to reach a specific number of bubbles (one at a

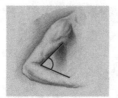
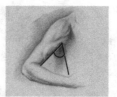

(a) Angle between arm and forearm

(b) Angle between arm and torso

Fig. 4. Measured angles in Chasing Bubbles and Space Lights

time) that keep appearing on the TV screen in the shortest amount of time. Depending on the difficulty level, the bubbles will appear randomly in a specific distance interval from the center of the screen. The idea is to promote wide arm movements and monitor the angle between the torso and the arm and the one between the arm and the forearm (Fig. 4).

Space Lights. This game is similar to the previous one and also aims at monitoring the aforementioned angles. The main difference is that now the game goal is achieved in two steps, since the user must first pick a light, standing his hand over it for roughly 1.5 s, and drag it into a black hole on a different position on the screen (Fig. 5). This leads to a bigger physical effort from the user.

Dragging Apples. Unlike the first two, this third game is played with the Leap Motion sensor and mainly targets the rehabilitation of the hand, trying to increase its opening range. With the 3D motion sensor is not possible to measure this but the Leap Motion sensor does a great job here. The goal of the game is to pick an apple standing on a specific position of the screen by opening the hand by a certain extent, drag the apple to a basket (still with the hand opened) and drop it by closing the hand. Leap Motion can provide the radius of a virtual sphere that fits the curvature of the hand (Fig. 6) and this value is

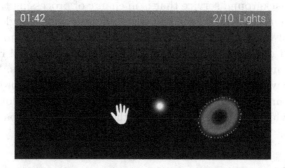

Fig. 5. Space Lights game

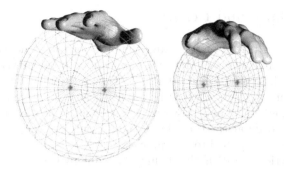

Fig. 6. Leap Motion virtual sphere (source: Leap Motion Developer Documentation)

used as the main metrics to assess the patient's evolution. The difficulty level is also proportional to the minimum sphere radius needed to open the hand.

Light Lamps. This game is played with two sensors simultaneously, the 3D motion sensor and Orbotix Sphero. The game is mainly targeted for the rehabilitation of the hand because it promotes and measures the rotation of the hand, while the user is holding the Sphero sensor in his hand. The 3D motion sensor is used to track the hand that is holding the Sphero and may again be used to measure the angles between the arm-forearm and arm-torso. The main goal of the Light Lamps game is to turn on the lamps that keep appearing in random positions of the screen by moving the hand cursor to them and then rotating the hand to an extent that depends on the selected difficulty level.

Posture Detection. This is still not exactly a game but more of a proof of concept. The goal is to have the user doing in the best possible way the body posture that appears on the screen. Several postures are shown and, by applying the algorithm described in [13], the system can validate, in real time, the current posture of the user and match it against the one that has been asked. After performing the correct posture, the user should keep his position for roughly two seconds.

3.3 PHR Integration

This type of solution can only achieve its main goal if used throughout the whole or a major part of the rehabilitation process. Its effectiveness can only be assessed if there is any mechanism to track the patient's evolution during the rehabilitation process. Therefore, the client application is currently integrated with eHealthCom [6], a Personal Health Record (PHR) that allows health professionals to manage patient profiles and their health status. At the end of each game, the results may be sent to this PHR and saved in the patient profile. The physiotherapist can then graphically visualize the evolution of the metrics used in each game, including the difficulty level used.

4   Performance and Results

Three sets of tests, two in one day and the other one four months later, were made with five impaired users (IU) with upper limb hemiparesis at Centro de Reabilitação Profissional de Gaia (CRPG) (Gaia's Professional Rehabilitation Center). In the first two sets, there were also five healthy users (HU) and only the first two games mentioned in Sect. 3.2 were tested, since the third one using Leap Motion was not ready at the time. From the IU, only one had some experience using motion sensors applied to interactive games.

In the first series of tests both sets had three different sessions, each one with different difficulty levels. The first set consisted in playing the Chasing Bubbles game. This game was easily understood by all participants considering there were no mistakes and not a single assistance was given in any of the sessions. The second set (Space Lights) was a bit more difficult to be understood and played due to its characteristics. 80 % of the users needed assistance with this game.

Despite those difficulties, the efficiency results for each game were good as well as the overall satisfaction. All ten users were able to achieve the goals for each game. The game results are detailed in Tables 1 and 2 and clearly reveal the increasing difficulty between the different test sets. It can be spotted on Table 2 the considerably longer time taken to pick the object when compared to the time taken to drag it, due to the extra effort needed to stand the arm for 1.5 s.

Table 1. Efficiency on Chasing Bubbles (ANB - *Average Number of caught Bubbles*; ATS - *Average Time Spent (secs)*

| | Chasing Bubbles | | | | | |
| | 1st Test | | 2nd Test | | 3rd Test | |
	ANB	ATS	ANB	ATS	ANB	ATS
IU	42	1.34	32	1.82	13	2.44
HU	61	0.80	61	0.96	25	1.02

Table 2. Efficiency on Space Lights (ANL - *Average Number of dragged Lights*; ATSP - *Average Time Spent Pickin (secs)*; ATSD - *Average Time Spent Dragging (secs)*

| | Space Lights | | | | | | | | |
| | 1st Test | | | 2nd Test | | | 3rd Test | | |
	ANL	ATSP	ATSD	ANL	ATSP	ATSD	ANL	ATSP	ATSD
IU	8	5.01	2.51	7	4.40	2.87	2	7.81	2.62
HU	15	2.94	1.16	15	4.05	1.00	6	3.25	1.09

Table 3. Usability questionnaire results

Participants	Avg. score (max. 100)
IU	87.5
HU	91.5

Regarding user satisfaction, each patient was asked to fill in a SUS (System Usability Scale) questionnaire at the end of the performed tests and the results are shown on Table 3.

The second series of tests took place in order to validate some improvements in the former games' design and to test the new ones that were developed in the mean time. The tests took place again at CRPG with five impaired users (IU) with upper limb hemiparesis and consisted of a series of tasks where they were asked to explore every functionality of the system using the three sensors and the GoogleTV remote controller. The main idea was to test the acceptance and usability of the new sensors and not really to measure accuracy and precision of the results.

The first task was just to have the user select a game in the main interface by using the hand tracking feature provided by the 3D motion sensor or through the GoogleTV remote controller. Four of the five participants performed the tasks without any problems and the fifth participant, due to the severity of her injury, was not able to perform the wave gesture needed to start tracking her hand. As for the remote controller, only two of the participants were able to use it with the hand in treatment and the other three had to use it with their healthy hand in order to complete the task.

As previously mentioned, the Chasing Bubbles and Space Lights game only had design modifications so the concept and rules were already known by the participants. Even so, there are two aspects that are worth mentioning: first, the participant that was not able to navigate in the system using the 3D motion sensor was also not able to play these games because they require a wave gesture too; second, even knowing how to play the game, the process of picking the light in the Space Lights game was still very challenging for the participants.

The second test was similar to the first one but this time using the Leap Motion sensor to navigate in the system and to play a new game (Dragging Apples). The goal of the game and how to use the sensor were easily understood but an explanation of when to close and open the hand during the game was needed. The participant that was not able to use the 3D motion sensor was also not able to play this game because she could not open her hand, not even with the help of the therapist. The other four participants completed the game but two of them experienced some difficulties related to the position of the hand and some failures of the sensor while tracking their hand.

The last sensor to be tested was the Sphero. At the time the tests were made, the Light Lamps game was still not ready so the Sphero was only used to control the UI. In this task, the results were less positive since only two of the

Table 4. Usability questionnaire results

Participant	Avg. score (max. 100)
P2	77.5
P3	57.5
P4	75
P5	87.5

five patients were able to hold and use the sensor with no limitations while the other three could not even open the hand enough to hold the Sphero without losing mobility in that hand.

Finally, the Posture Detection game was also tested by the participants. Once again, due to her rehabilitation stage, one participant was not able to do any of the existing postures. The other four participants were able to perform them with more or less difficulty, depending of their complexity. Since the game was still under development at the time, there were some false positives due to minor issues in the implementation of the algorithm, which are currently fixed.

After the evaluation, each participant, with exception of the one who was not able to perform the tests, was asked to answer a System Usability Scale questionnaire and the results are shown in the Table 4.

5   Conclusion and Future Work

The presented solution, as a whole, had a good reaction and feedback from the patients who tested it and, although there are still no quantitative data regarding the impact of the use of the solution on the rehabilitation process, there is now a clear road ahead. One of the issues found is the login gesture. Due to their condition, patients may have difficulties in making the login gesture (which may be a wave, a click/push or a hand raise gesture), which is needed to start the tracking with the 3D motion sensor. However, there is already a workaround for this issue that allows the user to interact with the system without performing any gesture, although it may happen that the user interacts with the application inadvertently.

The choice for an Android application running on Google TV also proved not to be quite practical in terms of deployment, since there is the need to have a second device running the server (the server does not run on Android devices) with a proper network setup. Therefore, one of foreseen developments is to implement the client application using the Unity framework, which will allow building releases for different platforms (including Android, which runs on Google TV), and will allow integrating the server and the client into the same application running in one device (Windows, Linux or Android).

To assess the feasibility and effectiveness of the solution in the rehabilitation process, long term tests are planned. There are also plans to widen the array of supported sensors, namely with the inclusion of the Myo sensor, as well as improving posture and gesture recognition algorithms. Also, the Nintendo Wii Balance Board (or similar) will be integrated and there will be new games designed with the help of therapists to improve standing balance in patients with acquired brain injuries through motivational and adaptative exercises. New games focusing on the rehabilitation of the lower limb will also broaden the spectrum of the solution.

Acknowledgments. The authors would like to thank CRPG, namely Dra. Cristina Crisóstomo and Dra. Alexandra Couto, for their support, and acknowledge the financial support from North Portugal Regional Operational Programme (ON.2 - O Novo Norte), Portuguese National Strategic Reference Framework (NSRF) and the European Regional Development Fund (ERDF) from European Union through the project "Fall Competence Center" NORTE-07-0124-FEDER-000041.

References

1. The world health report 2002 - Reducing Risks, Promoting Healthy Life. World Health Organization (2002)
2. Alankus, G., Proffitt, R., Kelleher, C., Engsberg, J.R.: Stroke therapy through motion-based games: a case study. TACCESS **4**(1), 3 (2011)
3. Bach-y-Rita, P., Wood, S., Leder, R., Paredes, O., Bahr, D., Bach-y-Rita, E., Murillo, N.: Computer-assisted motivating rehabilitation (CAMR) for institutional, home, and educational late stroke programs. Top. Stroke Rehabil. **8**(4), 1–10 (2002)
4. Chang, Y.-J., Chen, S.-F., Huang, J.-D.: A kinect-based system for physical rehabilitation: a pilot study for young adults with motor disabilities. Res. Dev. Disabil. **32**(6), 2566–2570 (2011)
5. Deutsch, J., Latonio, J., Burdea, G., Boian, R.: Post-stroke rehabilitation with the rutgers ankle system: a case study. Presence **10**(4), 416–430 (2001)
6. Ferreira, L., Ambrosio, P.: Towards an interoperable health-assistive environment: the ehealthcom platform. In: BHI, pp. 930–932. IEEE (2012)
7. Kitsunezaki, N., Adachi, E., Masuda, T., Mizusawa, J.-I.: Kinect applications for the physical rehabilitation. In: Medical Measurements and Applications Proceedings (MeMeA), pp. 294–299. IEEE (2013)
8. Kleim, J., Jones, T., Schallert, T.: Motor enrichment and the induction of plasticity before or after brain injury. Neurochem. Res. **28**(11), 1757–1769 (2003)
9. Langhorne, P., Coupar, F., Pollock, A.: Motor recovery after stroke: a systematic review. Lancet Neurol. **8**(8), 741–754 (2009)
10. Lotze, M., Cohen, L.G.: Volition and imagery in neurorehabilitation. Cogn. Behav. Neurol. **19**(3), 135–140 (2006)
11. Lozano-Quilis, J., Gil-Gómez, H., Gil-Gómez, J., Albiol-Pérez, S., Palacios, G., Fardoum, H.M., Mashat, A.S.: Virtual reality system for multiple sclerosis rehabilitation using kinect. In: Pervasive Computing Technologies for Healthcare (PervasiveHealth), pp. 366–369. IEEE (2013)
12. Matos, N., Santos, A., Vasconcelos, A.: Kinteract: a multi-sensor physical rehabilitation solution based on interactive games. In: Proceedings of the 8th International Conference on Pervasive Computing Technologies for Healthcare (PervasiveHealth 2014). Institute for Computer Sciences, Social-Informatics and Telecommunications Engineering (ICST) (2014)

13. Monir, S., Rubya, S., Ferdous, H.S.: Rotation and scale invariant posture recognition using microsoft kinect skeletal tracking feature. In: Abraham, A., Zomaya, A.Y., Ventura, S., Yager, R., Snásel, V., Muda, A.K., Samuel, P. (eds.) ISDA, pp. 404–409. IEEE (2012)
14. Öberg, T., Karsznia, A., Öberg, K.: Basic gait parameters: reference data for normal subjects, 10–79 years of age. J. Rehabil. Res. Dev. **30**, 210–210 (1993)
15. Saini, S., Rambli, D.R.A., Sulaiman, S., Zakaria, M.N., Shukri, S.R.M.: A low-cost game framework for a home-based stroke rehabilitation system. In: Computer & Information Science (ICCIS), vol. 1, pp. 55–60. IEEE (2012)
16. Shaughnessy, M., Resnick, B., Macko, R.: Testing a model of post-stroke exercise behavior. Rehabil. Nurs. **31**(1), 15–21 (2006)
17. VirtualWare Group. Virtualrehab, February 2014. http://virtualrehab.info/

Measuring Stereoacuity by 3D Technology

Angelo Gargantini$^{(\boxtimes)}$, Giancarlo Facoetti, and Andrea Vitali

Università degli Studi di Bergamo, Bergamo, Italy
{angelo.gargantini,giancarlo.facoetti,andrea.vitali1}@unibg.it
http://3d4amb.unibg.it

Abstract. This paper presents a novel method for measuring with great precision the stereoacuity, that is the smallest depth difference that can be detected in binocular vision. The proposed technique is implemented by a software program that runs on a PC with 3D capabilities. The 3D technology is exploited to provide two different images to the two eyes. The measurement is performed by a classical random dot test, but differently to other tests printed on paper or plastic, the images shown to the patient can vary and the disparity between the two images can be set in order to exactly measure the stereoacuity. Moreover, thanks to the exploited 3D technology, the test does not present any monocular clue. These features allow delivering the test also in groups (instead of individuals) like school classes, and to reduce the risk of undetected amlyopia. The system can be easily operated also by not specialized personnel and this may further increase the cost efficiency of the test. We present the experiments carried on with a large set of children of age between five and seven years. We discuss the results and compare our technique with some traditional approaches.

Keywords: Stereopsis · Randomdot test · Amblyiopia · 3D

1 Introduction

Amblyopia, otherwise known as 'lazy eye', is reduced visual acuity that results in poor or indistinct vision in one eye that is otherwise physically normal. It may exist even in the absence of any detectable organic disease. Amblyopia is generally associated with a squint or unequal lenses in the prescription spectacles. This low vision is not correctable (or only partially) by glasses or contact lenses. Amblyopia is caused by media opacity, strabismus, anisometropia, and significant refractive errors, such as high astigmatism, hyperopia, or myopia. This condition affects 2–3% of the population, which equates to conservatively around 10 million people under the age of 8 years worldwide [17]. Children who are not successfully treated when still young (generally before the age of 7) will become amblyotic adults. As amblyotic adults, they will have a normal life, with no proven losses in terms of education and occupation opportunities [5], except that they are prohibited from some occupations and they are exposed to a higher risk of becoming seriously visually impaired. The best described long term consequence of amblyopia is an increased risk of bilateral blindness, caused most

© Springer-Verlag Berlin Heidelberg 2015
H.M. Fardoun et al. (Eds.): REHAB 2014, CCIS 515, pp. 155–167, 2015.
DOI: 10.1007/978-3-662-48645-0_14

frequently by traumatic eye injury in younger people and age related macular degeneration in older people. The projected lifetime risk of vision loss for an individual with amblyopia is estimated around at least 1–2% [13].

For these reasons screening for amblyopia in early childhood is done in many countries to ensure that affected children are detected and treated within the critical period, and achieve a level of vision in their amblyopic eye that would be useful should they lose vision in their non-amblyopic eye later in life. However, there is no strong scientific evidence that preschool vision screening is cost-effective and some researchers suggest that health authorities should stop purchasing pre-school vision screening services [14].

One factor that weakens the effectiveness of amblyopia screening is that population-based screen tests can suffer from a very low sensitivity and specificity. Several methods are available for the measurement of stereopsis. The most common procedures are anaglyph (with use of red-green filters) and vectographic (with use of polarized filters) procedures. However, these tests since they have monocular clues [12] and may result difficult to pass even for normal people can have low sensitivity and specificity. In one proven case, screening for amblyopia by the local nurses using the visual acuity tests or random dot stereopsis test alone displayed a very low sensitivity (around 20 %) [4].

In this research work, we extend the approach of [11] and we present our research project that has the main goal of developing a method (called 3DSAT) for measuring with precision the stereoacuity of a patient with the main goal of avoiding the typical weaknesses of classical stereo tests. 3DSAT aims to be:

- Very **easy to deliver** at a **low cost**. Even unqualified personnel can perform the test, thus increasing the widespread use and reducing the cost of the test.
- With a very high **sensitivity** (also called the true positive rate, or the recall rate in some fields): its measure of the proportion of actual amblyopic positives which are correctly identified as such is equal to 100 %. In this way it reduces the risk of undetected amblyopia.
- With an acceptable **specificity** (sometimes called the true negative rate): its measure of the proportion of negatives which are correctly identified as such is near to 100 %. This has the goal of avoiding frequent visits with more qualified (and costly) personnel.

3DSAT exploits a 3D computer system, a modern technology able to reproduce stereo images on computer screens. There are already some works on using 3D monitor for stereotest and for amblyopia treatment [15]. Our method advances w.r.t. [7] because it implements Random dot instead of Wirt tests, and extends the work presented in [3] with more advances features (like use of active 3D glasses, use of multiple images instead of simple random dot circles).

In this paper, first we describe stereo acuity and its evaluation using random dot test through the development of an application exploiting the 3D technology. Then, we show the test procedure defined to execute the tests on a set of children using this application. Finally, we show and analyze the results of this experiment by highlighting pros and cons of our research work.

2   Related Work

In the last two decade, many researchers have developed different systems exploiting 3D technology to recreate virtual environments that can be very useful for traditional processes in different fields, such as industrial field and healthcare. In last years, many computer devices have been designed in order to create the emulation of five senses using classic computers. The emulation of eyesight is based on the use of digital shutter glasses which allow recreating depth sense by seeing the 2D screen of computer [2,6,16]. After different studies about this technology, some projects started to develop applications replicating medical work flows to treat eyes diseases, such as amblyopia and stereopsis deficiency. Among these applications, there are systems that only use typical technology in order to make available your solution at patients and medical personnel [15]. These applications can be subdivided in two categories. The first one is formed by applications that can permit to substitute traditional processes (e.g., occlusion for amblyopia treatment) with innovative techniques that are able to apply particular occlusion digital filters exploiting existent videos and video games [1]. In this way, young patients can do treatment with funny and peaceful approach [8]. Second category is formed by applications emulating traditional process made by oculists to make some measurements, such as stereoacuty and stereopsi [7,9,18]. The quality of stereopsis can be tested using the Lang stereotest. It subsist in a random-dot stereogram on which a series of parallel strips of cylindrical lenses are imprinted in several shapes, which separate the views seen by each eye in these areas. Without stereopsis, the image seems only a field of random dots, but the shapes become detectable with increasing stereopsis, and generally consists in several simple shapes,such as a cat, a star as well as a car. This last feature facilitates the use of Lang test in young children. In the next section, we present how the stereo acuity test can be emulated using standard technology and our research work will be introduced in order to understand different technical aspects about software development.

3   3DSAT: A 3D Stereo Acuity Test

3.1   Stereoscopic Acuity and Its Measurement

Having two eyes, as being humans and animals, located at different lateral positions on the head permits binocular vision. It allows seeing two different images that are used to provide a means of depth perception. Through complex brain processing, the human brain uses the binocular vision to allow some important features of sight, such as binocular disparity, discrimination of object size, and surface orientation to determine depth in the field of view. This particular brain skill is defined as *stereopsis.*

Stereopsis is tridimensional vision that is defined by simultaneous stimulation of retinal points that are horizontally disparate. The depth perception doesn't only depend by binocular vision, but it is also defined by different elaborations of mind, perceptive sensations and physiological phenomena whose knowledge

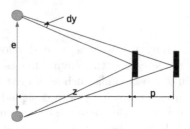

Fig. 1. Mathematical model for stereo acuity.

allows to recreate the sensation of distance and depth. The sense of stereopsis is acquired between the first three or four months of life by being humans.

The total or partial stereopsis absence is cause of some pathologies, such as blindness on one eye and strabismus. The examination of stereopsis ability can be evaluated by measuring stereoscopic acuity.

Stereoscopic acuity, also named stereoacuity, is the smallest measurable depth difference that can be observed by someone with two eyes and normal brain functions. It had been invented by Howard and Dolman who explained stereoacuity with a mathematical model as follows in Fig. 1. The observer sees a black column at a distance z of 6 m (=20 ft). A second columns, that is behind it, can be translated back and forth until it is just detectably nearer than the fixed one. Stereoacuity is the distance between the two positions, converted into an angle of binocular disparity. Equation 1 shows how to convert the depth p in order to obtain the angle of disparity δy in arc of minutes.

$$\delta y = c\, e\, \frac{p}{z^2} \tag{1}$$

In Eq. 1, e is the interocular distance of the watcher and z the space of the fixed column from the eye. To transfer δy into the unit of minutes of arc, a multiplicative constant c is inserted whose value is 3437.75 (1 rad in arcminutes). The 'arc of minute' unit permits to evaluate dimension of an object in degrees of angles (Fig. 2). This approach is very useful because it is possible manage perceived dimensions of objects according to distance of observer from the same objects.

The stereacuity of being humans is excellent when its value is between 15 and 30 seconds of arc.

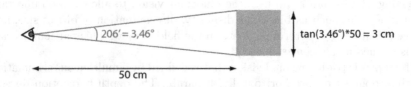

Fig. 2. Calculation of arcseconds

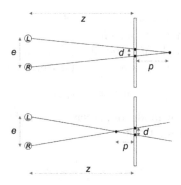

Fig. 3. Application of geometrical model using stereoscopic screen. In this image, the model only considers the middle line of screen.

At present, there are different procedures to measure stereoacuty without using cumbersome two-peg device. The difference between screening for the presence of stereopsis and a measurement of stereoacuity is very important. To establish that depth can be seen in a binocular views, a test must be easily managed and not subject to misunderstanding. These tests can measure stereacuity using either real stereogram or the emulation of stereogram using 3D technology. Furthermore, there are different factor that must to be avoided in order to measure the correct value of stereacuty:

- Low contrast.
- Brief duration exposures (less than 500 milliseconds).
- Pattern elements with small space between them.
- Errors due to uncorrected or unequally corrected refraction (monovision).

In order to get a good measurement of stereopsis by avoiding the described problems, the Random-dot stereogram (RDS) is widely used because it permits to obtain a test procedure, named Randot stereotest, that is easily administrated and not subject to deception. RDS consists in a stereo pair of random-dot images viewed either with the aid of a stereoscope or the eyes focused on a point in front of or behind the images. In this way, the RDS system produces a sensation of depth, with objects appearing to be in front of or behind the display level. Randot stereotest has been easily emulated using 3D technology in this research work, i.e. a 3D based software, named 3DSAT, has been developed by exploiting IT potentiality. In particular, the random small pattern elements are the pixels of PC screen forming digital images, one behind the other, showed to the patient using 3D glasses. Therefore, formula 1 has been adapted by substituting pegs with pixels and the geometrical models has been redefined according to the use of PC.

Figure 3 shows how to apply Howard and Dolman model using a 3D display. The observer's eyes, which are indicated with L (left) and R (right), have a binocular distance defined by e and they are away from screen plane with distance z. The value d is defined as pixels disparity between two stereoscopic images that are shown on stereo screen.

The disparity of a couple of stereo images, defined as x_l and x_r, is simply the difference along x-axis of screen that is measured in pixels.

$$d = x_r - x_l \tag{2}$$

Therefore, the geometric model of perceived depth is defined in following way (assuming that p is small w.r.t. z):

$$p = \frac{z \cdot d}{e} \tag{3}$$

In Eq. 3, it is important to highlight depth perception that is directly proportional at observers distance. Thus, a observed stereo image will allow to perceive different depths from different distances. By substituting the depth p in Eq. 1, we find that the stereo acuity can be computed as:

$$\delta y = c \frac{d}{z} \tag{4}$$

As desired, the Eq. 4 measures the stereo acuity in angles and it does not depend on the interocular distance. In the next subsection, we would introduce the way to apply this geometrical model using 3D technology and we describe the software system to emulate Random Dot test using this technology.

3.2   Using 3D for Stereo Acuity Test

3DSAT is a system based on a 3D computer system. The current version is based on the NVIDIA® 3D Vision™ technology, although other 3D technologies may be supported as well in the future. The NVIDIA 3D Vision technology is one of the most accessible 3D technologies available on the market today, it requires a standard personal computer with a NVIDIA graphic card, a monitor 3D Vision ready, which is capable of a refresh rate of 120 Mhz, and a NVIDA LCD shutter glasses. The NVIDIA 3D vision is based on active shutter technology. With this method, the left and right eye images are presented on alternating frames, but since these monitors are capable of 120 Hz, each eye still sees a full 60 Hz signal that is equivalent to the refresh rate on LCD monitors today. This offers a number of advantages with respect to other stereoscopic technologies like polarized or anaglyphs glasses or head-mounted displays:

- **Full image quality per eye:** In 3D mode, each eye receives the full resolution of the display for the highest possible image quality for text and objects. The colors are not altered and both eyes can receive images of the same quality.
- **Wide viewing angle for 3D:** Because full images are presented on alternating frames, there are no restrictions on the viewing angle in 3D mode. Users are free to move their heads vertically or horizontally within the full viewing angle of the display without losing the 3D effect or suffering increased ghosting which allowing for comfortable viewing for continuous gaming or movie watching.

- **Personalized fit:** The NVIDIA glasses have top-of-the-line optics, include adjustable nose pieces, and are modeled after modern sunglasses. They can be worn over prescription glasses.
- **Acceptable cost:** The cost of the glasses is around 140 USD, while the 3D ready monitors cost a little more than the traditional monitors but they offer a better quality also in 2D.

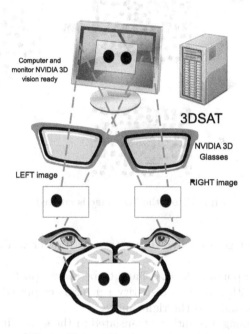

Fig. 4. Using 3D to separate the dots

In the context of amblyopia, 3D technology can be used also in the treatment with the goal of complementing the classical therapy of eye patching [10].

3.3   3DSAT

The system we have developed for 3DSAT consists in a normal PC desktop connected to a 3D monitor (3D Vision-Ready Display). The PC must be 3D capable and have all the 3DSAT software installed on it. The patient wears the NVIDIA active LCD shutter glasses that allow viewing a different image from the left and right eye. The scenario is depicted in Fig. 4. This principle is the separation of the images provided to the right and left eye.

The stereo image to show to the child is built by the following steps as depicted in Fig. 5.

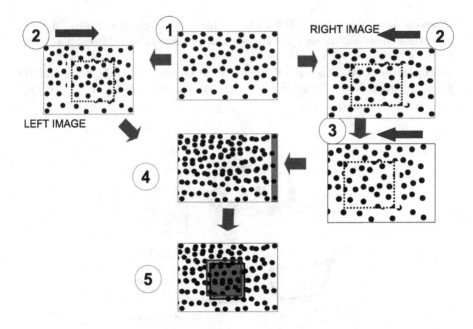

Fig. 5. How the 3D image is created

1. A random dot image is created (every time with different distribution of the dots)
2. The pixels corresponding to the shape to be shown (in the Fig. 5 a square) are translated with a desired disparity (in terms of pixels) in two opposite directions for the left and the right image.
3. One of the two images is entirely translated in the same direction.
4. The two images are composed in an unique 3D image shown to the child.
5. The child, in the presence of stereopsis and wearing the 3D glasses, perceives the shape in depth.

The shape is seen in depth because the left eye sees one set of dots and the right eye sees a second set of dots. The dots are identical, except for the dots within the square that have been horizontally displaced in order to try to emulate the distance of interocular disparity. Using this technique, our brain fuses the two 2D retinal images into single image in which displaced pixels define a shape that is perceived with a different depth. Through identifying corresponding points, 'matching primitives' in the slightly offset retinal images of the left and right eye, the images can be aligned in such a way as to reveal depth information. The nasal displacement produces the stereoscopic perception that the square of circles is raised off the screen [19].

The translation of one entire image (step 3) eliminates any clue of the shape one could have without the 3D glasses: if the two images are composed in the same position all the pixels except those translated are in the identical position and are completely overlapped. This would cause an increase in the composed

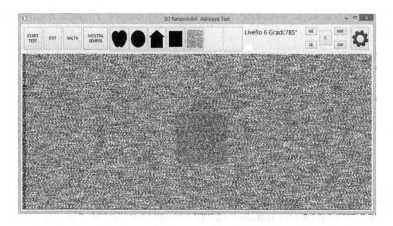

Fig. 6. User interface of 3DSAT application

image of the density of the pixels in correspondence of the shape. Wearing the glasses would eliminate the diversity of density but without the glasses one would have a clue of the shape. By translating one image we restore an equal density of the dots.

3.4   Software Development and Use of 3DSAT

The 3DSAT software has been implemented using Java and OpenGL and works under Microsoft Windows systems. A screenshot of the software is shown in Fig. 6. At the beginning the user inserts the patient data, selects an image set[1], the starting disparity, the distance of the child from the screen, the dimension of the screen and the dimension of the shapes. After a preview of what the shapes will look like (as shown in Fig. 6), the software randomly chooses a shape in the shape set and shows the 3D random dot stereotest for that shape. The child either says or indicates what it sees and if the guess is right then the software chooses another shape and decreases the angle of disparity. The software assesses a certain level of disparity if the child can guess the shapes for that level for three times with maximum one error. The minimum angle of measurement depends on the monitor and on the distance of the child, and some examples are reported in Table 1.

Policies. In order to reduce the number of false negative (i.e. amblyopic not correctly identified and falsely passing the test) and increase the test **sensitivity** we have devised the following policies: (i) the shape is randomly chosen every time, (ii) also the control null image (no shape is shown) can be inserted, (iii) either the user that delivers the test has no clue about which shape is currently displayed, (iv) we have checked the absence of any monocular clue by using the

---

[1] 3DSAT now provides set of images similar to those presented in the LANG stereotest I and II, TNO, LEA, pacman and letters. New image sets can be easily added.

Table 1. Minimum angle definition according to dimensions, resolution and distance of the PC screen.

Dim	Resolution	Distance	Minimum angle
23″	FHD 1920 × 1080	40 cm	136.8″
23″	FHD 1920 × 1080	80 cm	68.4″
27″	FHD 1920 × 1080	40 cm	160.5″
27″	FHD 1920 × 1080	120 cm	53.5″

software both without glasses and with glasses but with one occluded eye. In both cases we were unable to identify the images.

In order to reduce the number of false positives (i.e. non amblyopic falsely failing the test) and increase the test **specificity**, we have devised the following policies: (i) the shape is shown as image: if the child has difficulties to recognize the shape and identify its name, he/she can simply point his/her finger, (ii) the test has initial phase in which no measurement is taken and the images are shown colored: in this way the child understands what the shape will look like when the actual measurement is started and the color disappears, (iii) when a child fails the test, the test can be retried with a different set of images (after the equipment is checked for failures). Since the images are randomly chosen, the test can be repeated without loss of sensitivity (differently from the classical test on paper).

4   Experiments

We tested the system on a total population of 90 subjects with age between 5 years and 7 years (Fig. 7). In the group there was a small presence of amblyopic subjects (known before starting the tests). The main aim of the test was to verify the presence of false positives or false negatives results. Due the young age and the high number of the people taking the tests in the same session, we decided to organize the tests as a group game. Indeed, we planned that the aim of the game was to guess a given shape visualized on the screen, wearing the 3D glasses. Obviously, only the child with the glasses would be able to see what happens on the screen, while other children can see just a noisy image. Children were asked to guess the shapes wearing glasses one after the other. It turned out that this modality fits very well in a context of group screening, especially with young and lively children. With the traditional tests, such as Lang test, young patients would suggest each other the correct results, causing false negatives. With our computer-based system, shapes to be guessed change every time, making cheating very difficult. This could highly reduce the number of false negatives cases. Also, our approach permits to show a great number of different shapes (also possibly expandable and customizable), reducing further the number of false negatives caused by wild guesses. However, for the tests we just used shaped derived from LEA, TNO and LANG traditional tests. The

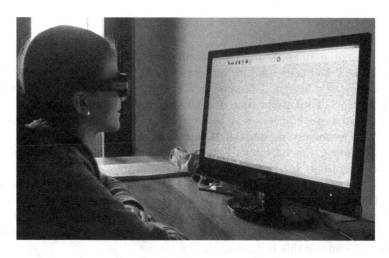

Fig. 7. A child is using 3DSAT with LCD shutter glasses.

group screening proved to be time effective: the mean time required to test one person is 2 min, faster than the traditional way. In total we tested 90 subjects for a total of 180 test results. We identified 8 potential positive cases, confirmed by previous medical diagnosis. We clustered test data grouping the distance from the screen and the data is shown in Table 2.

Looking at the collected data, we observe that the minimum and maximum stereo acuity values decrease linearly with the increasing of the distance. The mean values depend on the stereo acuity of the various subjects taking the tests, however they present too a decreasing trend with the distance increase. This is expected since by increasing the distance, the minimum measurable angle of stereopsis decreases (see Table 1).

Table 2. Distance from the screen, mean, minimum and maximun stereo acuity values.

Distance	Mean	Min	Max
40 cm	398.12″	139.12″	962.02″
50 cm	407.44″	128.27″	769.62″
60 cm	278.84″	106.89″	641.35″
80 cm	170.41″	79.49″	481.01″
100 cm	231.12″	64.13″	384.81″
120 cm	109.32″	53.44″	213.78″
150 cm	101.06″	42.75″	299.29″
160 cm	100.21″	40.08″	240.50″
200 cm	51.30″	25.65″	64.13″

5   Conclusions

We have presented an application that emulates random-dot test using 3D technology. 3DSAT has been used for our experiment on young children and early results have been considered promising. The test procedure has demonstrated the potentialities of our application compared to the traditional approach. Therefore, our research work proposes an innovative and better approach for this test, which is also frequently used for detecting amblyopia, strabismus and suppression, and to measure stereoacuity. Furthermore, we have wanted to demonstrate that is possible to get innovative solution in healthcare exploiting low cost technology and free software. Thanks to this approach, 3DSAT may be added into a bigger IT system that allows sharing patient information using web and mobile technology in easy way. About this issue, new developments have been planned in order to try the real potentiality according to needs of both physicians and patients who can use this technology in the future.

References

1. Achtman, R., Green, C., Bavelier, D.: Video games as a tool to train visual skills. Restorative Neurol. Neurosci. **26**(4–5), 435–446 (2008)
2. Aflaki, P., Hannuksela, M., Sarbolandi, H., Gabbouj, M.: Rendering stereoscopic video for simultaneous 2D and 3D presentation. In: 3DTV-Conference: The True Vision-Capture, Transmission and Dispaly of 3D Video (3DTV-CON), pp. 1–4, October 2013
3. Breyer, A., Jiang, X., Rütsche, A., Mojon, D.S.: A new 3D monitor-based random-dot stereotest for children. Invest. Ophthalmol. Vis. Sci. **47**(11), 4842 (2006)
4. Chang, C.-H., Tsai, R.-K., Sheu, M.-M.: Screening amblyopia of preschool children with uncorrected vision and stereopsis tests in eastern taiwan. Eye **21**(12), 1482–1488 (2006)
5. Chua, B.: Consequences of amblyopia on education, occupation, and long term vision loss. Br. J. Ophthalmol. **88**(9), 1119–1121 (2004)
6. Chyou, T., Clark, A., Meyer, J.: A 3D vision approach for correction of patient pose in radiotherapy. In: Engineering and Physical Sciences in Medicine and the Australian Biomedical Engineering Conference (EPSM ABEC 2011) (2011)
7. de Bougrenet, J.L., de la Tocnaye, B., Cochener, S., Ferragut, D., Iorgovan, Y.F., Lamard, M.: Supervised stereo visual acuity tests implemented on 3D TV monitors. J. Display Technol. **8**(8), 472–478 (2012)
8. Dixon-Woods, M., Awan, M., Gottlob, I.: Why is compliance with occlusion therapy for amblyopia so hard? a qualitative study. Arch. Dis. Child. **91**(6), 491–494 (2006)
9. Gadia, D., Garipoli, G., Bonanomi, C., Albani, L., Rizzi, A.: Assessing stereo blindness and stereo acuity on digital displays. Displays **35**(4), 206–212 (2014)
10. Gargantini, A., Bana, M., Fabiani, F.: Using 3D for rebalancing the visual system of amblyopic children. In: 2011 International Conference on Virtual Rehabilitation (ICVR), pp. 1–7, June 2011

11. Gargantini, A., Facoetti, G., Vitali, A.: A random dot stereoacuity test based on 3D technology. In: Proceedings of the 8th International Conference on Pervasive Computing Technologies for Healthcare (PervasiveHealth 2014), Brussels, Belgium, pp. 358–361. Institute for Computer Sciences, Social-Informatics and Telecommunications Engineering (ICST) (2014)

12. Hahn, E., Comstock, D., Connick, S., MacCarron, J., Mulla, S., Peters, P., LaRoche, R.: Monocular clues in seven stereoacuity tests. Dalhousie Med. J. **37**(1), 4–13 (2010)

13. Rahi, J.S., Logan, S., Timms, C., Russell-Eggitt, I., Taylor, D.: Risk, causes, and outcomes of visual impairment after loss of vision in the non-amblyopic eye: a population-based study. The Lancet **360**(9333), 597–602 (2002)

14. Stewart-Brown, S., Snowdon, S.: Evidence-based dilemmas in pre-school vision screening. Arch. Dis. Child. **78**(5), 406–407 (1998)

15. Vitali, A., Facoetti, G., Gargantini, A.: An environment for contrast-based treatment of amblyopia using 3D technology. In: International Conference on Virtual Rehabilitation, Philadelphia. PA, USA, 26–29 August 2013. (2013)

16. Waddingham, P.E., Butler, T.K.H., Cobb, S.V., Moody, A.D.R., Comaish, I.F., Haworth, S.M., Gregson, R.M., Ash, I.M., Brown, S.M., Eastgate, R.M., Griffiths, G.D.: Preliminary results from the use of the novel interactive binocular treatment (I-BiT^{TM}) system, in the treatment of strabismic and anisometropic amblyopia. Eye **20**(3), 375–378 (2006)

17. Webber, A.L., Wood, J.: Amblyopia: prevalence, natural history, functional effects and treatment. Clin. Exp. Optom. **88**(6), 365–375 (2005)

18. Westheimer, G.: Three-dimensional displays and stereo vision. Proc. Roy. Soc. B Biol. Sci. **278**(1716), 2241–2248 (2011)

19. Wright, K.: Handbook of Pediatric Strabismus and Amblyopia. Springer, New York (2006)

A Cloud-Assisted Wearable System
for Physical Rehabilitation

Giancarlo Fortino and Raffaele Gravina[(✉)]

Department of Informatics, Modelling, Electronics and Systems,
University of Calabria, Rende, Italy
`fortino@unical.it, rgravina@deis.unical.it`

Abstract. Wearable smart devices, ubiquitous Internet connectivity, and Cloud-computing are posing traditional health-care system against a disruptive revolution. The integration of Body Sensor Networks (BSN) systems and Cloud-computing technologies can effectively foster the spread of mobile-Health (mHealth) services in real life, such as physical rehabilitation assistance. The continuous remote monitoring of patients during rehabilitation exercises is one of the key aspect to follow the patients at all post-admission stages, to objectively assess their improvements, as well as to significantly reduce many of the costs associated with the whole process. In addition, patients can perform rehabilitation exercises at home and still be monitored - and followed - remotely, with clear benefit in terms of comfort, physical stress, and again economic costs. This paper describes *Rehab-aaService*, a hardware/software system for physical rehabilitation assistance. It is based on a three-tier architecture involving smart wearable motion sensor nodes, a personal mobile device, and a Cloud-computing infrastructure supported by the BodyCloud framework.

1   Introduction

Body Sensor Networks (BSNs) [3] are specific Wireless Sensor Networks (WSNs) for monitoring of humans. BSNs are potentially a disruptive technology in several human-centered applications, including medical monitoring, fitness and sport, large-scale events management and social networking. BSNs involves a broad range of wearable sensors for physiological measurements such as heart and respiratory rate, body temperature, blood glucose, limb motions, electrocardiogram (ECG), electromyography (EMG), and electroencephalogram (EEG). Physiological signals are processed to infer higher level knowledge to enable more complex services, including physical activity recognition, heart attack early detection, emotion detection, and neurodegenerative diseases monitoring.

However, to fully exploit this emerging technology, there is the need to deal with management of a large number of cooperative and non-cooperative BSNs. Supporting pervasive applications for large communities of users is in fact a critical and complex task. The massive data that BSN networks can generate, requires a scalable and flexible platform for their collection, secure storage and processing.

© Springer-Verlag Berlin Heidelberg 2015
H.M. Fardoun et al. (Eds.): REHAB 2014, CCIS 515, pp. 168–182, 2015.
DOI: 10.1007/978-3-662-48645-0_15

Effective and efficient management of networks of BSNs cannot be accomplished uniquely relying on their limited resources.

We tackle this problem using a Cloud computing infrastructure and providing an integrated platform, namely BodyCloud [7,17,18], built upon the following functional requirements:

- heterogeneous wearable sensing through personal mobile devices acting as local coordinators;
- scalability in terms of processing power for diverse medical analysis;
- scalability in terms of physiological signals collection and data storage;
- global access to processing and storage functionalities;
- simple and authenticated sharing of results.

This paper presents Rehab-aaService - a scalable motor rehabilitation research prototype based on BodyCloud [7] - which extends the preliminary work proposed in [16].

BodyCloud is a Software-as-a-Service (SaaS) platform that provides real-time storage, online/offline management of physiological signals, data processing and analysis using software plugins hosted in the Cloud. In particular, BodyCloud has been designed to effectively support diversified cross-disciplinary applications and processing tasks. It enables ubiquitous large-scale data sharing, collaborations among users and applications in the Cloud, and delivers Cloud-based services through sensor-rich mobile and wearable devices. In addition, BodyCloud includes data mining functionalities to enable high-level decision support based on the collected BSN data.

Rehab-aaService is a hardware/software system to assist the physical rehabilitation. It is built atop the BodyCloud platform so to support remote and ubiquitous collection, storage and processing of data streams from non-invasive sensors worn by patients during therapy and rehabilitation. During motor rehabilitation therapy, it is quite common to require repetitive physical exercises, for instance, to recover from a muscle strain, a limb fracture, or a surgery. Having real-time feedback about exercise performance quality allows users to independently exercise properly without the need of a continuous professional assistance. As a consequence, especially for certain types of motor traumas, the concept of *tele-rehabilitation* becomes strategic. Being able to perform rehabilitation independently (e.g. at home), is a benefit for patients in terms of physical stress and economic cost reductions. Thus, a strong motivation for this project is to optimize and manage the rehabilitation stages through hardware/software systems installed at the remote patient. Our system, therefore, proposes a novel contribution to the state-of-the-art by: (i) providing an integrated hardware/software system for continuous non-invasive monitoring patients undergoing rehabilitation; (ii) introducing of a Cloud-based management and analysis service, used by medical doctors and physiotherapists, with support for remote access to rehab exercises traces, improvement parameters, and other information throughout the whole rehabilitation process of their patients.

The rest of the paper is structured as follows. Section 2 discusses related work on physical rehabilitation aided by wearable sensors and, specifically, we propose a categorization in terms of methods, frameworks, and systems. Section 3 overviews the BodyCloud architecture. Section 4 describes the proposed cloud-based Motor Rehabilitation application service; we give details on the method we used, its accuracy and we provide insights of the performance evaluation of our system. Finally, in Sect. 5 conclusive remarks are drawn and directions of future work are briefly outlined.

2   Related Work

Literature on physical rehabilitation assistance supported by wearable sensors is being consolidating. For the sake of this work we propose a categorization of the related work in terms of methods, frameworks, and systems and we discuss some interesting studies in the following subsections.

Method refers to algorithmic and mathematical aspects. A related work is classified as a *Framework* if focuses on a customizable programming layer on top of which implementing end-user services. *System* is intended as a work focusing on hardware/software technical and functional aspects.

A comparison of the works that we took in consideration is summarized in Table 1. The table shows that, conversely to the related work, Rehab-aaService includes all the three aspects of the proposed categorization.

We anticipate that, to the best of our knowledge, none of them offers adaptable and customizable tele-rehabilitation of both upper and lower limbs. Rehab-aaService, instead, proposes an original contribution, responding to (i) the need for integrated hardware/software systems for the continuous monitoring and follow-up of patients under rehabilitation therapy and (ii) the lack of effective solutions for data collection, integration and analysis with support for data mining and statistical techniques for the management of the various rehabilitation stages. With Rehab-aaService, the stakeholders (e.g., physicians, physical therapists, patients, centers for rehabilitation and physiotherapy, gyms) are connected to each other and have integrated and interoperable access to data related to patients' rehabilitation process.

The interested reader can refer to interesting recent surveys [8,11].

2.1   Methods

An early research [1] focuses on the therapist perspective aiming at determining the physical activity stress and the energy expenditure of therapists while practicing using a portable accelerometer sensor placed on their waist belts. In [9] authors propose the use of wearable accelerometer sensors for objectively assessing motion capabilities and activity levels of patients affected by multiple sclerosis, so not to rely uniquely on self-reports and questionnaires. Combined use of inertial sensors and Kinect for rehabilitation robotics has been explored in [22]; trigonometry and Kalman filter framework have been used in the proposed joint angle estimation method. In [23] a complete model-based human motion analysis system is proposed, including estimation of both upper and lower limbs motion. However, the method is based on computer vision rather than wearable devices and there is the assumption that the limbs can bend only on certain 2-D planes. An interesting review [24] covers different techniques and methods for joint angles and limb rotations using inertial sensors (including accelerometer, digital compass and gyroscope). In [25] authors focus on upper limb joint angle tracking and propose the combined use of gyroscope and accelerometer with an estimation method based on the unscented Kalman filter.

2.2 Frameworks

RehabSPOT [19] is the only customizable BSN programming framework specifically tailored for physical rehabilitation. RehabSPOT is built on top of the SunSPOT sensor platform [20] originally from Sun Microsystems. The platform consists of a number of SunSPOT nodes attached to various parts of human body, and a SunSPOT basestation connected to a PC. To enforce a high degree of system configurability and reliability, both the wearable nodes and basestation are powered by a flexible software architecture. This framework has been used to prototype a system installed in a clinical center for testing and evaluation, with positive initial feedback from the patients under rehabilitation and their therapists. SPINE [6] is domain-specific software framework for the design and fast prototyping of BSN applications. It includes powerful, flexible and extensible libraries and functionalities to aid the implementation of mHealth systems, and it has been used to develop the embedded and mobile components of Rehab-aaService.

2.3 Systems

The specific problem of supporting patients during rehabilitation exercises with the aid of wearable sensing devices and real-time visual feedbacks is being investigated more systematically in recent times. In [12] authors describe a rehabilitation support system based on a smartphone and a bracelet to capture patient's rehabilitation exercises. Dynamic Time Warping is used to train and recognize movements. The system is fully customizable so it allows the therapist to choose the position of the device and other parameters in order to adapt to different exercises. The proposed system, however, by relaying on a single sensing device suffers of the problem that a number of exercises cannot be monitored and relevant parameters, such as elbow and knee flexion angles, cannot be measured. RIABLO [5] is a game system realized to specifically support physical orthopedic rehabilitation. Authors suggest the use of game elements to motivate and engage the patient, while providing feedback on the correctness of the performed exercises. The system is based on five wearable devices equipped with a 3-axial accelerometer and a gyroscope, positioned on the body with elastic straps, and a pressure sensor tile connected via Bluetooth with the game station. Another interesting project [15] uses two wearable motion sensors attached to the patient's arm or leg and a commercial Android tablet where a graphical application provides with a visual real-time feedback on the performed exercises

Table 1. A comparison of the related work.

Ref.	Method	Framework	System
[22]	•		
[23]	•		
[24]	•		
[25]	•		
[19]		•	•
[12]		•	•
[5]			•
[15]			•
[21]			•
[4]	•		•
[10]		•	•
Rehab-aaService	•	•	•

as well as an assessment on the practice quality with respect to a reference movement previously recorded. An interesting pre-commercial system is Rehabitic [21], a tele-rehabilitation service specifically designed for total knee arthroplasty patients. The aim of the service is to enable for rehabilitation at the patient's home. The system includes knee real-time motion tracking by means of Shimmer sensors and technologies to allow for distance education and video conference between the patient and the therapist. Finally, in addition to purely academic researches, CoRehab [4] and PamSys [10] are commercial solutions with similar functionalities to what described above.

3   BodyCloud

BodyCloud [7] is an open platform for the integration of BSNs with a Cloud Platform-as-a-Service (PaaS) infrastructure. It specifically supports remote sensory data storage, offline signal processing and custom-defined algorithms via a plug-in mechanism. Its design and implementation choices allow BodyCloud to flexibly be tailored, in a very effective manner, for supporting a broad range of smart-Health applications, focusing on mHealth services. As depicted in the simplified component diagram in Fig. 1, the architecture is composed of four main components:

– *Body*: the component that monitors the assisted living by means of wearable sensors, and forwards the collected data to the Cloud through a personal mobile coordinator device. Data acquisition is currently handled using Android-SPINE [2, 6, 13] and wireless communications with the sensors based on Bluetooth.

- *Cloud*: the component that gives full support for specific applications through data collection, processing/analysis, and visualization. In particular, applications are defined through specific software abstractions (Group, Modality, Workflow/Node, View). Such abstractions are supported by a RESTful web service (Server Servlet), programmed atop the Restlet Framework [14]. Every interactions is authenticated using OAuth 2.0 protocol. The Cloud-side runs on the Google App Engine (GAE) PaaS. GAE exposes the Datastore API, used by BodyCloud to store sensory and processed data generated by the application services, and the Task Queue API, through which BodyCloud supports asynchronous execution of tasks triggered by application requests.
- *Analyst*: the component supporting BodyCloud customization/extension, in terms of development of new application services (plugins). Specifically, new services are defined in terms of the aforementioned *abstractions*, and deployed using simple HTTP PUT requests to the corresponding Cloud-side resource, thus requiring only a simple HTTP client as Analyst-side supporting application. As the workflow requires new nodes to be developed, the Analyst-side also requires an appropriate development environment. Once developed, new nodes are also uploaded with a HTTP PUT request to the corresponding Cloud-side resource. A predefined set of nodes is natively available.
- *Viewer*: the component supporting graphical visualization of raw and processed data through flexible graphical reporting options. The graphical view is automatically generated by applying the View specification to the data.

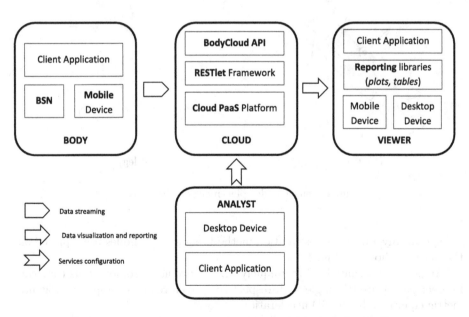

Fig. 1. A simplified architectural representation of BodyCloud.

4   Rehab-aaService

Rehab-aaService is a Cloud-assisted motor rehabilitation assistant application, currently optimized for elbow and knee. Limbs motion measurement is performed using two tiny and lightweight wearable devices equipped with 3-axial accelerometers. Sensors are attached by means of elastic bracelets in specific positions of the limbs for acquiring accelerometer data, which are eventually processed by the BSN coordinator to estimate medical-relevant rehabilitation information such as joint (e.g. elbow and knee) flexion and extension angles.

4.1   Method

To estimate the flexion and rotation information of the limbs, the proposed system uses SPINE-enabled wearable nodes [6] equipped with 3-axial accelerometer sensors. The application configures the nodes to sample the accelerometers at a rate of 30 Hz.

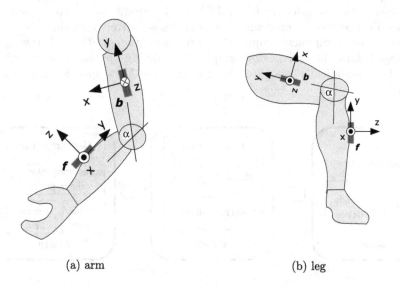

(a) arm   (b) leg

Fig. 2. Sensor nodes placement on the limbs.

Specifically, our angles estimation method requires the nodes to be placed on the body as shown in Fig. 2.

Angles are estimated using uniquely 3D inertial accelerometers, as they can indirectly measure tilt angle with respect to a given reference applying trigonometric equations to the 3D acceleration vector.

As shown in Fig. 2, **b** and **f** indicate the nodes placed respectively on the arm (or on the thigh) and on the forearm (or on the leg). The method is based on the assumption that both the elbow and knee joints can be considered as *hinge joints*, in which only flexion and extension rotation is allowed.

Under this assumption and by considering the sensor placement as in Fig. 2, only the following acceleration components are needed to estimate the flexion/extension angle (α):

$$\mathbf{b} = \begin{bmatrix} X_b \\ Y_b \end{bmatrix} \quad \mathbf{f} = \begin{bmatrix} Y_f \\ Z_f \end{bmatrix} \tag{1}$$

Since we are interested in the relative inclination of the forearm (leg) with respect to the arm (thigh), we need to express the reference system of one of the two accelerometers according to the other one. This is possible by applying a rototranslation of the first reference system. If we rotate the reference system of $\mathbf{f}$ and we translate it so to align its origin and axes with the reference system of $\mathbf{b}$ (clearly, the discussion is valid also the opposite way), we obtain a new reference system whose representation is rotated of an angle θ (see Fig. 3).

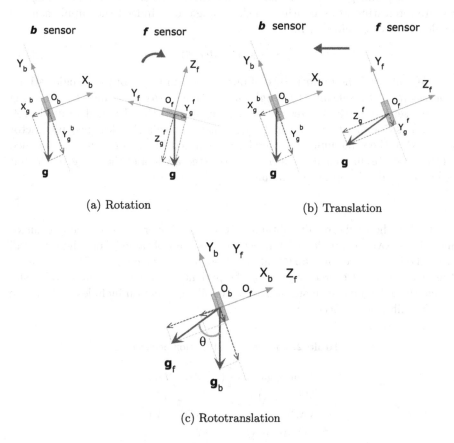

(a) Rotation   (b) Translation

(c) Rototranslation

Fig. 3. Rototranslation of the reference system.

We can calculate the angle θ between $\mathbf{g}_b$ and $\mathbf{g}_f$ using the following equation:

$$\mathbf{g}_b \cdot \mathbf{g}_f = Y_b Y_f + X_b Z_f \tag{2}$$

This can be rewritten as:

$$\mathbf{g}_b \cdot \mathbf{g}_f = \|\mathbf{g}_b\| \, \|\mathbf{g}_f\| \, cos(\theta) \tag{3}$$

where

$$\|\mathbf{g}_b\| = \sqrt{X_b^2 + Y_b^2} \, , \quad \|\mathbf{g}_f\| = \sqrt{Y_f^2 + Z_f^2} \tag{4}$$

The value of θ (expressed in radiants) can be obtained by the inverse equation in Eq. 3:

$$\theta = arccos\left(\frac{\mathbf{g}_b \cdot \mathbf{g}_f}{\|\mathbf{g}_b\| \, \|\mathbf{g}_f\|}\right) \tag{5}$$

If we pose $\mathbf{g}_f$ along the directrix so to let it consecutive to $\mathbf{g}_b$, the angle α between $\mathbf{g'}_f$ and $\mathbf{g}_b$ will be equal by construction to the *flexion joint angle* α we are interesting at estimating. Such an angle it is indeed the supplementary angle of θ; we therefore have:

$$\alpha = 180° - deg(\theta) \tag{6}$$

We evaluated the performance of our method in terms of joint angle estimation accuracy. Specifically, the angle measurement was performed by attaching the two sensors to the interested limb; we compared the obtained values in reference positions (with a step of 10°) against a specifically-designed protractor attached to the same limb. We therefore calculated the estimation error, defined as the absolute difference between the estimated angle and the one given by our reference medical-approved goniometer:

$$\epsilon_\alpha = |\hat{\alpha} - \alpha| \tag{7}$$

Table 2 shows the results obtained, in terms of average, variance and maximum error, over a sample of 50 measurements, half obtained from the arm, half from the leg. The results show that the average error is less than 5°. However, if the sensors are not correctly worn by the patient, the precision can decrease significantly. To handle such situation, the mobile application includes an intuitive sensor calibration procedure.

Table 2. Joint angle estimation accuracy

Joint angle error (°)	Arm	Leg
MEAN(ϵ_α)	4	3,5
VAR(ϵ_α)	3,76	3,24
MAX(ϵ_α)	7	5

4.2 Framework

Implemented according to the software abstractions (*Group, Modality, Workflow, View*) introduced by the BodyCloud framework, Rehab-aaService defines the following entities:

- *Rehab Group*: represents the group of monitored patients.
- *RehabDataFeed Modality*: allows the transmission of rehabilitation session data from the Body-side to the Cloud-side.
- *RehabDataAnalysis Modality*: based on the *RehabDataAnalysis Workflow*, analyzes individual data and provides (aggregated and statistical) information about the progress of the therapy.
- *RehabData View*: the graphical display (e.g. plots, diagrams, and tables) through which rehabilitation data are rendered at the Viewer-side.

To provide an exemplification, we report the XML definition of the Rehab-DataFeed modality:

```xml
<?xml version="1.0" encoding="UTF-8"?>
<modality>
    <inputSpecification>
        <column>
            <name>foreNode-accX</name>
            <type>INTEGER</type>
            <source>GENERIC</source>
        </column>
        <column>
            <name>foreNode-accY</name>
            <type>INTEGER</type>
            <source>GENERIC</source>
        </column>
        <column>
            <name>backNode-accY</name>
            <type>INTEGER</type>
            <source>GENERIC</source>
        </column>
        <column>
            <name>backNode-accZ</name>
            <type>INTEGER</type>
            <source>GENERIC</source>
        </column>
    </inputSpecification>
    <action>
        <uri>/group/rehab-aaservice/data</uri>
        <method>PUT</method>
        <repeat>true</repeat>
    </action>
</modality>
```

4.3 System

As discussed in the previous subsections, our system can monitor limb bending movements dynamically (*brown arm*, as in the application screen-shot shown in

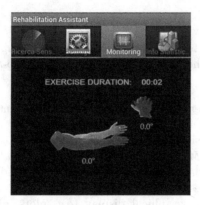

Fig. 4. Rehab-aaService: live rehabilitation exercise monitoring dashboard on the mobile device.

Fig. 4; it also allows to overlap the visual real-time feedback with the reference movement model, recorded by the physiotherapist during a set-up phase (*grey arm*, as in the application screen-shot shown in Fig. 4). The application scenario consists of two steps, namely setup and exercise phases. During the set-up phase, the user wears two sensors on either leg or arm that needs to be exercised and performs the correct exercise under the guidance of rehabilitation professional. Meanwhile, the system records the data and stores it as reference exercise. Then, during the exercise phase, the user repeats the bending movement and is provided with a real-time feedback about how the movement is done with respect to the stored reference exercise.

All the rehabilitation session data are also securely transmitted to a Cloud server using the BodyCloud infrastructure.

A number of improvement indices (such as range of motion, improvement trend, and training time) are reported in a separate panel, so to allow the patient to get quantitative information regarding his improvements throughout the rehab therapy. In addition, the application retrieves online the patient's rehab exercise scheduling.

The Cloud web-based front-end allows authenticated users, such as physiotherapists and doctors, to visualize detailed information about each patient's exercise sessions, to compare graphically their adherence to previously recorded reference exercise template, and to create or update individual exercise scheduling programs, that are seamlessly downloaded to the patient's mobile device.

In particular, the graphs depicted in Fig. 5 compares the knee flexion, thigh inclination, and leg torsion angles between the reference exercise (*blue line*) and the movement actually performed (*red line*).

To evaluate the performance of the mobile application of our system, we took into consideration several Android-based mobile devices with different characteristics in terms of computational power, firmware version, and battery capacity. In particular, we run Rehab-aaService onto the following devices:

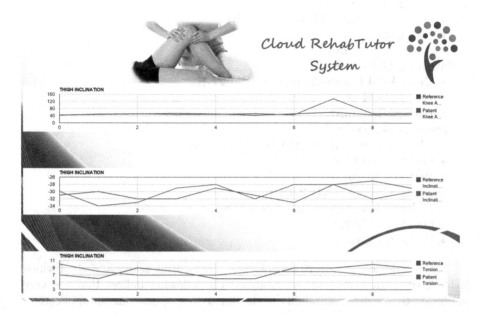

Fig. 5. Rehab-aaService: a graphical analysis of a recorded rehabilitation session on the Cloud side (Color figure online).

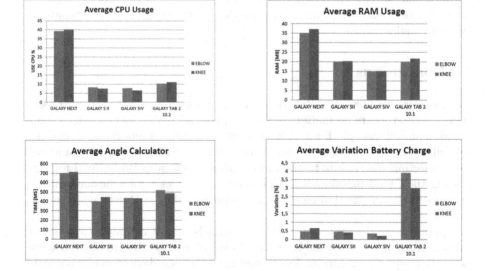

Fig. 6. Perfomance evaluation results.

- **Samsung Galaxy Next**
  - CPU: Qualcomm 7227T-1 - 600 MHz
  - OS: Android 2.3.6
  - Battery: 1750 mAh
- **Samsung Galaxy S II**
  - CPU: ARM Cortex-A9 dual-core - 1.2 GHz
  - OS: Android 4.0.4
  - Battery: 1800 mAh
- **Samsung Galaxy S IV**
  - CPU: Snapdragon 600 APQ8064T - 1.9 GHz
  - OS: Android 4.2.2
  - Battery: 2600 mAh
- **Samsung Galaxy TAB 2 10.1**
  - CPU: NVidia Tegra2 dual-core - 1 GHz
  - OS: Android 4.2.2
  - Battery: 7000 mAh

For each device, we run 20 rehabilitation monitoring sessions, each of which lasted 15 min. In particular, we analyzed the following indices that are very important to assess the suitability of the device to properly run our application:

- CPU usage;
- RAM usage;
- Execution time of angles estimation;
- Battery discharge.

Figure 6 summarizes the results of our analysis. It is worth noting that the execution time has been evaluated with the system configured to estimate all the joint angles locally.

5   Conclusions

In this paper we presented Rehab-aaService, motor rehabilitation digital assistant based on wearable motion sensors, a personal mobile device, and Cloud-based management platform. The current prototype supports arm and leg rehabilitation and has been programmed using the SPINE-Android framework for connecting the sensors to the mobile device, and atop BodyCloud for supporting the Cloud functionalities. The system includes a joint flexion/rotation angle estimation algorithm based on accelerometer data with average error less than $5°$.

An interesting lesson learned of this research is that, according to our preliminary performance evaluation in terms of execution time required by our angle estimation equations, current low-to-mid range mobile devices might not have enough computing power to execute, at regular periodic basis (the system has to estimate instantaneous joint angle values at a rhythm that is driven by the sensor sampling rate), the involved math within the sensor sampling period.

This alone is a strong motivation for us to have moved the algorithm on the Cloud. Currently, our prototype retrieves the device' CPU speed and executes the estimation algorithm locally on the mobile device (so to forward to the Cloud directly the estimated angles) if the mobile device is powerful enough, or enables Cloud-computing otherwise.

Ongoing works are currently devoted to re-engineering the system to allow for more flexibility in customizing it to different physical rehabilitation (e.g. the shoulder). We are also realizing a bidirectional audio/video communication feature to allow patients requesting a video chat with their physiotherapists while performing the rehab exercises, so to further improve the guided-exercise mode. Future works will mainly be devoted to perform a usability analysis by running an experimentation on real patients with the help of our rehabilitation center partner and physiotherapists. All involved actors, at the end of the field trial, will be requested to fill differentiated questionnaires with the aim of assessing the usability of our system (of both the wearable devices and the software).

Acknowledgments. Our thanks to Daniele Parisi and Vincenzo Pirrone for their efforts in implementing BodyCloud and to Fabrizio Granieri and Luigi Salvatore Galluzzi for their support with the Rehab-aaService prototype. This work has been partially supported by the "2007–2013 NOP for Research and Competitiveness for the Convergence Regions (Calabria, Campania, Puglia and Sicilia)" with code PON04a3_00238.

References

1. Balogun, J., Farina, N.T., Fay, E., Rossmann, K., Pozyc, L.: Energy cost determination using a portable accelerometer. Phys. Ther. **66**, 1102–1107 (1986)
2. Bellifemine, F., Fortino, G., Giannantonio, R., Gravina, R., Guerrieri, A., Sgroi, M.: SPINE: a domain-specific framework for rapid prototyping of WBSN applications. Softw. Pract. Exp. **41**(3), 237–265 (2011)
3. Chen, M., Gonzalez, S., Vasilakos, A., Cao, H., Leung, V.C.: Body area networks: a survey. Mob. Netw. Appl. **16**(2), 171–193 (2011)
4. CoRehab-Website (2014). www.corehab.it
5. Costa, C., Tacconi, D., Tomasi, R., Calva, F., Terreri, V.: RIABLO: a game system for supporting orthopedic rehabilitation. In: Proceedings of the Biannual Conference of the Italian Chapter of SIGCHI (2013)
6. Fortino, G., Giannantonio, R., Gravina, R., Kuryloski, P., Jafari, R.: Enabling effective programming and flexible management of efficient body sensor network applications. IEEE Trans. Hum. Mach. Syst. **43**(1), 115–133 (2013)
7. Fortino, G., Parisi, D., Pirrone, V., Fatta, G.D.: BodyCloud: a SaaS approach for community body sensor networks. Futur. Gener. Comput. Syst. **35**, 62–79 (2014)
8. Hadjidj, A., Souil, M., Bouabdallaha, A., Challal, Y., Owen, H.: Wireless sensor networks for rehabilitation applications: challenges and opportunities. J. Netw. Comput. Appl. **36**(1), 1–15 (2013)
9. Hale, L., Williams, K., Ashton, C., Connole, T., McDowell, H., Taylor, C.: Reliability of RT3 accelerometer for measuring mobility in people with multiple sclerosis: pilot study. J. Rehabil. Res. Dev. **44**(4), 619–627 (2007)
10. PamSys-Website (2014). www.biosensics.com

11. Patel, S., Park, H., Bonato, P., Chan, L., Rodgers, M.: A review of wearable sensors and systems with application in rehabilitation. J. NeuroEng. Rehabil. **9**(21) (2012)
12. Raso, I., Hervas, R., Bravo, J.: m-Physio: personalized accelerometer-based physical rehabilitation platform. In: Proceedings of the 4th International Conference on Mobile Ubiquitous Computing, Systems, Services and Technologies (2010)
13. Gravina, R., Alessandro, A., Salmeri, A., Buondonno, L., Raveendranafhan, N., Loseu, V., Giannantonio, R., Seto, E., Fortino, G.: Enabling multiple BSN applications using the SPINE framework. In: 2010 International Conference on Body Sensor Networks, BSN 2010, pp. 228–233 (2010)
14. Restlet-Website (2014). http://restlet.org
15. Nerino, R., Contin, L., da Silva Pinto, W.G., Massazza, G., Actis, M., Capacchione, P., Chimienti, A., Pettiti, G.: A BSN based service for post-surgical knee rehabilitation at home. In: Proceedings of the 8th International Conference on Body Area Networks (2013)
16. Fortino, G., Gravina, R.: Rehab-aaService: a cloud-based motor rehabilitation digital assistant. In: Proceedings of the 2nd Workshop ICT for Improving Patient Rehabilitation Research Techniques Workshop (REHAB 2014) jointly held with PervasiveHealth 2014 (2014)
17. Fortino, G., Di Fatta, G., Pathan, M., Vasilakos, A.V.: Cloud-assisted body area networks: state-of-the-art and future challenges. Wirel. Netw. **20**(7), 1925–1938 (2014)
18. Fortino, G., Pathan, M., Di Fatta, G.: BodyCloud: integration of cloud computing and body sensor networks. In: Proceedings of the IEEE 4th International Conference on Cloud Computing Technology and Science (CloudCom 2012), pp. 851–856 (2012)
19. Zhang, M., Sawchuk, A.: A customizable framework of body area sensor network for rehabilitation. In: Proceedings of the 2nd International Symposium on Applied Sciences in Biomedical and Communication Technologies, ISABEL 2009, pp. 24–27 (2009)
20. SunSPOT-Website (2014). http://www.sunspotworld.com
21. Rehabitic whitepaper (2014). http://www.imim.es/media/upload/arxius/oferta-%20tecnologica/REHABITICwebIMIM_EN.pdf
22. Lanari Bo, A.P., Hayashibe, M., Poignet, P.: Joint angle estimation in rehabilitation with inertial sensors and its integration with kinect. In: Proceedings of the 33rd Annual International Conference of the IEEE Engineering in Medicine and Biology Society (EMBC 2011) (2011)
23. Huang, C.-L., Chung, C.-Y.: A real-time model-based human motion analysis system. In: Proceedings of the International Conference on Multimedia and Expo 2003, vol. 2 (2003)
24. Naghshineh, S., Ameri, G., Zereshki, M., Krishnan, S., Abdoli-Eramaki, M.: Human motion capture using Tri-Axial accelerometers (2014). http://edge.rit.edu/edge/P10010/public/PDF/HME.pdf
25. El-Gohary, M., Holmstrom, L., Huisinga, J., King, E., McNames, J., Horak, F.: Upper limb joint angle tracking with inertial sensors. In: Proceedings of the 33rd Annual International Conference of the IEEE Engineering in Medicine and Biology Society (EMBC 2011), pp. 5629–5632 (2011)

Early Detection of Cognitive Impairments with the Smart Ageing Serious Game

Dani Tost[1]([✉]), Ariel von Barnekow[1], Eloy Felix[1], Stefania Pazzi[2],
Stefano Puricelli[2], and Sara Bottiroli[3]

[1] CREB-Technical University of Catalonia, Barcelona, Spain
dani@lsi.upc.edu, ariel.von.barnekow@upc.edu, s.pazzi@cbim.it
[2] CBIM-CBIM Consorzio di Bioingegneria E Informatica Medica, Pavia, Italy
{s.pazzi,s.puricelli}@cbim.it
[3] National Neurological Institute Mondino and University of Pavia, Pavia, Italy
sara.bottiroli@unipv.it

Abstract. This paper presents the design and usability validation of
a telematic test aimed at the early detection of Mild Cognitive Impairments in persons ageing between 50 and 80. The test represents a 3D
domestic environment in which users perform 5 daily life activities that
involve various cognitive skills: short-term and mid-term memory, attention, executive functions and spatial orientation. The test is also aimed
at assessing cognitive impairments in persons already diagnosed or having neurodegenerative dementia. In order to make it usable by seniors
without previous computer literacy, the test integrates different accessibility features: automatic navigation, assisted selection and feedback
mechanisms. The usability of the system has been tested with a set of
target users. The results show that users are able to understand the virtual environment and the tasks. In addition, they learn very quickly to
manoeuvring in it. Moreover, they find it attractive.

Keywords: 3D serious games · Mild cognitive impairments · Screening

1 Introduction

There is a general agreement on the idea that playing can boost brain functions
and improve well-being [2]. Playing is a pervasive cognitively demanding activity
that, as shown in a recent study [8], can yield to structural changes in the brain.
Serious Games (SG) designed on a hand-to-hand collaboration between game
developers and neuroscientists can have a more effective impact on cognitive
training than purely leisure games [1].

In particular, SG potentially represent new and effective tools in the management and treatment of cognitive impairments in the elderly [4]. Indeed, there
are evidences that adults engaged in computer activities have decreased odds
of developing Mild Cognitive Impairments (MCI) [13], and that virtual reality-
based memory training can contribute to prevent memory decline [14] and reduce
depressive symptoms [7] in elderly adults.

© Springer-Verlag Berlin Heidelberg 2015
H.M. Fardoun et al. (Eds.): REHAB 2014, CCIS 515, pp. 183–195, 2015.
DOI: 10.1007/978-3-662-48645-0_16

Our main hypothesis is that in addition to rehabilitation and training, SG can also be an effective tool for the detection of cognitive impairments and dementia. Therefore, they can be used to perform large-scale, cheaper screening of the population over 50 yielding to earlier detection of cognitive impairments and anticipated enrollment in rehabilitation programs. A secondary hypothesis is that the efficacy of this tool can be higher if it is based on daily life activities in a realistic 3D scenario in which the user's virtual skills are representative of the actual user skills.

On the basis of this hypothesis and with the ambition of partially substituting pen-and-paper-based tests, we have designed and implemented *SmartAgeing* [17], a web-based electronic test of Mild Cognitive Impairments (MCI) based on the SG technology. In the development of this new technology, we have faced various challenges to make it accessible to a diversity of users most of them without computer skills. We describe our solution in the next sections. A preliminary description of this work have been presented as an extended abstract [17] in Rehab2014. We herein describe it in depth and present and discuss the results of the usability tests.

2   Scenario

The scenario represents a 3D home-like space (loft) providing a diversity of ambiances in one room: dining room, sitting room, bedroom and kitchen, plus a separate bathroom. It is filled with furniture and objects that users can manipulate virtually (see Fig. 1).

The choice of the scenario is motivated by two major reasons: first to be a familiar place that anyone can recognize, and second to be an open space with specialized areas (room, kitchen, sitting room) where a variety of exercises can be done without having to navigate through doors and corridors, because navigation is difficult for most users unfamiliar with computers and games.

The objects that appear in the scenario are commonly used, as international as possible, so that anyone can recognize them. Their design is a trade-off between realism and shape. For many objects, such as food cans, the geometry is very simple and the identification of the product is based mostly on the texture mapped on the model. To make easier the internationalization of the test, we have avoided to overuse text in the textures, and have tried to apply images with a high iconic value, be them drawings or real-life pictures.

The location of the objects in the scenario is configurable, so that the task can be realized several times with different challenges. In all configurations, however, the location of the objects is of common sense in order to avoid unnecessary traps in the tasks of finding objects.

3   User Interface

3.1   Dimension

The game is designed in a first-person perspective so the player experiences the action through the eyes of an invisible avatar which reinforces his/her

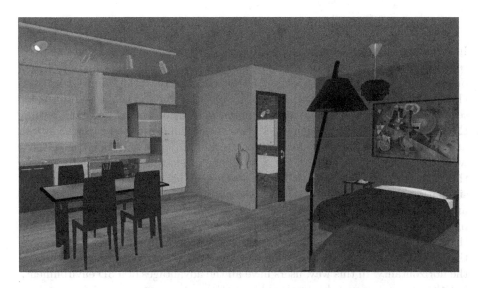

Fig. 1. A view of the virtual scenario

involvement in the game. The actions are dimensionally congruent [5]: navigation and manipulation are done in 3D, but actions that are inherently 2D such as reading and writing are done using 2D interfaces launched from the 3D virtual environment. As an example, in order to dial a telephone number, users interact with the 3D model of the telephone. This causes the display of a 2D view of the telephone where users can dial the numbers very easily (see Fig. 2). Once finished, the game comes back to the last view of the 3D scenario. In this way, the game naturally accommodates the two visualization and interaction models within a same framework.

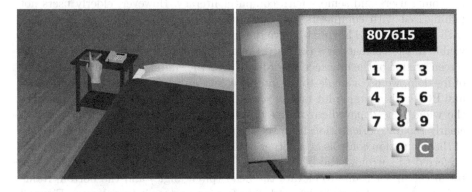

Fig. 2. An example of integration of 2D tasks in the 3D environment

3.2 Degrees-of-Freedom

In order to simplify as much as possible the interface, the interaction has been reduced to three degrees of freedom: two for camera orientation control and one for selection. Locomotion is semi-automatic, based on the Point Of Interest (POI) paradigm [9]. Users click on a POI. Since the scenario is a closed space, all selections fall onto a surface of an environment. If the object at the POI is within the user's avatar reach, the game performs the action associated with the object at that moment of the play, for instance picking, dropping or opening. Otherwise, the best path to reach the POI avoiding collisions is computed [10]. Then, the path is followed automatically at a constant height over the floor's plane simulating a smooth walking. During the automatic navigation, all interactions are disabled. At still positions, users can perform a view-around action implemented as rotations of the pitch and yaw angles (elevation and axial rotation of the head). To prevent exaggerate elevations, a maximum pitch angle is fixed so that at still positions and orientation, after a delay, the system smoothly recovers the horizontality. In this way, users have all the advantages of a 3D environment, but they are not required to master locomotion. More complex movements such as kneeling or stretching are not allowed, since they would complicate the interface unnecessarily. Objects too high for the user's reach are not accessible and just used for decoration.

3.3 Input Devices

Two types of input devices have been tested: with mouse and with a touch screen. In the mouse version, the cursor is always centered in the middle of the graphical area. The mouse movement is mapped to pitch and yaw rotations, and the selection is done by clicking the left mouse button. The object selected is, thus, always at the center of the screen. The preliminary user tests performed during the development of the project [11] showed that this navigation was very intuitive for young users and seniors with computer literacy. However, elderly users not familiarized with computers had difficulties in mapping the mouse movement with the cursor, and having to move the camera center to select an object already visible in the current view confused them. Therefore, we implemented a touch-screen version of the interface. In order to keep the simplicity of the three degrees of freedom, we use a single-touch interface. The cursor is free, so users can select any POI with a simple hit on the screen. For the camera orientation, we chose the widget-based paradigm rather than a gesture-only model [12] in order to clearly separate orientation from selection. Instead of the traditional mini-map of the navigation controls at a corner of the screen, that seemed too abstract, we preferred to surround the 3D view by a partially transparent 2D frame. Users touch the upper frame to elevate the head (pitch angle) and the bottom frame to lower it. They touch the left and right frame to rotate it (yaw angle). Figure 3 shows the interface with the two types of input devices.

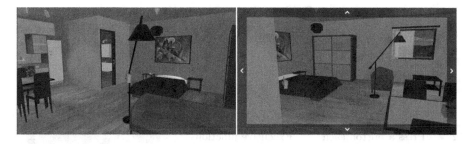

Fig. 3. Three-degrees of freedom interface. At left with a mouse input device: the cursor (shown as a hand) is centered, the mouse movement is mapped to the yaw and pitch angles, and selection is always done at the center of the window where the cursor is fixed. At right with single-touch screen, the frame is used for camera orientation, and the cursor is free for selection at any point of the window. Users do not need to change the orientation to select an object visible in the current frame.

3.4 Manipulation

The available actions with selected objects can be classified in two categories: instantaneous actions and time-lasting actions. The former ones are done immediately, when an interaction is detected. They are to pick, to drop, to turn on and off, to open and close doors. Time-lasting actions such as dragging an object, playing music or filling a can are also available. Picking yields to attaching to the cursor a miniaturized version of the objects that do not collide with the environment. Dragging an object is thus done implicitly through navigation and viewing around with a picked object attached to the cursor. Dropping is then achieved by clicking onto the desired surface.

4 Tasks

The test consists of five tasks addressing different cognitive aspects: executive functions (reasoning and planning), attention (selected and divided), memory (short and long term, perspective), orientation (visuo-spatial). Table 1 summarizes the tasks.

Before starting the tasks, the game presents a traveling through the environment to familiarize the user with it. During this traveling, all the doors and drawers of the cupboards and furniture of the loft are opened one after the other to show their content. Next, a familiarization task is proposed in which users practice the navigation and the selection of objects. They are asked to go to a specific place, to pick and drag objects and to drop them.

The first task consists of finding in the 3D environment the objects shown in a 2D panel at the left of the screen, in total 12 objects. The image in the panel is a representative view of the objects from which they are clearly identifiable. All the objects have been shown in their current location in the initial traveling. Some of them are visible at a simple glance, but most of them require to open

Table 1. Tasks of the test

Task	Description	Cognitive function	Image
1	Find in the 3D kitchen the objects shown in the 2D panel	Memory Spatial orientation Attention	
2	Press a button each time you listen a specific word. Meanwhile, water the flowers.	Executive function Spatial orientation Divided attention	
3	Call Mr. X. Look for his telephone number, learn it and dial. At the end, turn on the television.	Executive function Selective attention Short-term and long-term memory	
4	Identify in the 2D panel the objects you looked for in task 1.	Executive function Selective attention Short-term and long-term memory	
5	Find in the 3D kitchen the objects that you looked for in task 1.	Memory Spatial orientation Attention	

drawers or doors. The task requires memory, spatial orientation and attention at the same time.

In the second task, users are asked to turn on the radio and listen. They must perform a click each time they listen a specific word. With the mouse-driven input, the click is performed with the left button of the mouse, and in the touch screen version, a 2D button is shown at the bottom part of the screen, above the navigation bar. After a while, users are required to water the flowers while keeping clicking when they listen the word. Watering is a sequential activity: picking the watering can, filling it in the tap (which requires to first turn on the faucet and after having filled the can, recalling to turn it off), and finally, watering the flowers. Thus, the task involves divided attention and executive planning functions.

In the third task, users are first warned to turn on the television at the end of the task. Then, they must select the agenda that is on top of the table near the bed. The selection deploys a 2D interface where users must find open the agenda at the right page and then, click on the proper name. Then, the telephone number is shown. Users learn it during a maximum lapse of time that they can shorten freely. After that, the game comes back to the 3D environment where users select the telephone yielding to the deployment of a 2D interface for dialing. At the end of the task users must remember to turn on the television. This task involves short-term and long-term memory and executive functions and selective attention.

Finally tasks 4 and 5 are related to task 1. In task 4, a 2D panel with 20 objects is shown. Users must identify in the panel the 12 objects selected in task 1 among the impostors. This task tests memory. In task 5 the user must find the objects in 3D as in task 1, but without following any instruction. It is therefore a long-term memory exercise coupled with spatial orientation and attention.

5 Indices

The game records all users actions. From these data, it computes a set of indices for each task of the game separately. At the end of the game these indices are parsed to give an overall score of the patient's cognitive skills. Currently, clinicians are working on the evaluation model, with the goal of making it equivalent to standardized measures based on pen and paper screening tests. Recording all the indices provides flexibility in adjusting the model during the validation stage.

The parameters registered by the game are summarized in Table 2. We differentiate between correct and incorrect actions. Correct actions can be done on time or within a pre-defined delay. For instance, in task 1, identifying an object is correct and on time if the picture of the object is shown in the panel when the identification is done. It is correct but not in time when it is identified after

Table 2. Main indices registered for each task of the game

Interactions	Number of navigation interactions
	Number of interactions on 3D objects
	Number of interactions on 2D objects
	Number of interactions on 2D widgets (button)
Actions	Number of correct actions on time
	Number of correct actions out-of-time
	Number of incorrect actions
Navigation	Distance traveled
	Total
Time	Per action
	Void
	Between interactions

the object has been shown and within a given delay. It is incorrect if the object has never been shown before or when the delay has expired.

6   Validation

6.1   Usability Validation

The development of the game was done on the basis of a strong collaboration between clinicians and game developers and following a user-centric development paradigm. Thus, throughout the development of the project, the game was periodically evaluated by clinicians and tested by small groups of users including patients with cognitive decline.

At the end of the development we performed a usability test on 16 users aged from 55 to 82 (average age of 64.4), 7 women and 9 men, without any 3D computer game experience but with different computer skills. None of the participants were diagnosed of cognitive decline. The participants were volunteers, recruited in the social network of the team and had no relationship with the project. Each test was performed separately and conducted by a member of the team acting as facilitator. Seven of them used a touch screen, while the other ten used the mouse. At the beginning of the experiment, the facilitator clarified the aims of the experiment and stated clearly that only the usability of the game was going to be measured, not the cognitive skills of the participants. During the experiment the facilitator encouraged the participants to "think aloud" and freely comment on the interaction techniques. At the end, the participants filled a 10-questions SUS test [3] extended with 4 specific questions (SUS-E, see Table 3). The minimum, maximum and average values of each question are shown in Fig. 4. Table 4 shows the extended SUS scores for all participants, sorted by age. This SUS-E score corresponds to the 4 additional questions. It was computed similarly to the SUS score by giving for positive questions (P11, P12, P13 and P5) the selected value in the Likert scale minus one and, for negative questions, five minus the selected value. The sum of points has been multiplied by 5 to have a scale from 0 to 100. Finally, Table 5 shows the maximum, minimum average and standard deviation of the SUS and SUS-E scores.

All participants could finish the four tasks with only very few errors. The time needed to complete the tasks were rather similar, except for Task 4 that some users completed very quickly (see Table 6). Participants were nervous at the beginning, fearing not being able to play, but they felt quickly confident. Although none of them had any experience with 3D environments, they immediately understood the first-person perspective and had a feeling of immersion in the environment. In general, all users liked the game and found it usable and fun. The SUS and SUS-E scores are in general very high. Participants that were tested with the touch screen were invited to test also the mouse input version. All them referred to feel more comfortable with the touch screen that they found easier to master, even if they were used to the mouse. The average SUS and SUS-E scores of these users is higher that the score of the other users: 95.36 and 92.14 versus 85.83 and 85. This result coincides with the preliminary tests done

Table 3. The SUS test extended with 4 additional questions.

P1	I think that I would like to use this system frequently
P2	I found the system unnecessarily complex
P3	I thought the system was easy to use
P4	I think that I would need the support of a technical person to be able to use this system
P5	I found the various functions in this system were well integrated
P6	I thought there was too much inconsistency in this system
P7	I would imagine that most people would learn to use this system very quickly
P8	I found the system very cumbersome to use
P9	I felt very confident using the system
P10	I needed to learn a lot of things before I could get going with this system
Extra questions	
P11	I like the graphical design of the game
P13	The tasks are similar to daily life activities
P14	I understood the instructions
P15	I had technological difficulties in achieving the goals
P16	I think the game is fun

Table 4. Usability analysis results

Participant	1	2	3	4	5	6	7	8	9	10	11	12	13	14	15	16
Age	55	56	56	58	58	58	60	62	62	63	64	70	72	81	81	82
Gender	F	F	M	M	F	M	F	F	M	M	M	F	M	M	F	M
Computer skills	5	5	5	5	2	2	2	2	2	2	2	2	1	5	3	2
Device	T	T	T	T	M	M	M	M	M	M	M	M	T	T	T	M
SUS score	100	100	97.5	97.5	90	100	90	92.5	95	92.5	57.5	77.5	90	92.5	90	77.5
SUS-E score	95	100	90	95	95	100	75	95	80	70	65	100	100	75	90	85

Table 5. Usability test scores

	min	max	aver	stdev
SUS	57.5	100	90.00	3.54
SUS-E	65.0	100	87.33	14.14

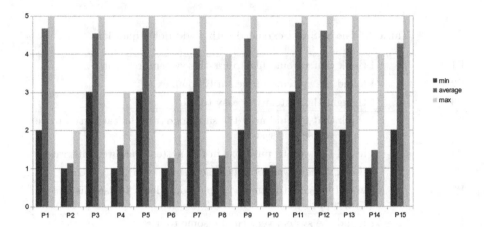

Fig. 4. Minimum, average and maximum values of the extended SUS quest.

Table 6. Time required to perform the tasks

	Task 1	Task 2	Task 3	Task 4
min	393.0	188.0	95.0	32.0
max	562.0	234.0	158.0	71.0
aver	476.2	209.7	117.4	59.4
stdev	68.6	4.2	7.1	24.7

on neuropsychological patients that yield to the development of the touch screen version. Some of touch screen users, that were familiar with tablet devices, tried to drag the objects with the finger and to apply gesture to rotate the camera. This may indicate that a gesture version of the game could also be useful. A few of them commented that the design of a couple of objects (banana and toasts) was not enough realistic. These objects have now been changed.

7   Scientific Validation

The scientific validation stage is currently in process with a primary target group represented by 1000, 50 years old and older persons, 50 to 80 of which are already diagnosed with MCI and/or neurodegenerative dementia. MCI patients are recruited from IRCCS Mondino and Don Gnocchi Foundation, which are two important centers for the diagnosis and treatment of neurological disorders. Subjects are already diagnosed as affected by MCI according to [15] criteria and selected from the institutions' patient registries. The inclusion criteria are a Mini Mental State Examination - MMSE [6] score > 24 and the memory domain subscale of the Clinical Dementia Rating Scale < 0.5.

The sample of 1000 users are recruited from aggregation centers, public entities as well as through newspaper advertisements. The sample will be stratified

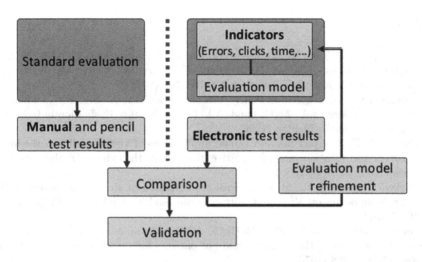

Fig. 5. Schema of the scientific validation process

according to gender (female/male), age (50–60, 61–70, 71–80), and education (primary, middle, high, university). The inclusion criteria are a negative history for neurologic and psychiatric diseases, a MMSE score > 24 and a performance within normative ranges for age and education at the pen and pencil tests. It is expected that at least 8 % [16] of these participants will be excluded from the validation stage failing to pass the inclusion criteria, and then resulting as potentially affected by any neurological disorders. As shown in Fig. 5 in the validation stage, the evaluation model will be refined to compute a score equivalent to standardized scores for pen and pencil test.

8   Conclusions

The *SmartAgeing* serious game is a novel methodology to detect cognitive impairments while performing 3D real-life tasks. It brings an automatic way of reporting the users performance through the registration of many run-time parameters. The usability results of the tests performed throughout the development of the game and at its end show that the game is easy-to-use and fun, specially the touch screen version. After the scientific validation stage, we expect to be able to show its efficacy and ecological value. Once deployed for large-scale screening campaigns, it will require less resources both in terms of time and human activity that current methodologies. Finally, the *SmartAgeing* scenario can also be used to perform rehabilitation tasks for diagnosed patients. In this case, it will provide a coherent environment that will allow a continuous tracking of the patients evolution. We are currently working on this extension of the system.

References

1. Bavelier, D., Davidson, R.: Games to do you good. Nature **494**, 425–426 (2013)
2. Bavelier, D., Green, C., Han, D., Renshaw, P., Merzenich, M., Gentile, D.: Brains on video games. Nat. Rev. Neurosci. **12**, 763–768 (2012)
3. Brooke, J.: SUS: a quick and dirty usability scale. In: Jordan, P.W., Thomas, B., Weerdmeester, B.A., McClelland, A.L. (eds.) Usability Evaluation in Industry. Taylor and Francis, London (1996)
4. Cherniack, E.: Not just fun and games: applications of virtual reality in the identification and rehabilitation of cognitive disorders of the elderly. Disabil. Rehabil. Assist. Technol. **6**(4), 283–289 (2011)
5. Darken, R., Durost, R.: Mixed-dimension interaction in virtual environments. In: ACM Symposium on Virtual Reality Software and Technology VRST 2005, pp. 38–45 (2005)
6. Folstein, MF., Folstein, SE., McHugh, PRG.: Mini-mental state. A practical method for grading the cognitive state of patients for the clinician. J. Psychiatr. Res. **12**, 189–198 (1975)
7. Fernández-Calvo, B., Rodriguez-Pérez, R., Contador, L., Rubio-Santorum, A., Ramos, F.: Efficacy of cognitive training programs based on new software technologies in patients with Alzeimer-type dementia. Psicothema **23**(1), 44–50 (2011)
8. Kühn, S., Gleich, T., Lorenz, R., Lindenberger, U., Gallinat, J.: Playing Super Mario induces structural brain plasticity: gray matter changes resulting from training with a commercial video game. Mol. Psychiatr. **19**, 265–271 (2014)
9. Mackinlay, J.D., Card, S.K., Robertson, G.G.: Rapid controlled movement through a virtual 3D workspace. In: ACM Computers and Graphics, Proceedings of SIGGRAPH 1990, pp. 171–176 (1990)
10. Moya, S., Grau, S., Tost, D.: The wise cursor: assisted selection in 3D serious games. Vis. Comput. **29**(6–8), 795–804 (2013)
11. Moya, S., Grau, S., Tost, D.: First-person locomotion in 3D virtual environments: a usability analysis. J. Univ. Comput. Sci. **20**(7), 1026–1045 (2014)
12. Marchal, D., Moerman, C., Casiez, G., Roussel, N.: Designing intuitive multi-touch 3D navigation techniques. In: Winckler, M. (ed.) INTERACT 2013, Part I. LNCS, vol. 8117, pp. 19–36. Springer, Heidelberg (2013)
13. Negash, S., Smith, G., Pankratz, S., Aakre, J., Geda, Y., Roberts, R., Knopman, D., Boeve, B., Ivnik, R., Petersen, R.: Successful aging: definitions and prediction of longevity and conversion to mild cognitive impairment. Am. J. Geriatr. Psychiatr. **19**(6), 581–588 (2011)
14. Optale, G., Urgesi, C., Busato, V., Marin, S., Piron, L., Priftis, K., Gamberini, L., Capodieci, S., Bordin, A.: Controlling memory impairment in elderly adults using virtual reality memory training: a randomized controlled pilot study. Neurorehabilitation and Neural Repair **24**(4), 348–357 (2010)
15. Petersen, RC., Stevens, JC., Ganguli, M., et al.: Practice parameter: early detection of dementia: mild cognitive impairment (an evidence-based review). Report of the quality standards subcommittee of the American Academy of Neurology. Neurology **56**(9), 1133–1142 (2001)

16. Ravaglia, G., Forti, P., Montesi, F., et al.: Mild cognitive impairment: epidemiology and dementia risk in an elderly Italian population. J. Am. Geriatr. Soc. **56**, 51–58 (2008)
17. Tost, D., Pazzi, S., von Barnekow, A., Felix, E., Puricelli, S., Bottiroli, S.: SmartAgeing: a 3D serious game for elderly detection of mild cognitive impairments. In: Proceedings of the 8th International Conference on Pervasive Computing Technologies for Healthcare (PervasiveHealth 2014), ICST, Brussels, Belgium, pp. 294–297 (2014)

Design and Evaluation of a Self Adaptive Architecture for Upper-Limb Rehabilitation

Alexis Heloir[1,2]([✉]), Fabrizio Nunnari[1], Sylvain Haudegond[2,3],
Clémentine Havrez[2,3], Yoann Lebrun[2,3], and Christophe Kolski[2]

[1] DFKI, Saarbrücken, Germany
[2] LAMIH-UMR CNRS 8201, Valenciennes, France
[3] Play Research Lab - CCI-Grand Hainaut, Valenciennes, France
alexis.heloir@univ-valenciennes.fr

Abstract. This chapter presents an intuitive user interface based on a self-adaptive architecture. It uses a consumer-range 3D hand capture device that allows its users to interactively edit objects in 3D space. While running, the system monitors the user's behaviors and performance in order to maintain an up-to-date user model. This model then drives the re-arrangement and reparameterization of a rule-based system that controls the interaction. A user study let us define the initial parameters of this self-adaptive system. This preliminary study was conducted in a 3D infographics and animation school on 15 students. The study was both qualitative and quantitative: the qualitative evaluation consisted of a SUMI evaluation questionnaire while the quantitative evaluation consisted of analysing manually annotated recordings of the subjects together with a fine-grained log of the interaction mechanics. We believe that the self-adaptive aspects of the system is well suited to the problematics of rehabilitation. This system could, from the beginning, adapt to both the user's impairments and needs, then follow and adapt its interaction logic according to the user's progress. Such a system would, for instance, enable a clinician or a therapist to design tailored rehabilitation activities accounting for the patient's exact physical and physiological condition.

Keywords: Training tools for rehabilitation · Motor rehabilitation · Virtual rehabilitation · Gesture based interaction · Self-adaptive architecture

1 Introduction

New possibilities offered by Information Technologies lead to the proposition and the massive deployment of new multimodal User Interfaces (UIs) [4,6,12,15,18]. These new types of UI allow new usages in various application domains, including healthcare and rehabilitation [2,7,13,17]. More precisely, recent advances in consumer-range interaction devices like the Kinect[1] or the Leap Motion[2] have

---

[1] http://www.xbox.com/kinect (10 September 2014).
[2] http://www.leapmotion.com (10 September 2014).

© Springer-Verlag Berlin Heidelberg 2015
H.M. Fardoun et al. (Eds.): REHAB 2014, CCIS 515, pp. 196–209, 2015.
DOI: 10.1007/978-3-662-48645-0_17

opened the door to an unpreceded range of new UIs, interaction modalities and metaphors where gesture and bodily interaction are the cornerstones [19].

Taking inspiration from these trends, we propose in this chapter a self adaptive architecture that has the potential to assist users in 3D authoring task. We believe that the interaction metaphors offered by such architecture can be used for building self-adaptive rehabilitation applications that focus on the upper limbs (arms and wrist). In this chapter, we extend our paper published in the REHAB 2014 conference [5] (extended introduction, conclusion, and state of art, revised design framework, detailed user study). Our contribution consists of a proposal for a self-adaptive architecture that has the potential to be used in the field of rehabilitation. We also detail the user study that we conducted in order to assess the usability and the efficiency of the proposed architecture. We evaluate the system by analysing the behavior and performance of fifteen subjects who have some experience in 3D editing and animation. The results of the evaluation suggest three categories of users that might be considered when designing the user model underlying the architecture. The remainder of this paper is organized as follows. The next section describes the self-adaptive architecture proposed and used in this research. Section 3 details the evaluation. Section 4 presents our conclusions and research perspectives.

2   Self Adaptive Architecture

In the literature, specific input devices and interactive user interfaces (UIs) are research topics which aim at improving the task of *authoring* in 3D modeling and animation softwares [8]. Some researches propose devices that are either better suited to live animation recording (by capturing the motion and the dynamics of the user [3]) or to static 3D editing [14] (by allowing the user to perform complex translation and orientation tasks in a 3D space). Only few system are actually suited to both interaction schemes [10], and the possibility to switch seamlessly between the two during an editing session have not really been exploited. We propose to extend the architecture presented in [5] and to evaluate it so we could use the evaluation result to tune the default parametrization of the system. The system we propose is innovative because not only it allows a large variety of users to naturally edit complex animations using natural input devices, it also adapts itself to the user's performance and experience profile. This system is designed upon the Leap Motion device. It represents a new way to track and record the position and orientation of the users hands. It permits to control an object that is manipulated in a 3D editing space. The overall architecture of this system is presented in Fig. 1. The architecture is composed of 3 components following a feedback-controlled loop model, each component is individually detailed in the following:

- *Motion Analyzer*: this component infers a set of mid-level motion primitives and sends them to the *Interaction Manager*.
- *Interaction Manager*: this component is a reconfigurable rule based system in charge of triggering the right interaction mode according to its input motion primitives. The interaction manager delivers a flow of edit actions.

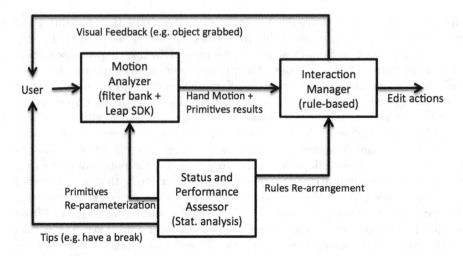

Fig. 1. Proposed architecture, inspired by a feedback controller pattern.

- *Status and Performance Assessor*: this component analyzes continuously the flow from the *Interaction Manager*.

2.1 Motion Analyzer

The Motion analyzer is a component that receives and interprets the data acquired directly from the Leap Motion device. This data, represented by a flow of frames, is filtered out and analyzed. This is achieved by a set of primitive functions stored in the component and applied over a two-second time-sliding window buffer. All these functions are predicates, and a selection of them can be viewed as anonymous functions that are to be instantiated, parametrized and combined according to the instructions delivered by the Status and Performance Assessor and stored in the ruleset of the interaction manager.

2.2 Interaction Manager

The Interaction Manager updates the interaction state depending on the set of motion primitives returned by the Motion Analyzer, as shown in Fig. 1. These primitives are analyzed by a dynamic rule engine, driving to one of the three following interaction states: (1) HOVER, when the user is not acting on an object but his or her hand is detected by the device, (2) GRAB, when he or she is acting on an object and (3) IDLE, when no user's hand is detected by the device.

Figure 2 visually depicts the states and transitions of the Interaction Manager. To move from one state to another, some primitives are defined, mostly based on the user's performance time and the distance of the hand. When a hand

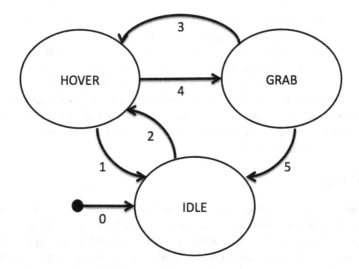

Fig. 2. The interaction mechanics of our system, presented as a state chart.

is newly detected, the state goes to HOVER (transition 1 on Fig. 2). On the contrary, when it is not detected anymore, the state becomes IDLE (transition 2). To move on GRAB state, the user has to stabilize his or her hand for some time in the tracked area (transition 4). The object is then considered as grabbed, and the user can move his or hand in order to move the object. Of course, the hand must stay in the detected action space throughout the desired move. Otherwise, the state will switch to IDLE (transition 5) and the user will have to re-grab the object, stopping the ongoing action and replacing his or her hand. To stop the action, the user has to stabilize one again his or her hand (transition 3).

2.3   Self-adaptivity – Status and Performance Assessor

The rules characterizing the state change we introduced in the previous section are not fixed. Indeed, the primitives on which the rules are based on can be dynamically modified so that the system is more easily usable for a user. These modifications of the primitives are handled by the Status and Performance Assessor.

The ability of the user to stabilize his or her hand, his or her velocity and his or her reactivity to visual clues are taken into account. The system can adapt itself permanently and does not try to stick to a fixed model of the user. Thus, it follows the performance of the user and assists him or her according to his or her current performance level. To sum up, our system can be viewed as a closed feedback loop systems where the output (user performance) is constantly monitored and influences the amplification (or attenuation) of the input signal (user actions) until the system reaches a stable state. If the user performance latter changes, the thresholds will be decreased or increased, in order to adapt the reactivity and sensitivity of the system to the user. On the contrary, if the user performance is decreasing, thresholds will be relaxed to make the system less prone to timeouts and movement range exceeding. Even if the system is capable of on-the-fly adaptation, the initial parametrization of the system is crucial: it should be consistent to the underlying user model and generic enough to partially fit all users capabilities. The following of this paper presents a user study that provides some initial cues on the user model we are currently building these cues will eventually drive us towards a satisfying initial parametrization of the system that fits most users.

3   Evaluation

Using a mouse-based interface or a multitouch screen, users can control at most three to four degrees of freedom at the same time ([X, Y, scroll] or [X, Y, pinch, rotate]). In contrast, a 3D input device provides a direct mapping between the physical space of the user's hand and the edit space along six degrees of freedom (Rotation and Translation). In theory, users could simultaneously move and rotate objects in the 3D space, thereby perform edit tasks faster. We thus expect direct 3D manipulation to perform better than the mouse and keyboard, at least for 3D object positioning. For single target selection, Sears and Shneiderman [16] have shown that direct-touch outperforms the mouse. We performed a qualitative and quantitative evaluation to assess the ease of use and the perceived quality of use of this application. The quantitative evaluation consisted of a user test with fifteen subjects. The goal of this empirical evaluation was to observe people using the system in order to test specific issues such as hand tracking, for example. For the qualitative evaluation, all the subjects were asked to complete a SUMI questionnaire (Software Usability Measurement Inventory) [11] at the end of the user test. The goal of this subjective evaluation was to measure some scores related to their experience with the system they have just used.

3.1   Task and Experiment Design

The task we asked users to perform consisted of a docking task, as illustrated in Fig. 3. Users had to place and align the grey box inside a semi-transparent red box. When the grey box was correctly docked, the semi-transparent red box turned green. The experimental session has been split into three scenes of increasing complexity: translation only, rotation only, translation and rotation. The subject had to accomplish ten tasks per scene. Box size was set to $40 \times 20 \times 10$cm, the external size of the container box to $56 \times 28 \times 14$cm. Location and rotation tolerance have been imposed by the authors according to preliminary tests. Location tolerance was set to 6 cm (15 % of the longer edge), rotation tolerance to 0.2 rad ($\sim$11.5 degrees).

We compared the performances of users in the 3D positioning task by comparing two input conditions:

1. Mouse and keyboard (Mouse),
2. Our novel input system based on hand-tracker (Leap).

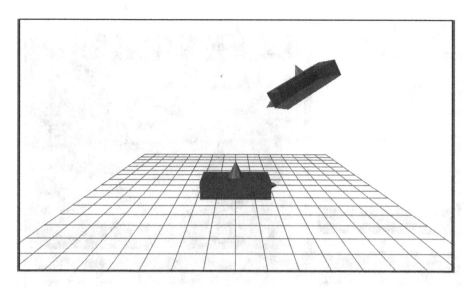

Fig. 3. This is what the user views when performing the task: a target brick and a brick that needs to be docked

3.2   Subjects and Apparatus

We conducted the evaluations with fifteen subjects. They all knew how to animate a 3D object, which requires high skills acquired over a long period of time. Subjects were animation students in third or fourth year of a renowned 2D&3D animation school located in Valenciennes, France, called Supinfocom, from the Rubika group[3]. These students can be considered as skilled 3D modeller and animators. They use softwares like 3D Studio Max[4] and Maya[5] daily. Subjects accomplished the tasks with both traditional mouse and keyboard (Mouse condition) input system and with the Leap Motion based system (Leap condition). The panel of the 15 subjects was made up of 11 men and 4 women. The evaluation process was the same for every participant and the session lasted approximately one hour each. The session was supervised by two experimenters. All the participants received verbal instructions from one experimenter and the other was present to assist in case of difficulties with the questionnaire.

The study was carried out on a Laptop PC connected to a 22 in. monitor (resolution 1680 × 1050). The screen was standing at about 60 cm of distance from the subject. One evaluator was sitting next to the subject, supervising the advancement of the experiment over the shoulder, switching between tasks and the (de)activation the logging system. The 3D environment was Blender[6] version 2.66.1. We developed a set of Python language scripts to map the Leap Motion

---

[3] http://supinfocom.rubika-edu.com/ (10 September 2014).

[4] http://www.autodesk.fr/products/3ds-max/overview (10 September 2014).

[5] http://www.autodesk.fr/products/maya/overview (10 September 2014).

[6] http://www.blender.org/ (10 September 2014).

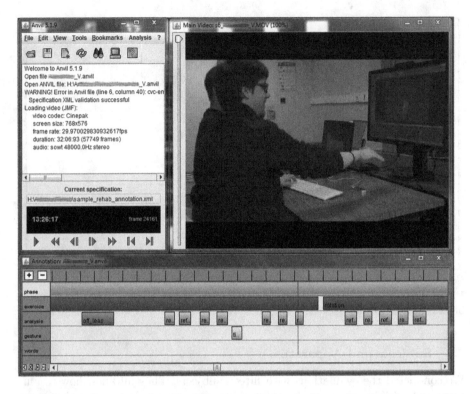

Fig. 4. Screenshot of the Anvil annotation tool whit the log and annotation channels synchronized.

input onto 3D objects position. The sources that are necessary to build and reproduce the described experiment are published on-line[7].

3.3 Quantitative Evaluation

In order to retrieve the interaction data, we instrumented the Blender software to keep track of and log all the actions performed by the users. We later processed the log, synchronized them with the video and imported them back into the Anvil annotation tool [9]. Figure 4 shows the Anvil user interface featuring the multiple tracks imported and the tracks used for manual annotations. Signs of fatigue and moments when the arm was down were annotated manually in the Anvil software. These annotation were stored in two separated tracks. For three users (#2, #4, and #5), the logger didn't start and no interaction data could be collected.

Figure 5 shows, for each task (translation only, rotation only and combined), the completion times between a keyboard/mouse and our system. This figure

---

[7] http://slsi.dfki.de/software-and-resources/ (10 September 2014).

suggests that the performance is, for most users comparable for the translation-only task and for the translation + rotation task. Users seem to perform worse in the orientation only task. This difference might be explained by the relatively unstable tracking of the sensor that was available at the time we conducted the experiment. At the time, the SDK provided by the manufacturer couldn't cope well with hand orientation changes. For translation and orientation tasks, performances are similar between our system and a classical mouse and keyboard solution. The fact that our hand tracked solution does not outperform the mouse and keyboard modality might be explained by two things: first, the tracking was not yet perfect, as for the orientation only task. Second, in this setup, there is no on the fly adaptation, the interaction does not account for the user's capabilities. Therefore, the system might be "out-of-tune" for the user. We can see, for instance that user #6 exhibits outstanding performance when using our system. This might be explained by the fact that the default (and static) configuration of the system was well-suited to this user.

Figure 6 shows additional results obtained through the manual annotation. It presents, for each user (represented as a circle, an horizontal triangle or a vertical triangle) the amount of time he or she spent his or her arm up and down (resting position). These results provide hints about how usable is our Leap-based system. Users where clustered using the K-mean algorithm and the elbow method [1]. Furthermore, we performed a linear regression on the data after having removed the outliers. We found strong regression coefficients (> 0.83). It appears that there is a strong linear relationship between the frequency of arm down events and the time spent wile having the arm up or down.

Two insights might be drawn from these results. First (Fig. 6 right), the more often the arm is down, the shorter time it is kept in mid-air (up). This suggests that subjects who are more likely to perform quick interactions have the tendency to rest their arm more often. Second (Fig. 6 left), the more often he or she puts his/her arm down, the longer the arm is down. Also readable as: the less often the arm is down, the shorter it is kept in a resting position. The latter result seems rather counter-intuitive: one would instead expect that subjects who put less their arm in a resting position would also rest their arm longer, and we would also expect that users who rest their arm more frequently would also keep their arm for a shorter period of time in a resting position. One can only speculate about the reason why users have this tendency to either rest their arm longer and more frequently or to keep their arm in mid-air, even if they end up to be tired. Further studies involving motion capture and inverse dynamics might be necessary. This would give us the possibility to precisely infer the amount of muscular energy spent – and thus the fatigue level – of each user. Also, the fact that users could be clustered into four categories suggests that we might consider some form of user-categorization to build our user adaptive model.

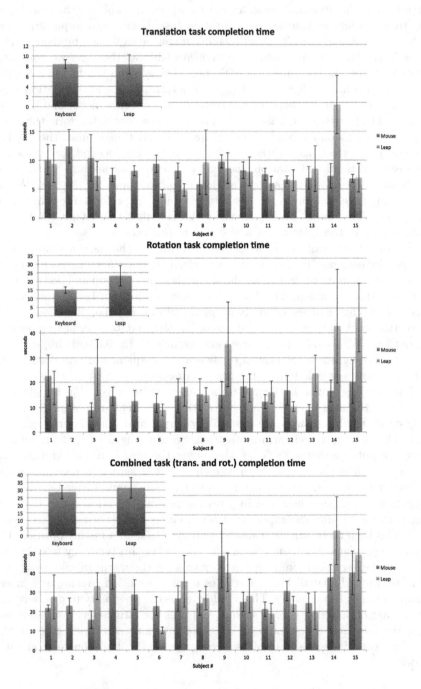

Fig. 5. Completion times along the three tasks.

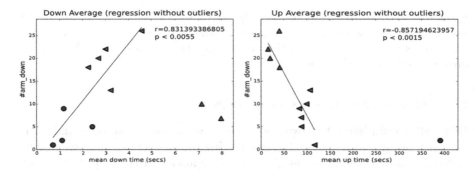

Fig. 6. The clusters inferred from our annotation data, for hand up (mid-air) and hand down (hand on the table) behavior.

3.4 Questionnaire Methodology

After the test, each user was asked to fill-in a questionnaire related to the usage of the self-adaptive architecture system. We used the SUMI questionnaire[8] [11] and translated it into French. The questionnaire includes 5 subscales which have been referenced in ISO 9126 and ISO 9241 international standard on usability and quality of use. These 5 subscales are related to:

- Efficiency: degree to which the user can directly achieve the goals of his/her interaction with the system;
- Affect: measures the users general emotional responses to the system;
- Helpfulness: degree to which the system user feels that the system assists him/her;
- Control: measures the extent to which the user feels in control of the system, not the other way;
- Learnability: measures the ease to which the user feels that he/she has been able to get started and the speed at which he/she has been able to master the system acquiring new features.

The questionnaire also provides a global usability score which is a mean of the 5 subscales. For each statement the subject can choose between three possible answers ("agree", "undecided", "disagree"). Here are two examples of the statements that were given:

- "The way that system information is presented is clear and understandable;"
- "I sometimes wonder if I am using the right command."

There are 50 statements in total, 10 of which are related to the subscales. The wording of the question may be affirmative or negative. Therefore, the right answers are not necessarily positive ("agree" responses). It really depends on each question. For example, if the question is "This system responds too slowly

---

[8] http://sumi.ucc.ie/ (10 September 2014).

to inputs", the correct response is "disagree", so a negative response. If the user responds negatively to this question, his/her response is considered a good one. Scores are calculated from the percentages of good responses obtained to questions related to the subscale.

3.5   Questionnaire Results and Analysis

Right after completing the tasks with the system, the 15 subjects individually filled in the questionnaire. In the following, we enumerate some conclusions and comment on one important observation we made during the test. First, we noticed that the proportion of "undecided" responses was important. A lot of subjects seem to be confused with some of the questions. If the subject thinks the question is not appropriate or consistent with what he/she did during the test, the point is to answer "undecided". 22% of the subjects replied "undecided" compared to 69.8% of positive responses and 8.2% of negatives ones. Table 1 shows the overall scores for the various subscales of usability.

Table 1. Questionnaire scores

	Global	Efficiency	Affect	Helpfulness	Controllability	Learnability
Mean	61.2	61.4	65.6	59.6	53.6	63.7
St Dev	5.4	7.5	8.8	5.3	6.4	5.8

The various scores are fairly high. There are all above 50% representing the acceptance criteria. The global scale is equal to 61.2% which indicates that the system is globally usable according to the questionnaire (see Table 1). This score represents the number of positive appreciations regarding the gestural user interface tested by the subjects. No major corrective action seems to be needed.

As we can see in Fig. 7, one subscale is below the other, close to 50%: Controllability (i.e. the extent to which the user feels in control of the system) with the mean value of 53.6%. It seems to indicate that the users feel that they are not totally in control of the system. This finding is consistent with the observation made during the test. Indeed, in order for the system to work properly, the user must keep his/her hand inside a limited area over the hand tracker. This effective area is similar to an invisible detection cone, above the Leap Motion device placed on the desk. Since there is no visual feedback, it is challenging for the user to know whether the hand is inside the detection cone or not. In fact, we observed that the user's hand often moves out of the detection limits. The consequence is that the user has the impression of not having complete control over the system. The lack of visual feedback might also impair the Helpfulness subscale, which is relatively low compared to the other subscales (59.6%).

The user seems to feel that the system does not provide enough help when needed. The participants experienced some frustration with the hand tracker,

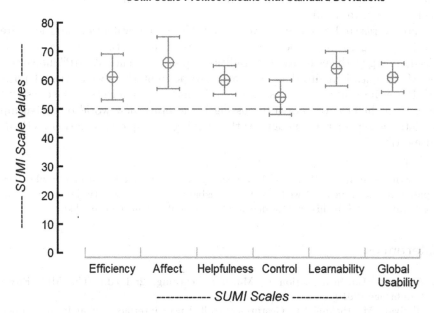

Fig. 7. Profile showing questionnaire subscales

being sometimes unable to move and rotate 3D objects. They sometimes suggested a visual feedback to help them relocate their hand correctly above the hand tracker.

4 Conclusion and Future Work

Potentially, the self-adaptive system that we presented can help injured patients to perform rehabilitation exercises remotely from their home. Their progress and their performance towards recovery would be assessed in real-time by the system and adapted guidance would be provided at the right time. For example, the system can call a trained clinician for assistance if the system detects that the patient is not progressing. The user interface we proposed in this chapter is designed for the upper limbs (hands and wrists). There is good reason to believe that the self-adaptive architecture we described would also be suited to the rehabilitation of other body parts.

The protocol presented in this chapter involved users who have experience with regard to 3D editing. As a consequence, the set of generic rules that we would infer from this user study might not fit users that are novice with regard to 3D editing. Indeed, in this system, user adaptation is enforced by tuning the variables and rules driving the interaction according to the parameters of a basic user model that is adapted from the user's behavior and performance. Even if the system is supposed to converge towards an optimal set of rules, inferred at runtime from the user's behavior, it needs to start with a set of rules that is generic enough to fit all users.

Another research perspective would be to design an evaluation questionnaire that is specific to multimodal user interfaces. The questionnaire we used, is indeed aiming at the evaluation of traditional point and click WIMP[9] interfaces. The SUMI questionnaire does not take into account the specificities of post-WIMP user interfaces, as it was expressed by many respondents of the questionnaire. It might however worth discussing if the brave new world of post-wimp user interfaces is mature enough for the defining principled evaluation methods and metrics.

Acknowledgment. Authors would especially like to thank the students who participated to the study as well as Azad Lusbaronian, head of studies at Supinfocom / Rubika SAS for his involvement and the essential help he provided.

References

1. Alpaydin, E.: Introduction to Machine Learning, 2nd edn. The MIT Press, Cambridge (2010)
2. Bhuiyan, M., Picking, R.: Gesture-controlled user interfaces, what have we done and whats next. In: Proceedings of the Fifth Collaborative Research Symposium on Security, E-Learning, Internet and Networking (SEIN 2009), pp. 25–29. Darmstadt, Germany (2009)
3. Chai, J., Hodgins, J.K.: Performance animation from low-dimensional control signals. In: Proceedings of ACM Transactions on Graphics (2005)
4. Hale, K.S., Stanney, K.M.: Handbook of Virtual Environments: Design, Implementation, and Applications. CRC Press, New York (2014)
5. Heloir, A., Haudegond, S., Lebrun, Y., Nunnari, F., Kolski, C.: Description of a self-adaptive architecture for upper-limb rehabilitation. In: 2nd ICTs for improving Patient Rehabilitation Research Techniques Workshop REHAB 2014, in conjunction with PervasiveHealth 2014. Oldenbourg, Germany (2014)
6. Jacko, J.A.: Human-Computer Interaction Handbook: Fundamentals, Evolving Technologies, and Emerging Applications. CRC Press Inc, Boca Raton (2012)
7. Kim, D., Kim, D.: An intelligent smart home control using body gestures. In: International Conference on Hybrid Information Technology 2006, ICHIT 2006, vol. 2, pp. 439–446 Nov 2006
8. Kin, K., Agrawala, M., DeRose, T.: Determining the benefits of direct-touch, bimanual, and multifinger input on a multitouch workstation. In: Graphics Interface 2009, GI 2009, pp. 119–124 (2009)
9. Kipp, M.: Anvil - a generic annotation tool for multimodal dialogue. In: Dalsgaard, P., Lindberg, B., Benner, H., Tan, Z.-H. (eds.) INTERSPEECH, pp. 1367–1370. ISCA (2001)
10. Kipp, M., Nguyen, Q.: Multitouch puppetry: Creating coordinated 3d motion for an articulated arm. In: ACM International Conference on Interactive Tabletops and Surfaces, ITS 2010, pp. 147–156. ACM, New York (2010)

---

[9] "windows, icons, menus, pointer".

11. Kirakowski, J., Corbett, M.: SUMI: the software usability measurement inventory. Br. J. Educ. Technol. **24**(3), 210–212 (1993)
12. Kolski, C.: Human-computer Interactions in Transport. John Wiley & Sons, Hoboken (2011)
13. L'Abate, L., Kaiser, D.A.: Handbook of Technology in Psychology, Psychiatry and Neurology: Theory, Research, and Practice. Nova Science Publishers, New York (2012)
14. Lin, J., Igarashi, T., Mitani, J., Liao, M., He, Y.: A sketching interface for sitting pose design in the virtual environment. IEEE Trans. Vis. Comput. Graph. **18**(11), 1979–1991 (2012)
15. Mitra, S., Acharya, T.: Gesture recognition: a survey. IEEE Trans. Syst. Man Cybern. Part C Appl. Rev. **37**(3), 311–324 (2007)
16. Sears, A., Shneiderman, B.: High precision touchscreens: design strategies and comparisons with a mouse. Int. J. Man-Mach. Stud. **34**(4), 593–613 (1991)
17. Stephanidis, C.: The Universal Access Handbook. CRC Press, Boca Raton (2009)
18. Tzovaras, D.: Multimodal User Interfaces: From Signals to Interaction. Signals and Communication Technology, 1st edn. Springer, Heidelberg (2008). doi:10.1007/978-3-540-78345-9
19. Wigdor, D.: Brave NUI World: Designing Natural User Interfaces for Touch and Gesture. Morgan Kaufmann, Burlington (2011)

Designing New Low-Cost Home-Oriented Systems for Monitoring and Diagnosis of Patients with Sleep Apnea-Hypopnea

Sara Balderas-Díaz[1]([✉]), Kawtar Benghazi[1], José Luis Garrido[1], Gabriel Guerrero-Contreras[1], and Elena Miró[2]

[1] Software Engineering Department, E.T.S.I.I.T. C/Periodista Daniel Saucedo Aranda S/n, University of Granada, Granada, Spain
sarabd@correo.ugr.es, {benghazi,jgarrido,gjguerrero}@ugr.com
[2] Department of Personality, Assessment and Psychological Treatment, School of Psychology Campus Universitario de Cartuja S/n, University of Granada, Granada, Spain
emiro@ugr.com

Abstract. The Sleep Apnea Hypopnea Syndrome (SAHS) is a symptomatology that affects between 2–5% of world populations and from which a high percentage have not been diagnosed. This syndrome presents serious consequences in daily life of the people who suffer it. Its detection requires an analysis in a hospital with specialized professionals and medical equipment, which entails long waiting lists. The new trends in Bring your Own Device (BYOD) and communication technologies allow designing new alternatives to current systems of diagnosis. In this paper a low-cost home-oriented system for remote monitoring and diagnosis of SAHS is presented. This system is based on the Service Oriented Architecture (SOA) approach and it is made up by different role-oriented subsystems, following a modular design in order to facilitate an incremental number of patients (scalability) and add new functionalities (extensibility). This system is proposed as a low-cost alternative to other detection methods currently implemented, with the main objectives of allowing a greater outreach to the population and reducing waiting lists in hospitals.

Keywords: Wireless and mobile computing · Multiple sensory devices · Service Oriented Architecture (SOA) · eHealth · Sleep Apnea Hipopnea Syndrome (SAHS) · Patients monitoring

1 Introduction

The current economic recession has a direct impact on the lives level of people. Healthcare is one of the sectors most affected by this situation and also one of the most worrying factors for the future [13], mainly for three reasons, the ageing of the population, the demographic downturn and the steady reduction in health system funding. In order to provide a high-quality, accessible

© Springer-Verlag Berlin Heidelberg 2015
H.M. Fardoun et al. (Eds.): REHAB 2014, CCIS 515, pp. 210–221, 2015.
DOI: 10.1007/978-3-662-48645-0_18

and sustainable healthcare systems, governments are investing a great deal of resources in research. In this context, new information and communication technologies (ICT) play a key role by providing the capabilities needed to deliver more efficient, effective, reliable and fast services, achieving an improvement in the diagnosis and treatment of patients, reducing waiting times and saving costs [8]. It will favour access to health care of the general population and especially the most vulnerable groups (elderly or disabled, among other). However, the implementation of these new systems spending could be a profitable long-term economic.

In particular, a common problem in the people's daily life is not getting a non-restful sleep. In this case, person may be suffering some sleep disorder from among the more than 90 cases that exist [19]. Specifically, the Sleep Apnea-Hypopnea Syndrome (SAHS) [5] is classified in the dyssomnias group and is characterized by drowsiness, cardiorespiratory and neuropsychiatric disorders, that lead to repeated episodes of obstruction in the upper airway during sleep. All this implies high blood pressure, a serious decrease in quality of life, traffic and workplace accidents or even die asleep.

Nowadays, between the 2–5 % of the world's population suffer from this syndrome and from which close to 90–95 % have not been diagnosed. This disorder affects people of all ages, children and adults, but the symptoms and treatments are different for both. In general, the probability of developing this disease in adulthood is higher in the case of men. When men reach the age of 40 and woman reaches menopause, tends to equalize the probability. Other factors that increase the probability of developing this disease are overweight, hypertension, abnormalities or defects that can affect the upper airway, among others. Some of the most common symptoms of SAHS are asphyctic episodes, observed apnea, abnormal movements and frequent awakenings.

Usually, for diagnosis of SAHS it is necessary to perform a test in a specialized room called Sleep Room (nocturnal polysomnography). One of the great disadvantages is that such installations are scarce for the high demand that exists, therefore, it leads to a long waiting list of patients. The sleep test requires that the patient remains asleep for several hours. Likewise, the patient is in a strange environment so in many cases makes it more difficult for sleeping, which requires to repeat the test with the repercussions that this have on the own patient and on the waiting list. Furthermore, the sleep room has a sophisticated, static, heavy and expensive medical equipment which allows detailed studies of patients. In addition, a specialized medical staff is required to place the sensors in the body of the patient. This medical staff also monitor the patient while he or she sleeps, and in the case that there are any problem with the equipment or the patient needs an urgent medical attention, because he/she is in a critical state, the medical staff can intervene. At present the nocturnal polysomnography is the most reliable study used to detect whether a person suffers from this disease [3].

Currently, it is important the good acceptance that the new technologies and trends as Bring your Own Device (BYOD) [12], are having between the population. Moreover, the cloud infrastructure is increasingly popular owing to the advantages offered, such as scalability or accessibility. The cloud may be the solution to the limited resources of mobile devices. This combination allows creating portable systems, with low economic cost and wireless connections, which implies a more feasible distribution of the system among users, it is possible to dispose more units for the same price and it is more comfortable to use, due to the reduced wiring and connections between system elements. This research work makes use of this type of system, thus medical specialists can realize a diagnosis and monitoring of the patient's status, as well as to specify a treatment and to control his/her evolution. Furthermore, the tests can be repeated as many times as necessary, owing to availability and low cost of the equipment. Moreover, the patient would be in a familiar environment e.g. (at home) and then more comfortable, which may help the effectiveness of test performed.

In this paper, a system for remote monitoring and diagnosis is presented. This system aims to facilitate the analysis, monitoring and diagnosis of patients who could suffer the sleep apnea-hypopnea syndrome. The system aims to reach a major to reach to a major number of people at the same time, to offer a more attainable service to people who have certain difficulties, for example, elderly or handicap people, who could have difficulties to move to medical center. In addition this could reduce the long waiting-lists for the test of polysomnography.

The rest of this paper is structured as follows. Section 2 presents related work. In Sect. 3, the design of the system for monitoring and diagnosis of patients with SAHS symptoms is presented. Finally, conclusions and future work are summarized in Sect. 4.

2   Related Work

The acceptance of technology among the population, favours the appearance of new health care systems, which are intended to improve the daily life of the patients. Such systems have great potential, since they offer new functionalities and provide support to medical specialists, patients and families [11]. There are currently several platforms for monitoring patients at home, these platforms are used by people with different needs (health and physical), such as elderly or disabled people, and/or with chronic diseases, among other.

Hygehos Home [18] is a system of remote monitoring and patient tracking that allows monitoring the different diseases, measuring of vital signs, controlling medication intake, providing information of the disease and establishing direct contact with medical specialists. In [14] a platform, called NOCTURNAL, for monitoring the rooms of the house of a person with dementia is presented. The aim is to extend the stay of people with this disease in their homes to improve their quality of life. In [16] a framework for analyzing the optimal deployment of services and applications of an eHealth monitoring system is proposed. This framework is based on the use of the cloud and mobile devices as a computing combined unit. In [17] a platform for remote monitoring of patients with brain injury is presented. The system allows to carry out a track of daily activities that the patient performed and to perform rehabilitation exercises.

Regarding the sleep apnea, in [2] a system for the monitoring and detection of sleep apnea which makes use of the patient's mobile device and sensors is proposed. The application processes the information received by the sensor, applies a personalized classifier and sends the gathered information to a server, where a general classifier (independent of a specific patient) is applied. The general classifier is deployed on a server, owing its high resource consumption. In the patient's device, a sub-classifier is generated from the general classifier, on the basis of patient's profile and the most representative characteristics. It is a lighter classifier which can be executed in a mobile device. In [4] the creation of a Virtual Sleep Unit, as the extension of a real Sleep Unit, is proposed. To this end, in a hospital, a room will be enabled, where some patients will be monitored from a remote Sleep Unit. A cardiorespiratory polygraph is used to collect the information about the patient's state and it is sent, along with the images captured by a webcam, in real time to the Sleep Unit. Patients are supervised by a locally nurse, who has been instructed to solve any problems that might arise during the study and with the use of biosensors. In [20] it is proposed an intelligent self-adjusting pillow for detecting and perform an apnea treatment. To detect sleep apnea a blood oxygen sensor is used and according to the parameters captured by that sensor, the pillow is adjusted automatically both in height and form, in order to fit the position of the patient body adequately. In [15] a sound monitoring system is proposed, in order to quantify the snoring sound and the severity of Obstructive Sleep Apnea (OSA), through a smartphone. NOWAPI [9] is a system that provides a remote control of CPAP treatment. It detects the efficiency of treatment, the time of use and events occurred.

However, some of this works do not deal directly with the problems of sleep apnea syndrome. The others more related to this disease, only provide local mechanisms to try to mitigate their symptoms. This proposal aims to design a system of remote diagnostic for sleep apnea, in order to facilitate and expedite the work of specialists, and provide comfort to patients.

3   Design of a Service-Based System for SAHS Symptoms

In this section a system for monitoring and diagnosis of patients is presented [1]. The main objectives of the system is to provide benefits such as:

- To offer the possibility of continuous monitoring and in real-time, i.e., the patient will be monitored or as long as necessary.
- To reduce costs in monitoring patients, in order to repeat the test as many times as necessary.
- To use low economic cost devices that allow performing the test successfully, with the aim of acquiring a greater number of devices, allowing a greater outreach to the population. This feature, together the previous point, could help to decrease the lists of patients which are waiting to be attended.
- To establish a continuous and committed relationship between patients and medical specialists.

– To perform the monitoring in a familiar environment for the patient could help
him/her to improve his/her quality of sleep. Moreover, the tests performed
will be more reliable, owing to the patient's status shall not be affected by the
nervousness of being in a strange place.
– To improve the quality of life and safety of patients. Thus, it is possible that
increase the safety by monitoring his health.

The system seeks for offering the possibility to perform a remote monitoring,
without the need, for the medical staff and patients, to be in the same physical
space or in a nearby place.

3.1 Architectural Design

This system is based on the service-oriented architecture (SOA) to guarantee interoperability, platform independence and reusability, among others quality attributes. This facilitates the coupling and integration of various services,
in order to build composite services of high level, so that the initial system
is extended without the need to develop new services which perform specific
functions.

The system is made up of four independents subsystems. Figure 1 shows the
architecture of the proposed system. Three of these subsystem are targetting
users with different roles (patient, specialist medical and relative of the patient),
in order to provide a joint attention to improve monitoring and continuous control. The another remaining subsystem provides support for these subsystems
and is made up of two main services ("Database Management" and "Patient
Information Management" services).

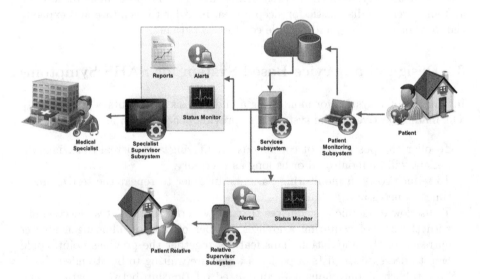

Fig. 1. Monitoring and diagnosis system architecture.

The three role-oriented subsystems cooperate among each other: (1) monitoring subsystem, which is located at patient's home, i.e., a home-oriented subsystem. This subsystem allows carrying out measurement of the patient's vital signs, taking into account the requirements of a specific patient. To do this, the patient makes use of a medical equipment (biosensors) that he/she should place in his/her own body. The sensors act as nodes that should be strategically positioned to capture the medical data and communicate among themselves. In this way, monitoring system use emerging wearable wireless body area networks (WBANs), following one of the most promising approaches [10]. (2) A subsystem for a relative, which receives information from monitoring subsystem about patient's status, in order to allow a collaborative supervision from relative. This subsystem aims to offer the possibility to relatives of the patient of collaborating in the monitoring of the patient, whenever they want to get involved. The relative of the patient can be at home or at patient's house. Finally, (3) medical subsystem, which allows a medical specialist to supervise the patient from his or her workplace or access the reports generated from the studies conducted in each sleep session. Both, medical specialist and relative of the patient can access to these information through a mobile device. Therefore, the system design ensures, through different subsystems, an intuitive and customizable environment for different users and devices that share information. In this way, a modular design approach has been followed in order to facilitate scalability in terms of numbers of patients who can use the system, and functional extensibility.

The support subsystem provides two main services, which has been designed and implemented, taking into consideration that the security in the management of the data (gathering, storing, communicating, querying, modification and deleting) should be guaranteed in every moment. This is because these are personal data and other health information, i.e., patient's sensitive information. (1) "Database Management" service is responsible of storing the information about patients and provides a query service. Furthermore, this service acts like an intermediate layer for security purposes, since it provides restriction mechanisms in data access and modification. (2) "Patient Information Management" service provides complex information through processing of the basic information, in order to reduce the workload of mobile devices and to allow code reusability, the same information will be accessed by different subsystems. It is important to mention that these services can be deployed in a local server, which ensures information control, or on the contrary, in a cloud infrastructure.

3.2   Subsystems Design

In this section, the four subsystem mentioned above (Fig. 2) are described in detail by defining the main objectives and the responsibilities of each subsystem.

Patient Monitoring. The objective of the Patient Monitoring subsystem is to emulate the sleep room of the medical center. It is made up of biosensors and a central component. Biosensors are devices of low economic cost (compared to the

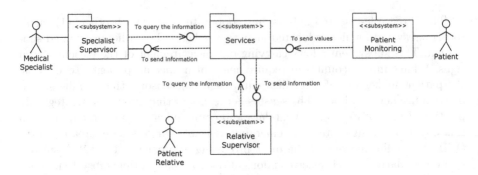

Fig. 2. The system design.

equipment used in a sleep room), however, they guarantee reliable measurements, which allows the correct monitoring of the patients. This central component is a gateway which receives and filters the data from the sensors and sends it to Database Management service. Moreover, if a disconnection occurs during the monitoring session, and it has no connection available with the service, it stores the information collected locally, to subsequently send it, when the connection is reestablished, applying synchronization defined in [7]. This central component can be the patient's computer or an embedded system specifically designed for this task.

Monitoring is carried out each time the patient goes to sleep, however, even if it is for a brief period of time, in order to analyze, a correct treatment, and any potential representative data that could occur during sleep. Information collected by biosensors during each monitoring session, is associated with a sleep study, for future reference and analysis.

Regarding to biosensors, it is necessary that patients learn to use them, before taking them home, in order to obtain correct measures. When the patient goes to sleep, he or she must place the sensors in his/her body as indicated by the medical specialists. Subsequently, biosensors must connect with the central unit in order to start a new monitoring session and sending data. Thanks to the reduced price of the biosensors used and the performance of the sleep study at the patient home, it is possible to repeat the study as many times as necessary, (without causing any delays in waiting lists). The system makes use of wireless and ergonomics devices to guarantee patients' comfort and not unduly interfere his or her sleep.

Specialist Supervisor. Through the subsystem Specialist Supervisor, the medical specialist can monitor the patient in real-time, consult the reports generated from conducted the studies (Fig. 3, left), access the patient's personal data and manage biosensors registered in the system; assign/unassign biosensors to patients in real time and remotely (from his or her workplace). Note that this allows specialist to monitor more than one patient at a time, without having to visit each patient's location. Furthermore, in complex cases, where one medical

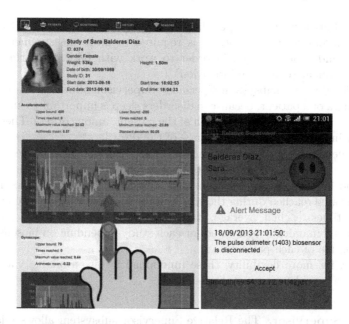

Fig. 3. (Left) Example of a study performed to a patient. (Right) Example of an alert message in "Relative Supervision Subsystem" application.

opinion is needed, it is possible that a group of medicals can work together and collaboratively, each one from their respective workplace, in order to obtain the best result in the monitoring and diagnosis of the patient.

The monitoring of a patient in real-time, allows the medical to perform a control of the vital signs of the patient and other relevant information that determines health status of the patient at each particular time instant. Part of the information is displayed in a set of graphs which allow to view and compare captured values in each time instant, it is also possible to view values in individual graphics. In both cases, the graphical representation facilitates detection of the peak values that could be related to other values corresponding to other measurements. Besides the graphical representation, other more complex information appears. This information is the result of processing the values captured by the biosensor, such as, maximum, minimum, and average values and number of occurrences, among other, which are relevant for the medical supervision.

The subsystem is provided with an alarm system. The medical specialists can activate the alarms for each biosensors independently. He/she can establish the limits of the alarm values (maximum and minimum) and if captured values by the biosensors exceeds the limit, a notification (audible and written signals) will be sent to the medical specialist. The notification contains some information about the patient who is at risk situation when threshold is exceed. While this situation continues or recurs, the notification will be sent periodically. Also, volume and sound type can be customized, and these notifications can be enabled or disabled in general. Furthermore, it is possible to assign/unassign biosensors to patients in real-time and remotely, when it is required to make measurements of new biosensors and other sensors, in order to work with patient information and their environment (context information).

Additionally, the subsystem Specialist Supervisor allows to managing the personal data of a patient, because in disorders sleep is important to know factors such as age, sex, physical constitution of the patient, among others. These factors can be an important part of the causes of the disorder.

Once the monitoring session is ended, the study of the patient's sleep contains the following information: date and time of procurement (start and end), patient weight and height, and for each biosensor connected to patient: maximum and minimum value reached during the study, upper and lower limits specified by the specialist, times reached, average, standard deviation and an interactive graph. This view is dynamically generated for each study depending on biosensors used and the profile of each patient.

Finally, for more flexibility, these functionalities are available via a mobile device, such a tablet or smartphone.

Relative Supervisor. The Relative Supervisor subsystem allows relatives of the patient to collaborate in his or her monitoring. This subsystem operates on the mobile device of the patient's relative and allowing, his or her to monitor the patient condition in real-time.

The subsystem displays the values captured by the biosensors and indicates if patient's condition is normal or a condition of risk is detected (Fig. 3, right). Additionally, the subsystem is endowed by an alert service connected to the specialist subsystem, if the values captured by the biosensors exceed the values established by the specialists, the system sends an audible notification to the patient's family, which allows the patient's family to react to a critical case.

Services. This subsystem provides support and facilitates the information exchanged between the role-oriented subsystems. It provides two main services:

– **Database Management.** This service provides an abstraction layer between data and application, offering functionalities that allow manage data at high level, reducing the efforts of the developers. The Database Management will be responsible to guarantee the security in access and management to external databases. Moreover, standards of web services, such as SOAP and WSDL, are being used for uniform access and to provide independence from platform, in this way, different devices with different properties, at hardware and software level, can access to this service. Furthermore, thanks to this services the system could interoperate with other systems, services or different applications, i.e., it is allowed exchange and access to information of other independent systems, services or applications.
– **Patient Information Management.** This service allows to perform a processing of the information with objective to provide complex information

that may require an intensive computing. Operation is as follows, this service receives a request of an application, it processes the request and determines the basic queries that compose it. Then, it is contacted with the Database Management Service, which sends the requested information, and the Patient Information Management Service processes the information received in order to obtain the request high level information. As in the previous case, this service also ensures security, interoperability and platform independence.

Services can be run on a local server, in the cloud or on a mobile device, but each case have their advantages and disadvantages. On the local server, the data is stored in a private location on which security mechanisms are established for ensuring the inaccessibility of the data by unauthorized users. The cloud server, provides flexibility, accessibility to information, promotes system scalability, offers large computational and storage capacity (on demand), but the problem is the difficulty in ensuring data privacy, something fundamental in e-health systems. Mobile devices have a performance unthinkable a few years ago, but their resources are limited (computing capacity, storage capacity, bandwidth network and battery or autonomy, among others) [6] for continuous control, so that local and cloud servers provide performance benefits, possibly most appropriate for such environments. Furthermore, for the deployment of services is essential to analyze the service quality requirements.

4   Conclusions and Future Work

In this paper a service-based system which enables remote home-oriented monitoring and diagnosis of patients with possible symptoms of SAHS has been presented. The system has been designed and implemented with the aim to improve health care for patients and is mainly composed of four different subsystems, three role-oriented subsystem and a support subsystem. Biosensors and devices of low economic cost used allow performing correct measurements to the patients which allows a greater outreach to the population. In this way the system that has been created allows monitoring of patients in their own homes, while the specialist in charge of treating them is in the hospital. This system is proposed as a possible alternative to other detection methods currently implemented. Thus, it aims to reduce waiting lists, that can reach up to two years, to repeat the test easily and to improve the health and the quality of life of patients. The proposal promotes continuous monitoring in a non-intrusive manner and avoids the movement of patients to the hospital, promoting better and faster patient recovery, economic savings in the health system and greater flexibility in the management and care of patients.

The system has been designed and implemented under the Service-Oriented Architecture (SOA) approach, providing advantages such as platform independence, scalability, reusability and autonomy. Finally, the system stems from a modular design which facilitates scalability and allow adding new biosensors and new functionality easily in the future.

As future work, the diagnostic system will be extended, with the incorporation of new services and biosensors. It is exploring the possibility of providing capabilities to the services, such as adaptivity, adaptability, extensibility and configurability, in order to get the most appropriate system at any time and improving performance. It is intended to use sensors that capture information of the patient environment to combine with values corresponding to the vitals signs of the patient, with the objective of providing to medical specialist a better support from the utilization of data mining tools that allow to generate a possible diagnosis. Finally, the system has been already developed and also informally validated, an experimental evaluation is being carried out with different users in order to analyse benefits more formally and address potential improvements.

Acknowledgment. This research has been partially supported by the Spanish Ministry of Economy and Competitiveness with European Regional Development Funds (FEDER) under the research project TIN2012-38600 and by the Granada Excellence Network of Innovation Laboratories (GENIL) under project PYR-2014-5. The authors would also like to acknowledge contribution from COST Action AAPELE1303.

References

1. Balderas-Díaz, S., Benghazi, K., Garrido, J.L., Miró, E.: A service-based platform for monitoring and diagnosis of patients with sahs symptoms (2014, in press)
2. Bsoul, M., Minn, H., Tamil, L.: Apnea medassist: real-time sleep apnea monitor using single-lead ECG. IEEE Trans. Inf. Technol. Biomed. **15**(3), 416–427 (2011)
3. Chesson Jr, A.L., et al.: The indications for polysomnography and related procedures. Sleep **20**(6), 423–487 (1997)
4. Coma-del Corral, M.J., Alonso-Álvarez, M.L., Allende, M., Cordero, J., Ordax, E., Masa, F., Terán-Santos, J.: Reliability of telemedicine in the diagnosis and treatment of sleep apnea syndrome. Telemed. e-Health **19**(1), 7–12 (2013)
5. Gould, G., Whyte, K., Rhind, G., Airlie, M., Catterall, J., Shapiro, C., Douglas, N.: The sleep hypopnea syndrome. Am. Rev. Respir. Dis. **137**(4), 895–898 (1988)
6. Guerrero-Contreras, G., Garrido, J.L., Rodríguez-Domínguez, C., Balderas-Díaz, S.: Self-adaptive service deployment in context-aware systems. In: 8th International Conference on Ubiquitous Computing Ambient Intelligence (UCAmI) (2014, in press)
7. Guerrero-Contreras, G., Garrido, J.L., Rodríguez-Domínguez, C., Noguera, M., Benghazi, K.: Designing a service platform for sharing internet resources in MANETs. Advances in Service-Oriented and Cloud Computing, vol. 393, pp. 331–345. Springer, Heidelberg (2013)
8. Hill, J.W., Powell, P.: The national healthcare crisis: is ehealth a key solution? Bus. Horiz. **52**(3), 265–277 (2009)
9. Isetta, V., Montserrat, J.M., Thiebaut, G., Weber, C., Navajas, D., Farré, R.: A new device for sleep apnea treatament telemonitoring: a bench study. Int. J. Adv. Life Sci. **5**(3–4), 250–259 (2013)
10. Jovanov, E., Milenkovic, A., Otto, C., De Groen, P.C.: A wireless body area network of intelligent motion sensors for computer assisted physical rehabilitation. J. NeuroEng. Rehabil. **2**(1), 6 (2005)

11. Kreps, G.L., Neuhauser, L.: New directions in ehealth communication: opportunities and challenges. Patient Educ. Couns. **78**(3), 329–336 (2010)
12. Kulkarni, G., Shelke, R., Palwe, R., Solanke, V., Belsare, S., Mohite, S.: Mobile cloud computing-bring your own device. In: Communication Fourth International Conference on Systems and Network Technologies (CSNT) 2014, pp. 565–568. IEEE (2014)
13. Lionis, C., Petelos, E.: The impact of the financial crisis on the quality of care in primary care: an issue that requires prompt attention. Qual. Prim. Care **21**(5), 269–273 (2013)
14. McCullagh, P.J., Carswell, W., Mulvenna, M.D., Augusto, J.C., Zheng, H., Jeffers, W.P.: Nocturnal sensing and intervention for assisted living of people with dementia. In: Healthcare Sensor Networks: Challenges Toward Practical Implementation pp. 283–303. CRC Press, Boca Raton (2011)
15. Nakano, H., Hirayama, K., Sadamitsu, Y., Toshimitsu, A., Fujita, H., Shin, S., Tanigawa, T.: Monitoring sound to quantify snoring and sleep apnea severity using a smartphone: proof of concept. J. Clin. Sleep Med. JCSM Official publ. Am. Acad. Sleep Med. **10**(1), 73–78 (2014)
16. Naqvi, N.Z., Preuveneers, D., Berbers, Y., et al.: Walking in the clouds: deployment and performance trade-offs of smart mobile applications for intelligent environments. In: 9th International Conference on Intelligent Environments (IE) 2013, pp. 212–219. IEEE (2013)
17. Ruiz-Zafra, A., Noguera, M., Benghazi, K., Garrido, J.L., Urbano, G.C., Caracuel, A.: A mobile cloud-supported e-rehabilitation platform for brain-injured patients. In: 7th International Conference on Pervasive Computing Technologies for Healthcare (PervasiveHealth) 2013, pp. 352–355. IEEE (2013)
18. Hygehos, S.L.: Hygehos home (2013). http://www.hygehos.com/hygehos-home/
19. American Academy of Sleep Medicine: International classification of sleep disorders: diagnostic and coding manual (2005)
20. Zhang, J., Zhang, Q., Wang, Y., Qiu, C.: A real-time auto-adjustable smart pillow system for sleep apnea detection and treatment. In: Proceedings of the 12th International Conference on Information Processing in Sensor Networks, pp. 179–190. ACM (2013)

A Pilot Study Using Tactile Cueing for Gait Rehabilitation Following Stroke

Simon Holland[1(✉)], Rachel L. Wright[2], Alan Wing[2],
Thomas Crevoisier[1], Oliver Hödl[1], and Maxime Canelli[1]

[1] The Music Computing Lab Centre for Research in Computing, The Open
University, Milton Keynes MK7 6AA, UK
{simon.holland,thomas.crevoisier,oliver.hodl,
maxime.canelli}@open.ac.uk
[2] School of Psychology, University of Birmingham,
Edgbaston Birmingham B29 6HZ, UK
{r.wright.l,a.m.wing}@bham.ac.uk

Abstract. Recovery of walking function is a vital goal of post-stroke rehabilitation. Cueing using audio metronomes has been shown to improve gait, but can be impractical when interacting with others, particularly outdoors where awareness of vehicles and bicycles is essential. Audio is also unsuitable in environments with high background noise, or for those with a hearing impairment. If successful, lightweight portable tactile cueing has the potential to take the benefits of cueing out of the laboratory and into everyday life. The Haptic Bracelets are lightweight wireless devices containing a computer, accelerometers and low-latency vibrotactiles with a wide dynamic range. In this paper we review gait rehabilitation problems and existing solutions, and present an early pilot in which the Haptic Bracelets were applied to post-stroke gait rehabilitation. Tactile cueing during walking was well received in the pilot, and analysis of motion capture data showed immediate improvements in gait.

Keywords: Haptic bracelets · Stroke · Gait rehabilitation · Tactile metronome · Haptic metronome · Parkinson's disease · Fall prevention · Walking · Hemiparesis

1 Introduction

The Haptic Bracelets are devices for tactile communication and co-ordination, originally designed and built by the Open University for musical purposes, such as learning and teaching multi-limbed rhythms. This paper considers an early pilot study in which the Haptic Bracelets were applied to gait rehabilitation following stroke.

2 Gait Rehabilitation Following Stroke

2.1 Characteristics of Post-stroke Gait

According to the World Health Organisation, approximately 15 million people experience a stroke each year. In the majority of cases, stroke results in some degree of

© Springer-Verlag Berlin Heidelberg 2015
H.M. Fardoun et al. (Eds.): REHAB 2014, CCIS 515, pp. 222–233, 2015.
DOI: 10.1007/978-3-662-48645-0_19

one-sided muscle weakness or hemiparesis. Impairment of gait following a stroke can have a major impact on an individual's life [1], and can impose substantial costs on health and social services [2]. Although the majority of stroke patients eventually recover an independent gait, many never regain a level of walking that allows common daily activities [3]. Thus, improvement of gait is a major goal of post stroke rehabilitation.

Walking after a stroke is characterized by decreased speed [4], increased variability [5], and spatial and/or temporal asymmetry [6]. As a result, the non-paretic limb is regularly exposed to higher vertical forces [7]. Over time, this can lead to further problems, such as joint pain [8] and degeneration [9]. An asymmetrical gait is associated with worse performance on clinical balance tests [10] and therefore may be linked to the increased risk of falling observed after stroke. Understanding and rehabilitating these features of hemiparetic gait is of vital importance, since walking affords a high level of independence, and thus a better quality of life for stroke survivors in general [11].

2.2 Existing Gait Rehabilitation Approaches

Hollands et al. [12] presented a systematic review of gait rehabilitation techniques after stroke, and identified external rhythmic cueing as a technique showing great promise for walking rehabilitation. Immediate effects of an auditory metronome have been reported, with chronic stroke patients able to synchronise to a metronome during treadmill walking [13]. Improvements in spatial [14] and temporal symmetry [15] and step time variability [16] were observed with auditory pacing, as was the ability to make gait adjustments in response to changes in the cue [17]. Auditory cueing has also been used in gait rehabilitation programmes, with significantly greater improvements in walking speed and stride length with auditory cueing compared to conventional gait training [18] and Bobath training [19].

Other modalities appear to have considerable promise for external cueing. Therapists routinely use touch to help stabilise patients and reduce postural sway. Visual spatial cues in the form of projected stepping-stones have also been used, and perturbation of the spatial phase of these cues shows promise [20]. However, these approaches can be intrusive, or can require laboratory installations, or both, whereas touch can be covert and more practical to apply in everyday life. It is known [21] that tactile cues can lead to an increase in stride length, without disrupting the natural gait rhythm in healthy participants.

3 The Haptic Bracelets

The Haptic Bracelets, designed and built at the Open University, are self-contained lightweight devices for wrists and ankles [22]. Each bracelet contains a computer, Wi-Fi chip, accelerometers and powerful, low-latency vibrotactiles with a wide dynamic range. The bracelets were originally designed for musical purposes, to be worn in sets of four (on each wrist and each ankle) – though, as in the present case, wearing fewer also has many useful applications. Bracelets can be coordinated and communicate together via laptop or smart phone. It is possible for sets worn by two or more people, whether co-located or remote, to be used for synchronization or communication in various ways. Synchronised use by two wearers is a feature of one of the therapeutic applications outlined below. The vibrotactiles are very low latency, and can be felt 6 ms after activation. The wireless Haptic Bracelets evolved out of the earlier Haptic Drum Kit [23] and our wider investigations of haptic technologies [24].

In Fig. 1, the vibrotactiles (two per unit) are visible as blue caps at the tip of the black leads. The third black lead on each unit connects to an external battery pack. Separation of the vibrotactiles from the main unit allows flexible placement of the vibrotactiles to suit individual wearers. This feature also helps to avoid feedback between vibrotactiles and accelerometers in applications that combine two way haptic communication. Given that parts of the ankles are generally less sensitive than the wrists, this flexibility of placement is also useful when bracelets are worn on the ankles. The vibrotactiles are typically tucked under the strapping in positions to suit the individual wearer.

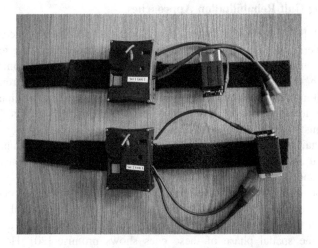

Fig. 1. Two haptic bracelets.

The wide dynamic range of the vibrotactiles means that while they can be set to as vibrate gently as preferred on wrists, they can also be adjusted to a higher level if strapped outside socks or trousers. In early design trials (Sect. 4) haptic cues could be clearly felt even when strapped on the outside of knee length boots. This is particularly useful, since the ease of perceiving cues on hemiparetic limbs can vary considerably amongst stroke survivors.

Also visible in Fig. 1 are a multipurpose rotary control and a multi-purpose button. In the present applications these may be used to set the level of the vibrotactiles, and to switch them off. These and other functions can also be controlled where appropriate from an external computer.

3.1 Modes of Use of the Haptic Bracelets in Gait Rehabilitation

We are currently prototyping three principal modes of tactile cueing in gait rehabilitation. The simplest mode constitutes a portable tactile metronome (the focus of this paper). If tactile cueing demonstrates similar benefits to auditory cueing [14–17] this approach would offer the benefit of being usable in a wide range of contexts, for example in the street, while avoiding the inconvenience and dangers associated with wearing earphones when awareness of motor vehicles, bicycles and other pedestrians is needed. The bracelets can at the same time collect gait data via the in-built accelerometers for live streaming via Wi-Fi, or for storage and later analysis. When used as a tactile metronome, one can be worn on each leg, with each bracelet cuing the leg on which it is worn. Alternatively, where preferred, a single bracelet can be worn on one wrist, with cues on the single wrist cueing both left and right footfalls. A second mode of use is flexible interactive pacing, with the aid of a carer, therapist or partner. The motivation in this second mode of use is that in situations where stumbles, environmental obstacles, changing slopes or other irregularities might make it impractical for the participant to keep in phase with a fixed beat, a partner wearing a communicating pair of bracelets could flexibly beat an appropriate pulse, either by beating with their hands, or simply by walking. The third mode of use is autonomous gait monitoring. In this mode, aimed at post-care, a pair of bracelets worn on the ankles continually monitor gait speed or gait asymmetry when the participant is walking, and give gentle tactile metronomic guidance when speed or symmetry falls below a pre-chosen limits. Prototype versions of all three of these applications have been implemented and are being piloted with stroke survivors. In this paper we focus on the first application alone.

4 Preliminary Views of Practitioners

As part of the system design process, before conducting a pilot test with a stroke survivor, we carried out participative demonstrations of the bracelets with two distinct meetings of physiotherapists with interests in neurology. Firstly, a brief invited talk, and participative demo, of the Haptic Bracelets was presented to a meeting of some fifty members of the professional Association of Chartered Physiotherapists with Interests in Neurology (ACPIN). This group (http://www.acpin.net/) has special interests in the neuro-rehabilitation of conditions such as Stroke, Parkinson's disease (PD), Ataxia and Head injury. Three potential applications of the Haptic Bracelets in rehabilitation were outlined as noted above: the tactile metronome, flexible therapist-driven tactile cueing, and post-care live gait monitoring and feedback. The first two of these applications were demonstrated. In order to inform design work, as well as collecting detailed comments, survey feedback from some fifty ACPIN participants was evaluated to find out initial general views on the likely relative value of the three approaches (Table 1).

Comments from members included:

> *'Great for Parkinson's disease - Cueing to enable stepping - PD patients tend to "freeze" and use visual/audio cueing to trigger stepping - tactile cueing could assist this.'*

'Stroke patients tend to have unequal stride length - the use of a metronome to encourage equal stepping by patients.'
'Use of feedback would assist therapists analysing gait and for patients to see their gait pattern.'

Table 1. General views of meeting of Physiotherapists with Interests in Neurology

Proposition	Agree	Agree strongly
The tactile metronome has the potential to influence practice	89 %	55 %
Live monitoring and feedback on gait symmetry has the potential to influence practice	83 %	50 %
Flexible tactile cueing has the potential to influence practice	93 %	27 %

Secondly, a presentation and participatory workshop was run for some seventeen physiotherapists from the Wye Valley NHS Trust. The workshop was part of a research day organised by a research facilitator from the West Midlands Stroke Research Network (http://www.crncc.nihr.ac.uk/about_us/stroke_research_network/in_your_area/west_midlands). The participatory workshop examined the pros and cons of cueing the gait or arm movements of patients with conditions such as Stroke, Parkinson's disease, Cerebral Palsy, Head injury, Ataxia, and others, using the Haptic Bracelets, as compared with other approaches. All participants were able to try out the Haptic Bracelets. Situations were identified where the Haptic Bracelets are not suitable for therapy (e.g. rehabilitation of grasp and reach, and in some Parkinson's disease cases where spasticity might be increased). Again, in order to inform design refinements, as well as collecting detailed comments, survey feedback from participants was evaluated to gain an impression of practitioners' initial views on the likely relative value of the three approaches (Table 2).

Table 2. General views of physiotherapists at participative workshop

Proposition	Agree	Agree strongly
The tactile metronome has the potential to influence practice	91 %	50 %
Live monitoring and feedback on gait symmetry has the potential to influence practice	91 %	50 %
Flexible tactile cueing has the potential to influence practice	49 %	33 %

Comments from attendees included:

'Maybe not appropriate for musculoskeletal patients with gait re-training in higher levels such as sporting injuries.'
'May help with children and developmental problems, for tapping etc.'
'Consider how therapists use, sensory input to facilitate neurological rehabilitation & the effects sensory stimulation can have on aspects such as tone/spasticity/muscle activation.'

5   Pilot Study with Stroke Survivor

5.1   Aims

The preliminary pilot study investigated the immediate effects of tactile cueing during walking with the Haptic Bracelets in a participant with hemiparesis.

5.2   Method

We recruited a female participant with chronic right hemiparesis (aged 69 years, height 1.66 m, mass 63.8 kg, Fugl-Meyer lower limb assessment = 29, 12 years post-stoke), who provided written informed consent. Testing took place in the large (17 × 12 × 4.5 m) gait laboratory in the Motion and Performance Centre at the University of Worcester. Whole body motion data were collected at 60 Hz using a fifteen camera Mcam2 Vicon system (Vicon Peak, Oxford Metrics Ltd., UK), according to standard clinical gait analysis procedures. The participant wore a single bracelet on her left (non-paretic) wrist (Fig. 2).

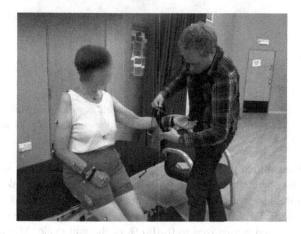

Fig. 2. Preparing for the pilot study

During pre-test, the participant performed 5 standard gait trials for baseline measures. Her cadence was averaged from these trials to generate the inter-response interval for the tactile cue. The participant had a 5-minute familiarization period of walking to the tactile cue. She was instructed to time her footfalls to the cue. This was followed by 5 walking trials with steps cued by the tactile device worn on her left wrist (Fig. 3), followed by a final 5 un-cued walking trials. Seated rest was taken between each walking condition to minimize fatigue effects.

Marker position data were filtered using the Woltring cross-validity quintic spline routine [25]. Step time asymmetry was determined using a step time ratio where the paretic step time was divided by the non-paretic step time. Similarly, step length

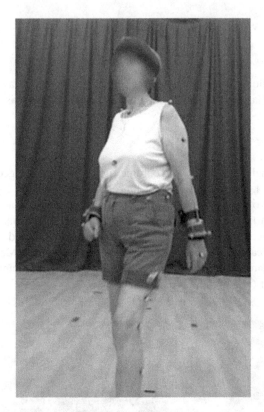

Fig. 3. Tactile cued walking of a stroke survivor. As well as wearing a haptic bracelet on the paretic (right arm), the participant is wearing optical markers on the body for motion tracking.

asymmetry was quantified using a step length ratio where the paretic step length was divided by the non-paretic step length [26]. Sagittal hip, knee and ankle angles were calculated from the kinematic marker data using the Plug-in Gait model (Vicon Peak, Oxford Metrics Ltd., UK) and reported in degrees. Joint angles were segmented into discrete gait cycles and normalized to 0–100 % of the gait cycle. Minimal detectable change values for gait variables in a within-session setting were used to identify functional differences between conditions [27, 28].

5.3   Results

The participant's normal walking speed was 0.82 m.s^{-1}, increasing to 0.85 m.s^{-1} when cued by the tactile bracelet. She displayed a mild level of temporal asymmetry at baseline, and a normal level of spatial symmetry. Her step length increased with the tactile cue, and the 3 cm increase for the paretic step was above the minimum detectable change threshold.

Analysis of the lower limb joint angle data (see Table 3) showed that the participant's paretic lower limb joint motion was reduced in all conditions compared to the laboratory's

Table 3. Gait variables in the three walking conditions

	Baseline	Cued	Post-cueing
Walking speed (m.s^{-1})	0.82	0.85	0.81
Non-paretic step time (s)	0.52	0.54	0.52
Paretic step time (s)	0.63	0.63	0.63
Step time ratio	1.21	1.17	1.21
Non-paretic step length (m)	0.47	0.48	0.47
Paretic step length (m)	0.46	0.49	0.45
Step length ratio	0.98	1.02	0.96
Paretic hip angle at toe off (°)	−5.8	−8.3	−7.3
Peak paretic knee flexion during swing (°)	32.3	39.8	37.8
Paretic ankle range of motion (°)	24.5	27.6	25.1

normal database. Her paretic, hip angle at toe off (Fig. 4) peak knee flexion during swing (Fig. 5) and ankle range of motion (Fig. 6) increased above the minimum detectable change threshold when cued with the tactile device compared to her baseline values.

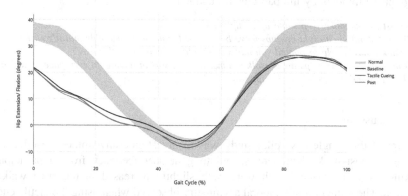

Fig. 4. Paretic hip angles across the gait cycle. The grey band shows the normal range; the black trace is baseline, the red trace is with tactile cueing and the blue trace is post cueing.

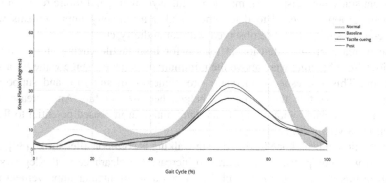

Fig. 5. Paretic Knee angles across the gait cycle.

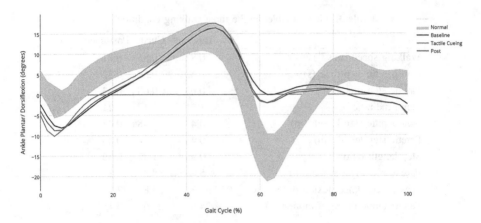

Fig. 6. Paretic ankle angles across the gait cycle.

The participant reported that she felt the tactile bracelet helped to generate an even walking pace, and that she felt she was using her hip more to swing her leg through straighter. Comments by the participant included:

"I must say its makes you stand up straighter"
"When I stand up straight my hips move better and I walk more smoothly and it's easier."
"I think it might help to remind you that you should be walking in this way"
"it does help.... this helps me to walk in time. It's just sort of having an even pace ... which helps me stand up straight and walk properly."

5.4   Discussion

The aim of this single case pilot study was to investigate any immediate effects on walking in post-stroke hemiparesis, and to gain user feedback from a participant. Walking speed and step length were both slightly increased in the cued walking condition. The reduction in temporal asymmetry observed when using the tactile cue is of a slightly lower magnitude than previously reported for auditory cueing when treadmill walking [18] or stepping in place [19]. This may be due to the participant in the current study only displaying mild temporal asymmetry, and future research with a participant group is needed to determine whether asymmetry improvements with a tactile cue are similar to those observed with an auditory cue.

The increase in hip extension at toe off for both tactile cueing and post-cueing conditions from baseline were above the minimum detectable change value for a stroke population. This suggests the increases are clinically meaningful, and supports the participant's views that the tactile cue helped her use her hip. An increase in hip extension is associated with a longer step length and an increased potential to flex the knee during swing [29].

A reduction in peak knee flexion during walking is common after stroke [30], and is associated with compensatory measures to increase toe clearance as the leg is swung through in this phase of the gait cycle [7]. Even a small angular improvement at the knee reduces the risk of tripping and falling [31]. The 7.5 ° and 5.5 ° increases in knee flexion for the cued condition and immediately post-cueing are not only clinically meaningful for walking function, but could also have benefits for reducing fall risk after stroke. Further research is needed to determine whether these improvements can be sustained.

Tactile cueing during walking was viewed positively by the participant in this study, and produced immediate improvements at the hip, knee and ankle on the paretic limb. This single case study indicates that a larger study investigating tactile cueing in hemiparetic gait is warranted.

6 Conclusions

Recovery of walking function is a paramount goal of rehabilitation after stroke. Existing therapies using audio metronomes have been reported to have valuable immediate effects, but gait asymmetry can be very resistant to long term improvement [21]. Audio cueing can be unsuitable outside the lab, due to dangers associated with earphone use near to motor vehicles, bicycles or even other pedestrians. Tactile cueing has potential to offer similar benefits to an auditory cue. In portable form, this approach could be used outside the lab for long periods without the potential problems associated with audio cueing. We have outlined three potential applications of the Haptic Bracelets in gait rehabilitation post-stroke, and have reported on an initial pilot study with an individual with post-stroke hemiparesis. The preliminary data suggests that a tactile device may have immediate benefits for walking in individuals post-stroke and warrants further investigation.

Acknowledgements. We acknowledge generous funding support from Janet Harper to SH, and from the Stroke Association (Grant code TSA2009/06) to AMW. A preliminary report on this work appeared as [32].

References

1. Belda-Lois, J.-M., et al.: Rehabilitation of gait after stroke: a review towards a top-down approach. J. Neuroeng. Rehabil. **8**(1), 66 (2011)
2. Evers, S.M., Struijs, J.N., Ament, A.J., van Genugten, M.L., Jager, J.C., van den Bos, G.A.: International comparison of stroke cost studies. Stroke **35**, 1209–1215 (2004)
3. Flansbjer, U.B., Holmbäck, A.M., Downham, D., Patten, C., Lexell, J.: Reliability of gait performance tests in men and women with hemiparesis after stroke. J. Rehabil. Med. **37**, 75–82 (2005)
4. Olney, S.J., Richards, C.: Hemiparetic gait following stroke. Part I: characteristics. Gait Posture **4**(2), 136–148 (1996)
5. Balasubramanian, C.K., Neptune, R.R., Kautz, S.A.: Variability in spatiotemporal step characteristics and its relationship to walking performance post-stroke. Gait Posture **29**, 408–414 (2009)
6. Chen, G., Patten, C., Kothari, D.H., Zajac, F.E.: Gait differences between individuals with post-stroke hemiparesis and non-disabled controls at matched speeds. Gait Posture **22**(1), 51–56 (2005)

7. Kim, C.M., Eng, J.J.: The relationship of lower-extremity muscle torque to locomotor performance in people with stroke. Phys. Ther. **83**(1), 49–57 (2003)
8. Norvell, D.C., Czerniecki, J.M., Reiber, G.E., Maynard, C., Pecoraro, J.A., Weiss, N.S.: The prevalence of knee pain and symptomatic knee osteoarthritis among veteran traumatic amputees and nonamputees. Arch. Phys. Med. Rehabil. **86**(3), 487–493 (2005)
9. Nolan, L., Wit, A.: Dudziñski, K., Lees, A., Lake, M., Wychowanski, M.: Adjustments in gait symmetry with walking speed in trans-femoral and trans-tibial amputees. Gait Posture **17**, 142–151 (2003)
10. Lewek, M.D., Bradley, C.E., Wutzke, C.J., Zinder, S.M.: The relationship between spatiotemporal gait asymmetry and balance in individuals with chronic stroke, J. Appl. Biomech. (in press)
11. Richards, C.L., et al.: Task-specific physical therapy for optimization of gait recovery in acute stroke patients. Arch. Phys. Med. Rehabil. **74**(6), 612–620 (1993)
12. Hollands, K.L., Pelton, T.A., Tyson, S.F., Hollands, M.A., van Vliet, P.M.: Interventions for coordination of walking following stroke: systematic review. Gait Posture **35**(3), 349–359 (2012)
13. Roerdink, M., Lamoth, C.J.C., Kwakkel, G., van Wieringen, P.C.W., Beek, P.J.: Gait coordination after stroke: benefits of acoustically paced treadmill walking. Phys. Ther. **87**(8), 1009–1022 (2007)
14. Prassas, S., et al.: Effect of auditory rhythmic cuing on gait kinematic parameters of stroke patients. Gait Posture **6**(3), 218–223 (1997)
15. Roerdink, M., Lamoth, C.J.C., Kwakkel, G., van Wieringen, P.C.W., Beek, P.J.: Gait coordination after stroke: benefits of acoustically paced treadmill walking. Phys. Ther. **87**(8), 1009–1022 (2007)
16. Wright, R.L., Masood, A., MacCormac, E.S., Pratt, D., Sackley, C.M., Wing, A.M.: Metronome-cued stepping in place after hemiparetic stroke: comparison of a one- and two-tone beat. ISRN Rehabil. **2013**(157410), 1–5 (2013)
17. Pelton, T.A., Johannsen, L., Chen, H.Y., Wing, A.M.: Hemiparetic stepping to the beat: asymmetric response to metronome phase shift during treadmill gait. Neurorehabil. Neural Repair **24**(5), 428–434 (2010)
18. Thaut, M.H., McIntosh, G.C., Rice, R.R.: Rhythmic facilitation of gait training in hemiparetic stroke rehabilitation. J. Neurol. Sci. **151**(2), 207–212 (1997)
19. Thaut, M.H., Leins, A.K., Rice, R.R., et al.: Rhythmic auditory stimulation improves gait more than NDT/Bobath training in near-ambulatory patients early poststroke: a single-blind, randomized trial. Neurorehabil. Neural Repair **21**(5), 455–459 (2007)
20. Bank, P.J.M., Roerdink, M., Peper, C.E.: Comparing the efficacy of metronome beeps and stepping stones to adjust gait: steps to follow! Exp. Brain Res. **209**(2), 159–169 (2011)
21. Sejdić, E., et al.: The effects of rhythmic sensory cues on the temporal dynamics of human gait. PloS One **7**(8), e43104 (2012)
22. Bouwer, A., Holland, S., Dalgleish, M.: The Haptic Bracelets: learning multi-limb rhythm skills from haptic stimuli while reading. In: Holland, S., Wilkie, K., Mulholland, P., Seago, A. (eds.) Music and Human-Computer Interaction. Springer Series on Cultural Computing. Springer, London (2013)
23. Holland, S., Bouwer, A., Dalgleish, M., Hurtig, T.: Feeling the beat where it counts: fostering multi-limb rhythm skills with the haptic drum kit. In: Proceedings of TEI 2010, Boston Cambridge, Mass (2010). Oro ID 18
24. Bird, J., Holland, S., Marshall, P., Rogers, Y., Clark, A.: Feel the force: Using tactile technologies to investigate the extended mind. In: Proceedings of Devices that Alter Perception, 21 September 2008, Seoul, Korea (2008)

25. Woltring, H.J.: A fortran package for generalized, cross-validatory spline smoothing and differentiation. Adv. Eng. Softw. Workstations **8**(2), 104–113 (1986)
26. Balasubramanian, C.K., Bowden, M.G., Neptune, R.R., Kautz, S.A.: Relationship between step length asymmetry and walking performance in subjects with chronic hemiparesis. Arch. Phys. Med. Rehabil. **88**(1), 43–49 (2007)
27. Kesar, T.M., Binder-Macleod, S.A., Hicks, G.E., Reisman, D.C.: Minimal detectable change for gait variables collected during treadmill walking in individuals post-stroke. Gait Posture **33**, 314–317 (2011)
28. Wilken, J.M., Rodriguez, K.M., Brawner, M., Darter, B.J.: Reliability and minimal detectable change values for gait kinematics and kinetics in healthy adults. Gait Posture **35**, 301–307 (2012)
29. George-Reichley, D.G., Higginson, J.S.: Potential muscle function during the swing phase of stroke gait. J. Appl. Biomech. **26**(2), 180–187 (2010)
30. Olney, S.J., Griffin, M.P., McBride, I.D.: Temporal, kinematic, and kinetic variables related to gait speed in subjects with hemiplegia: a regression approach. Phys. Ther. **74**(9), 872–885 (1994)
31. Levinger, P., Lai, D.T.H., Menz, H.B., Morrow, A.D., Feller, J.A., Bartlett, J.R., Bergman, N.R., Begg, R.: Swing limb mechanics and minimum toe clearance in people with knee osteoarthritis. Gait Posture **35**(2), 277–281 (2012)
32. Holland, S., Wright, R.L., Wing, A., Crevoisier, T., Hödl, O., Canelli, M: A gait rehabilitation pilot study using tactile cueing following hemiparetic stroke. In: REHAB 2014. European Union Digital Library. (2014). http://dx.doi.org/10.4108/icst.pervasivehealth.2014.255357

Assistive Smart Sensing Devices for Gait Rehabilitation Monitoring

O. Postolache[1(✉)], J.M.D. Pereira[3], M. Ribeiro[2], and P. Girão[2]

[1] Instituto de Telecomunicações/ISCTE-IUL, Lisbon, Portugal
opostolache@lx.it.pt
[2] Instituto de Telecomunicações/DEEC-IST-UL, Lisbon, Portugal
[3] Instituto de Telecomunicações/ESTSetúbal-IPS, LabIM, Setúbal, Portugal

Abstract. Smart sensing devices are nowadays part of the ambient assisted living architectures and may be adapted and personalized for gait rehabilitation assessment. Aiming an objective evaluation of patient progress during the physiotherapy sessions, the design and implementation of a set of sensing devices were carried out. Thus, it was considered a wearable solution materialized by a smart inertial measurement unit (IMU) and/or a set of walking aid objects characterized by embedded unobtrusive sensing units based on microwave Doppler radars. The data delivered by the smart sensing units designed for gait rehabilitation purpose are wireless transmitted to an advanced processing server that provides synthetic information to the physiotherapist that use a mobile device to access the available services. Elements of IMU sensor network and smart rollator design and implementation for gait assessment, as well as sensor signals digital processing, are included in the chapter.

Keywords: Microwave Doppler radar · Inertial measurement system · Gait monitoring · Time frequency analysis

1 Introduction

In gait-related clinical practice, the knowledge of the accelerations and velocities associated with the gait performed by the monitored patient are very important to diagnose gait patterns and to evaluate therapeutic interventions [1]. The analysis of the human body movement is commonly done in so-called 'gaits laboratories'. In these laboratories, body movement is measured by a camera system using optical markers [2], the ground reaction force (GRF) using a force plate fixed in the floor [3], and the muscle activity using EMG [4]. From the body movements and ground reaction forces, joint moments and powers can be estimated by applying inverse dynamics methods [5] providing estimate of the rehabilitation progress. Considering the lack of application of this kind of systems for real environments where physiotherapist and doctors assist the people under physiotherapy, an important challenge is to design and implement, reliable, easy to use, and low cost systems for gait measurement and analysis that can be used by physiotherapist during normal physiotherapy sessions or can be easily included as part of remote physiotherapy services [6]. At the same time, the developed systems

© Springer-Verlag Berlin Heidelberg 2015
H.M. Fardoun et al. (Eds.): REHAB 2014, CCIS 515, pp. 234–247, 2015.
DOI: 10.1007/978-3-662-48645-0_20

for gait measurement and analysis might be prepared for the particular case of patients that are using walking aids during motor rehabilitation.

Frequent solutions used for objective evaluation of rehabilitation processes are based on the use of inertial sensors attached to the human body [7, 8]. A set of wearable solutions developed by Postolache et al., characterized by Bluetooth connectivity as part of a smart system was used for motor and cardiac activity monitoring [9]. Interoperability and modularity were considered as important requirements for the latest developments in the smart sensors for vital signs and motor activity monitoring that conducted to a flexible multiprocessor plug-and-play architecture characterized also by multiple wireless connectivity capabilities [10]. The use of smart sensing solutions imposes the necessity to fix the sensing module in an appropriate way, which requires preparation from the physiotherapist to perform that task. In the case of remote physiotherapy, in addition to discomfort associated with long period of use, it could require special knowledge and motor ability from the user part, which limits the use of this type of systems. Taking into account that many patients use walkers or rollators during the physiotherapy, we designed unobtrusive solutions for gait rehabilitation monitoring by embedding sensors in this kind of equipment to extract the patient's motion information. Several authors reported the developing of walkers or rollators with capabilities to sense the motion and forces that should characterize the users gait during the physiotherapy sessions and provide this information to the physiotherapist in appropriate way [11–14].

In this chapter are presented as set of solutions for physical rehabilitation monitoring that include MEMS and microwave Doppler radars associated with human body as accessories or embedded in walking aids expressed by walkers and rollators.

The chapter is organized as follows: we start by presenting the IMU (inertial measurement unit) body area network, special attention being granted to the end-nodes that include 3D accelerometers and gyroscopes. Then, use of microwave Doppler radar to provide motion sensing capabilities for a rollator is introduced. In Sects. 4 and 5 the software aspects related with the system operation and with digital signal processing for gait analysis are detailed and some illustrative results presented. A short conclusion ends the chapter.

2 IMU – Wireless Network

The latest developments in micro-electro-mechanical systems (MEMS) makes possible to integrate multiple sensors, including gyroscopes, accelerometers and magnetometers, in a compact inertial sensor module, which may also include a digital processing unit for data fusion. This type of implementation is known as inertial measurement unit (IMU) and provides all the information needed for the detection of human movement [15].

The IMU applications were developed in the field of pedestrian dead reckoning (PDR). Step detection, walking speed and step length measurement are proper to the PDR and, at the same time, are considered as important elements to evaluate the gait during rehabilitation sessions. To measure these quantities we propose here a motion wireless node based on an IMU board developed in our laboratory (Qk motion) [16].

2.1 Inertial Measurement Module

To extract the gait information during a physiotherapy session an IMU expressed by a tri-axis gyroscope, accelerometer and magnetometer is employed. The L3G4200D gyroscope from STMicroelectronics was considered to measure the angular velocity. It includes a sensing element and an IC interface capable of providing the measured angular rate to the external world through a digital interface (I2C/SPI). Considering the necessity to assure the digital communication with a 3D accelerometer and 3D magnetometer, the I2C communication interface was chosen. Based on this interface the data from the gyroscope is transmitted to a PIC24F32KA302 microcontroller, the I2C protocol being implemented considering the functionalities of its SSL (Synchronous Serial Port) port, SDA and SCL lines. The Qk motion reduced schematics including the microcontroller and the IMU is presented in Fig. 1.

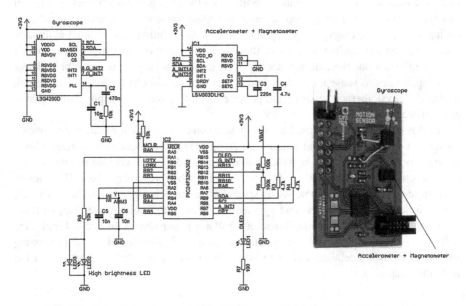

Fig. 1. Qk motion: microcontroller, IMU connection scheme and IMU board.

In Fig. 1 is also presented the physical implementation of the printed circuit board (PCB, green board)that includes the gyroscope, accelerometer and magnetometer and a specific connector that permits the interfacing between the Qk motion and communication module (Qk module) [10]). They were placed on the PCB so their X and Y axes are aligned and a drawing on the board's silkscreen indicates the direction of each axis. The specifications of each device are presented in Table 1.

The communication interface has the U2RX and U2TX communication lines that permit the data exchange between the microcontroller of the Qk motion board with IMU board and the microcontroller associated with the communication module that provide IEEE 802.15.4 or Bluetooth compatibility.

Table 1. Gyroscope, accelerometer and magnetometer specifications

	Gyroscope	Accelerometer	Magnetometer
Range/Sensibility	± 250°/s	± 2 g	± 1.3 to ± 1.8 gauss
	± 500°/s	± 4 g	
	± 2000°/s	± 8 g	
		± 16 g	
Resolution	16 bits		

2.2 Wireless Network

Taking into account the necessity to receive the information related to the feet motion during the gait rehabilitation, an IMU body wireless sensor network was designed and implemented. The implemented architecture is presented in Fig. 2, where is shown also the network coordinator IEEE 802.15.4 compatible and USB connected to a personal computer(PC) or tablet. The wireless network end-nodes include each of them a Qk motion board characterized by an IMU and a communication board characterized by XBee modem [17]. Each of the boards contains a microcontroller to implement a common protocol stack (the Qk protocol) that allows the data exchange between coordinator and the end-nodes. The gait motion is captured using two end-nodes disposed on the left-foot and right-foot. All boards can be remotely configured enabling different functionally without requiring firmware updates. For example, a sensor can be configured to send raw data or processed data. Taking into account the current supported technologies, ZigBee boards are the only ones that require the use of a Qk network board. This is the main element of a gateway since it allows collecting data from all networked sensor nodes being used. However, the final objective is to access

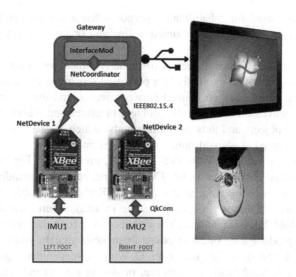

Fig. 2. IMU wireless network architecture (QkCom – Qk communication protocol) for gait rehabilitation.

nodes data from a computer, smartphone or tablet with limited connectivity options. Zigbee or IEEE 802.15.4-based protocols are currently not supported on these devices, which require the use of external adapters characterized by USB Bluetooth or WiFi communication protocols that correspond to smartphone or tablet wireless communication capabilities. In other words, the gateway transmits the data from all the network sensor nodes to the computing device (e.g. smartphone, tablet). This is a very important abstraction feature because the computer does not need to distinguish data coming from different network addresses and possibly carrying different information; instead it is all contained into a single structure sent in a packet. The packets are addressed and computer will know that they come from different sensors.

3 Smart Rollator

The walkers are usually used by people characterized by poor balance or join stiffness that limit the displacement. The walker can have no wheels or two or four wheels (rollator). All of these models commercially available can be used as walking aids also during the gait rehabilitation process.

To perform the unobtrusive monitoring of the user gait during the walker/rollator use a modular sensing, processing and communication unit, based on a microwave Doppler radar array, is proposed. Together with the radar array that allow the acquisition of gait signals, the modular unit includes a multifunction board MyDAQ that is USB connected to a compact battery powered computer with Wi-Fi connection capabilities.

3.1 Microwave Doppler Radar array

The smart rollator used for rehabilitation purposes has a sensing module with two microwave Doppler radar sensors mounted in line and oriented properly to catch the gait (Fig. 3).

Sensing using the Doppler Effect is particularly suited for unobtrusive sensing. Ultrasound sensing is not an alternative for pervasive sensing of physiological signals, particularly if the purpose is no contact between sensor and the person to monitor. Electromagnetic waves do not have the problem of ultrasound waves; they penetrate well non-metallic objects and thus the human body, which means that the source and receiver may be placed at some distance from the examinee.

The used Doppler radar sensors IVS-162 DRS, presented in Fig. 3b), are of the frequency modulated continuous wave (FMCW) type, each one including a transmitting (TX) and a receiving(RX) antenna. An FSK/FMCW-capable K-Band VCO transceiver, controlled through a tuning voltage (Vtune), assures a transmitting frequency in the 24-24.250 GHz interval. The signal coming from the receiving antenna is demodulated to produce a set of intermediate frequencies signals, which correspond to signal in phase, I, and signal in quadrature, Q, with the transmitted signal.

During the gait rehabilitation procedure, or during the normal utilization of the rollator, the motion of the user's legs is captured by an array of radars. The I1 and I2

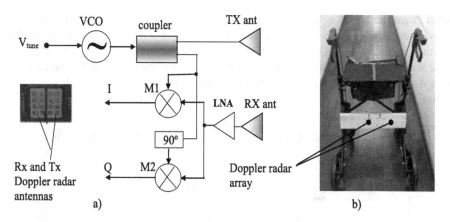

Fig. 3. The smart four wheel rollator based on Doppler radar sensor array: (a) Doppler radar sensor unit implementation and block diagram; (b) smart rollator implementation including the ruler of Doppler radar array, the multifunction board, and the embedded PC.

signals are acquired and used to calculate features that can highlight the evolution of the gait during periodic physiotherapy sessions, which can be used to evaluate the effectiveness of the applied training exercises and also can to perform the gait recognition.

3.2 Acquisition, Signal Processing and Communication

The acquisition of the signals from the Doppler radar sensors and the Vtune generation was performed for the smart rollator prototype using a multifunction board NI MyDAQ that is USB connected to the embedded PC mounted also on the rollator. The acquired signals are processed in order to extract the gait features. The values of the features and the motion wave captured by the Doppler radar array is Wi-Fi transmitted to a client application installed in a tablet that is used by the physiotherapist.

4 Pervasive Computing

Software for a Windows 10′ Tablet materialize the HMI used by the physiotherapist to visualize the signals coming from the IMU wireless network or from the smart rollator using ZigBee or Wi-Fi wireless communication protocol.

4.1 IMU – GUI Through Qk Viewer

Referring to the IMU wireless network software, the Qk Viewer application was developed using the Qt creator [18]. The software allows adding many plots as needed to the plotting area and each plot has its own waveforms selected according to the gait monitoring needs. Each waveform corresponds to a single sensor output data, and the sensor manager allows selecting data from a given IMU node (e.g. right foot node). The Waveform Manager can be used to set the plot's time window and it enables other features such as auto scale, stop plotting when the values reach the end on the chosen time window (e.g. 30 s time window was considered during the experimental tests). In Fig. 4 are presented the acceleration and angle variation associated with gyroscope delivered values.

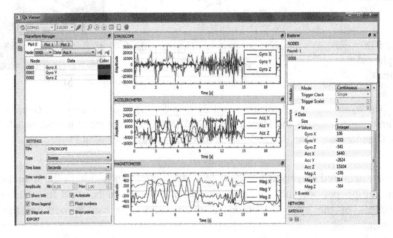

Fig. 4. The GUI associated with the Qk Viewer software.

4.2   IMU Data Processing for Gait Characterization

An IMU (Inertial Measurement Unit) consists of gyroscopes and accelerometers enabling the tracking of rotational and translational movements. A MARG (Magnetic, Angular Rate and Gravity)sensor, also known as AHRS (Attitude and Heading Reference System), is a hybrid IMU which incorporates a tri-axis magnetometer and allows for magnetic distortion compensation. These sensors are able to provide a complete measurement of orientation relative to the direction of gravity and the earth's magnetic field. In the following paragraph the principle of operation of the used IMU and the fusion algorithm implemented to extract useful information that can be used for objective evaluation of rehabilitation effectiveness is presented.

In a three-dimensional space, an object has six degrees of freedom: translation (linear motion) along rotation about each of the three axes: X, Y and Z. Hence, a tri-axis gyroscope and accelerometer are required to measure linear and angular motions and thus orientation. A gyroscope measures angular velocity and an accelerometer measures acceleration forces. These forces may be static, like the constant force of gravity, or they could be dynamic, caused by moving or vibrating the accelerometer. Hence, the accelerometer can also be used to measure linear acceleration. Because the movement and rotation along the three axes are independent of each other, such motion is said to have "six degrees of freedom" or 6DOF. In the case a magnetometer is also used, for magnetic distortion compensation, there are three additional degrees of freedom and the sensor is said to have 9DOF ("nine degrees of freedom"). Regarding the IMU, the angular velocity provided by a gyroscope may be integrated over time to compute the sensor's orientation. However, the integration of gyroscope measurement errors will lead to an accumulating error in the calculated orientation, commonly called drift. Therefore, gyroscopes alone cannot provide an absolute measurement of orientation. An accelerometer and magnetometer will measure the earth's gravitational and magnetic fields respectively and so provide an absolute reference of orientation. However, they are likely to be subject to high levels of noise, for example, accelerations due to motion will corrupt measured direction of gravity. The task of an orientation filter is to compute a single estimate of orientation through the optimal fusion of gyroscope, accelerometer and magnetometer measurements [19]. This process is also called as a data fusion algorithm. Such data fusion algorithms have complex implementations. Many companies and research projects use Kalman filters (or extended Kalman filters, its nonlinear version) [20–22].

As mentioned, data fusion algorithms can be very complex and demand large computational load. The linear regression iteration, fundamental to the Kalman process, demand sampling rates far exceeding the subject bandwidth, for example, a sampling rate between 512 Hz and 30 kHz may be used for human motion capture applications. The state relationships describing rotational kinematics in three-dimensions typically require large state vectors and an extended Kalman filter implementation to linearize the problem. S.O. Madgwick purposes an alternative approach, a novel orientation algorithm designed to support a computationally efficient, wearable inertial human motion tracking system for rehabilitation applications which is presented in [19]. The filter calculates the orientation by numerically integrating the estimated orientation rate. It is computed as the rate of change of orientation measured by the gyroscopes. The magnitude of the gyroscope measurement error is removed in the direction of the estimated error, which is computed from accelerometer and magnetometer measurements. To implement the algorithm, the following ANSI C function, *MadgwickAHRSupdate ()* provided by X-IO technologies, which is a reference software routine in this area, can be used.

```
void MagdwickAHRSupdate (float gx, float gy, float gz,  // Gyroscope values (rad/s)
            float ax, float ay, float az,              // Accelerometer values
            float mx, float my, float mz);             // Magnetometer values
```

Unlike the magnetometer and accelerometer output values, which are normalized by the algorithm, the gyroscope values need to be converted to rad/s. The gyroscopes outputs values are represented in two's complement and have 16 bits of resolution. Hence, its maximum value is $(2^{15}-1)$ and the angular velocity in radians per second is given by

$$G = \frac{G_{raw}}{2^{15}-1} \cdot s \cdot \frac{\pi}{180}$$

where Graw is the two's complemented 16 bit value, s is the scale of the gyroscope in degrees per second (by default is 2000°/s) and G is the angular velocity in radians per second. The algorithm uses a quaternion representation that corresponds to a four-dimensional complex number that is used to represent the orientation of a ridged body or coordinate frame in a three-dimensional space [5]. In each iteration of the algorithm, the quaternions are updated in order to obtain the best evaluation of the angular velocity. However, the QkMotion can also compute the Euler angles (yaw, roll and pitch). It should be noted that Euler angles always have an order in which they are applied. The order for the QkMotion is: pitch, yaw, roll. The Euler representation has the advantage that the angles may be more easily interpreted or visualized. However, its calculation can reach a singularity which results in two rotational axis point in the same direction so one degree of freedom is lost. The algorithm purposed by S.O. Madgwick has a single adjustable parameter, β ($0 < \beta < 0.5$) that is used minimize errors due to integral drift.

4.3   QkDSP: Fixed-Point Digital Signal Processing Algorithms

Biomedical signals are affected by noise and, in many cases, the use of DSP algorithms, such as digital filters, is mandatory for accurate extraction of physiological parameters. Filters are used for noise reduction but also to extract meaningful information from digital signals. Some implementations may be complex and require considerable computational power and memory. Hence, small and low power embedded systems present some challenges due to their lack of processing power and scarce memory. A library that makes digital filters easy to use and implement at the embedded level was implemented and is called QkDSP. This library not only allows the developer to abstract from the implementation details, but also helps to keep the code more orga-nized, since several filters may be implemented by using the same structures and functions. QkDSP provides data structures and functions for the following filters: i) Moving Average (MA), ii) Exponential Moving Average (EMA), iii) Finite Impulse Response (FIR), iv) Infinite Impulse Response (IIR).

All filters, except the MA filter, which does not use fractional numbers, are implemented in fixed-point format. The coefficients of EMA and FIR filters use Q15 format representation, which means that the fractional part of the fractional number is represented with 15 bits while the remaining bit is the sign bit. On the other hand, the format representation of the coefficients of IIR filters should be specified by the developer.

5   Signals and Digital Processing for Gait Characterization

In order to extract information from the smart rollator Doppler radar array sensing channels, different tests were carried out in laboratory conditions using a NI MyDAQ module characterized by a set of two differential analog inputs (AI0 and AI1) and a set of two analog outputs that work as the outputs of a virtual signal generator which are connected to the Vtune radar input. The GaitRadTest software was developed in LabVIEW and permits to generate the Vtune signals and to acquire the Ii (direct), Qi (quadrature) IF signals delivered by i-th sensor of the Doppler radar array. The acquired signals are stored in an embedded PC that materialize the server component of the implemented client-server architecture and the acquired and processed data is accessed through the LabVIEW "Shared variable" technology on the level of mobile devices (smartphone or Tablet) running Android OS or iOS. In this way a user friendly interface to be used by physiotherapist or by the accompanying person to assess the rehabilitation process was implemented.

5.1   Time Analysis

The tests were carried out using as volunteer one physiotherapist that simulates regular gait and also analgesic gait, hemiparetic gait and arthrogenic gait. As an example, Fig. 5 represents the evolution of VI1_n and VI2_n signals acquired from the DRad1 and DRad2 radar sensors using a data acquisition sampling rate equal to 500 S/s.

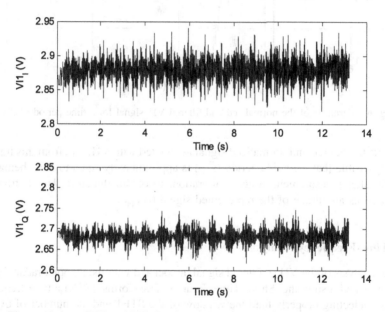

Fig. 5. Time variation of VI1 and VI2 signals acquired from the DRad1 and DRad2 mounted on the rollator.

As it is visible from the figure there exist, in both signals, periodic amplitude variations that are surely related with the gait of the rollator user. As a matter of fact, the period of the signal and peak to peak amplitude variations are related with the stride period and stride length, respectively.

In order to clarify this point, a time sub-interval of the acquired signal, between 6 and 8 s, was selected and filtered. For filtering purposes a finite impulse response filter (FIR) was considered in order to obtain a linear phase response. Moreover, the amplitude of the signal was normalized against its maximum amplitude value. Figure 6

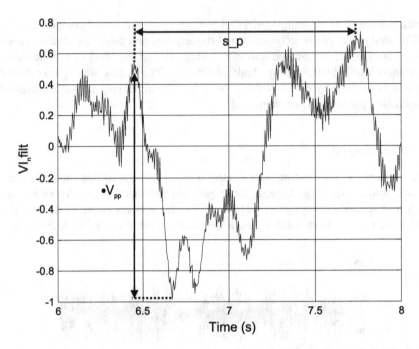

Fig. 6. Variation of the normalized and filtered VI1 signal for a time period of 2 s.

represents the filtered and normalized signal associated with VI1, and from this figure it is clearly visible that the stride period (s_p) is approximately equal to 1.3 s being also possible, after measurement system calibration, to obtain the stride length from the peak to peaks amplitude of the represented signal (ΔV_{pp}).

5.2   Time-Frequency Analysis

Spectral analysis of the VI1_n filtered signal, associated with the Doppler radar signals, was performed using the Short Time Fourier Transforms (STFT) time-frequency operator. Selecting properly the time window of the STFT and the number of overlap points used in the FFT evaluations, it is also possible to obtain in the frequency domain some gait parameters. Regarding the main drawback of the STFT time-frequency operator regarding the compromise that always exists between spectral resolution and time resolution [23], the time window length must be selected according to the patient gait speed, namely the time window must be lower than the stride period but high enough to assure an acceptable frequency analysis resolution. As an example, Fig. 7 represents the evolution of the STFT spectrogram associated with VI1_n for a time window of 2 s.

From the graph it is visible that the power spectrum of the signal is concentrated in a frequency range between 0 and 5 Hz and that the higher amplitude values of the spectral signal are distributed over time according to the step period value.

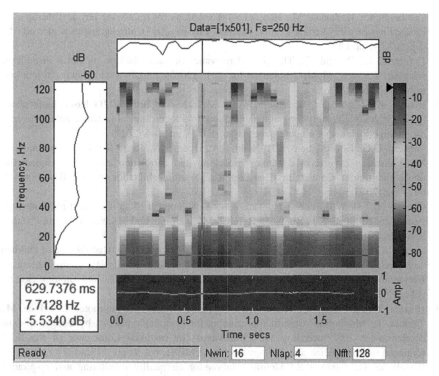

Fig. 7. The evolution STFT spectrogram associated with VI1_n normalized voltage for a time window of 2 s.

6 Conclusion

This work presents a smart rollator architecture based on a 24 GHz FMCW Doppler radar array that captures the gait information during physiotherapy sessions, permitting an objective and unobtrusive evaluation of gait rehabilitation progress, through gait assessment. The proposed system includes elements of the IMU sensor network design that captures kinematic walking parameters and hardware modules that support wireless communications. A particular attention was dedicated to several details related with the implementation and development of software modules to process measurement data and to evaluate gait parameters.

References

1. Wittwer, J., Goldiel, P., Matyas, T.A., Galea, M.P.: Quantification of physiotherapy treatment time in stroke rehabilitation - criterion-related validity. Aust. J Physiotherapy **46**, 292–298 (2000)

2. Campores, C., Kallmann, M., Han, J.J.: VR solutions for improving physical therapy. In: Proceedings of IEEE Virtual Reality, Orlando, Florida (2013). http://graphics.ucmerced.edu/papers/13-vr-pt.pdf
3. Prosperini, L., Pozzilli, C.: The clinical relevance of force platform measures in multiple sclerosis: a review. Multiple Sclerosis Int. 2013 (2013). http://www.hindawi.com/journals/msi/2013/756564/
4. Biswas, K., Mazumder, O., Kundu. A.S.: Multichannel fused EMG based biofeedback system with virtual reality for gait rehabilitation. In: Proceedings of International Conference on Intelligent Human Computer Interaction (IHCI), pp. 1–6 (2012)
5. Western, D.G., Ketteringham, L.P., Neild, S.A., Hyde, R.A., Jones, R.J.S., Davies-Smith, A. M.: Validation of inverse dynamics modelling and correlation analysis to characterise upper-limb tremor. Converging Clin. Eng. Res. Neurorehabilitation Biosyst. Biorobotics 1, 697–702 (2013)
6. Chen, S.L., Lai, W.B., Lee, T.H., Tan, K.K.: Development of an intelligent physiotherapy system. In: Billingsley, J., Bradbeer, R. (eds.) Mechatronics and Machine Vision in Practice. Springer, Heidelberg (2008)
7. Dunne, A., Do-Lenh, S., Laighin, G.O., Shen, C.: Upper extremity rehabilitation of children with cerebral palsy using accelerometer feedback on a multitouch display. In: Proceedings of International Conference of the IEEE on Engineering in Medicine and Biology Society (EMBC 2010), pp. 1751–1754 (2010)
8. Higashi, Y., Sekimoto, M., Horiuchi, F., Kodama, T., Yuji, T., Fujimoto, T., Sekine, M., Tamura, T.: Monitoring rehabilitation training for hemiplegic patients by using a tri-axial accelerometer. In: Proceedings of 23rd Annual International Conference of the IEEE Engineering in Medicine and Biology Society (EMBS), vol. 2, pp. 1472–1474 (2001)
9. Postolache, O., Girão, P.S.: Mobile solution for air quality monitoring and respiration activity monitoring based on an Android OS smartphone. In: Proceedings IMEKO TC19 Symposium, Cavtat, Croatia, vol. 1, pp. 1–4 (2011)
10. Ribeiro, M.R., Postolache, O., Girão, P.S.: A novel smart sensing platform for vital signs and motor activity monitoring. In: Mason, A., Mukhopadhyay, S.C., Jayasundera, K.P., Bhattacharyya, N. (eds.) Sensing Technology: Current Status and Future Trends I. Springer, Heidelberg (2014)
11. Postolache, O., Ribeiro, M., Girão, P., Pereira, J., Postolache, G.: Unobtrusive sensing for gait rehabilitation. In: Proceeding of REHAB 2014 Workshop, Germany (2014)
12. Postolache, O., Girão, P., Ribeiro, M., Carvalho, H., Catarino, A., Postolache, G.: Treat me well: affective and physiological feedback for wheelchair users. In: Proceedings of IEEE International Symposium on Medical Measurements and Applications, Budapest, Hungary (2012)
13. Postolache, O., Girao, P.S., Dias Pereira, J., Pincho, J., Moura, C., Postolache, G.: Smart walker for pervasive healthcare. In: Proceedings of Fifth International Conference on Sensing Technology, Palmerston North, New Zealand (2011)
14. Chan, A.D.C., Green, J.R.: Smart rollator prototype. In: Proceedings of IEEE International Workshop on Medical Measurement and Applications (2008)
15. Lin, J.F., Kulić, D.: Human pose recovery using wireless inertial measurement units. Physiol. Meas. 33, 12 (2012)
16. Ribeiro, M.R., Postolache, O., Girão, P.S.: Modular platform architecture for fast prototyping of vital signs and motor activity monitors. In: Proceedings of IEEE International Instrumentation and Technology Conference - I2MTC, Minneapolis, United States, vol. 1, pp. 1–6 (2013)
17. Farahani, S.: ZigBee Wireless Netwoks and Transceivers. Newnes, Elsevier, Amsterdam, Boston (2008)

18. KDE Techbase: Development/Tutorials/Using Qt Creator (2014). https://techbase.kde.org/Development/Tutorials/Using_Qt_Creator
19. Madgwick, S.O.H., Harrison, A.J.L., Vaidyanathan, R.: Estimation of IMU and MARG orientation using a gradient descent algorithm. In: IEEE International Conference on Rehabilitation Robotics (ICORR), pp. 1–7 (2011)
20. Mirzaei, F.M., Roumeliotis, S.I.: A kalman filter-based algorithm for imu-camera calibration: observability analysis and performance evaluation. IEEE Trans. Rob. **24**(5), 1143–1156 (2008)
21. Won, S.H., Melek, W., Golnaraghi, F.: Position and orientation estimation using kalman filtering and particle diltering with one imu and one position sensor. In: Industrial Electronics, 34th Annual Conference of IEEE, pp. 3006–3010 (2008)
22. Sabatelli, S., Galgani, M., Fanucci, L., Rocchi, A.: A double stage kalman filter for sensor fusion and orientation tracking in 9D IMU. In: Proceedings of IEEE Sensors Applications Symposium (SAS), pp. 1–5. IEEE (2012)
23. Allen, J.B., Rabiner, L.: A unified approach to Short-Time Fourier analysis and synthesis. In: Proceedings of IEEE, vol. 65, Issue. 11, pp. 1558–1564 (1997)

Blind User Perspectives on a Navigational Autonomy Aid

Saleh Alghamdi, Ron van Schyndel$^{(\boxtimes)}$, and Margaret Hamilton

School of Computer Science and IT, RMIT University, Melbourne, Australia
s3299407@student.rmit.edu.au,
{ron.vanschyndel,margaret.hamilton}@rmit.edu.au

Abstract. In previous papers, we presented a navigational autonomy aid system, which was tested by sighted people and reached a high level of satisfaction. However our new positioning technique is suitable for blind users as well as sighted since the user is able to wear or carry the reader. The system consists of a line-of-sight QR-code detector and the signal attenuation of active RFID tags using a wearable reader, which is non-line-of-sight. The aim of this chapter is to present user feedback from the perspectives of blind people. A significant outcome of the usability test on blind participants is that to meet the requirements of blind users, the system must work in an integrated manner.

Keywords: Blind user interface · RFID · QR-code · Blind user experience

1 Introduction

We have developed a system to guide blind people and assist them to reach their destinations. In this chapter we explain our usability testing of this system to produce a more usable navigation system for blind people. Therefore, the aims of this usability testing are to uncover the limitations of the system from the perspectives of actual blind users and to evaluate the satisfaction of real users in relation to further development of the navigational system.

This chapter is a complement to a publication presented in the workshop of the 8th International Conference on Pervasive Computing Technologies for Healthcare (Per-vasiveHealth '14) [15] taking into consideration the previous work, we present a concrete scenario of how the system works.

One important rehabilitation step for people who have recently become blind, or had their vision reduced, is to regain their autonomy and to feel that they are in control of their movement and lives again [1]. The ability to navigate and react to their immediate environment is central to their independence and hence autonomy. Since the levels of blindness vary among users and even in the one user from time to time, we decided to build a system which is both passive and active, relying on using both line-of-sight and non-line-of-sight technologies to give the user feedback about their current position.

The scenario for our system is summarised in Fig. 1, where the cubes represent the hardware components—active RFID, QR-code and Kinect—and the rounded rectangles represent the main service algorithms of the system. The navigation process

© Springer-Verlag Berlin Heidelberg 2015
H.M. Fardoun et al. (Eds.): REHAB 2014, CCIS 515, pp. 248–259, 2015.
DOI: 10.1007/978-3-662-48645-0_21

follows three steps: (1) the system indicates the initial position of the user as a start point using an RFID algorithm based on the technique of attenuation control; (2) the user is recommended to scan the surrounding area using a camera to detect QR-codes using a built-in QR-code reader application; and (3) the navigation application determines the most preferable route for the user and then starts providing voice instructions. Route calculation is based on Dijkstra's algorithm [2], which identifies the shortest path between two points (the current position and the destination).

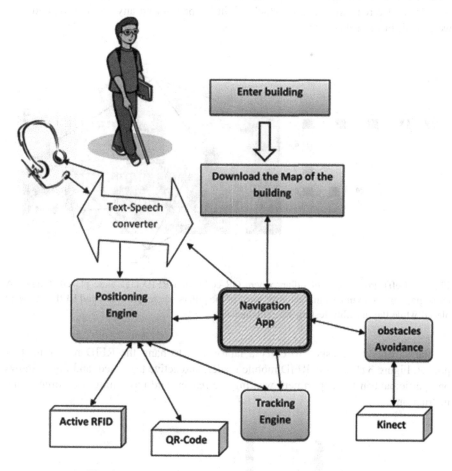

Fig. 1. The scenario of the proposed navigational system

An initial testing was performed in the office area. The system achieved excellent results in identifying the realtime position of the user and in guiding that user to various destinations within the domain of the Distributed Systems Department. Therefore, the author was enthusiastic about applying the system on real blind participants, and this represents the second stage of usability testing. Human Ethics approval for this part of the study, to be conducted on real blind subjects in Saudi Arabia, was provided by RMIT.

The participants who volunteered for the usability testing were eight males aged between 17 and 20 years. The path they were required to navigate took them around their indoor school gymnasium which was large enough to require significant navigation, but enclosed and protected enough for them not to run into other students or staff during testing. The QR-codes were printed on A4-size paper and attached to pillars at various points in the room (see Fig. 2(Left) and (Right). RFID tags were installed above the QR-coded sheets of paper. The distances between pillars were measured and recorded and so the system was fully adapted for that environment. All tests were conducted as a real-life scenario which might happen during any school day, and they were held during school time.

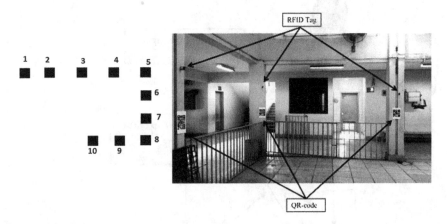

Fig. 2. (Left). Positioning of pillars where QR-codes and RFID tags were placed. **(Right)** A photograph of the gymnasium, featuring some of the pillars where QR-codes and RFID tags were placed while the usability testing was conducted.

Participants were asked to carry a laptop and to hang the RFID reader in their pocket. Figure 3 shows the RFID mobile reader, and active tags used, and Fig. 4 shows one participant in the experiment wearing the reader, and navigating according to the instructions.

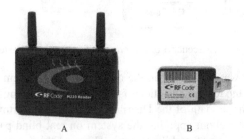

Fig. 3. (Left), RFCode M220 mobile reader. **(Right),** M175 active rugged tag.

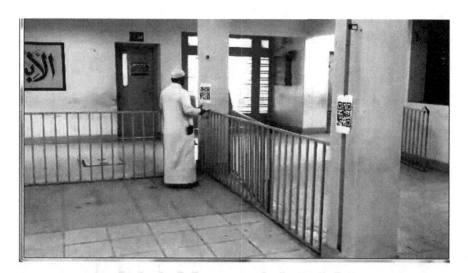

Fig. 4. One of the participants during the experiment, showing the RFID reader hanging from his pocket.

2   Related Work

In the past there have been several navigational technologies developed to aid blind and vision-impaired (BVI) people [3–10]. Many researchers have considered computer scene understanding both at high and low levels, and implemented systems using different modalities such as the navigational tool proposed by Mihajlik et al. [11], which is based on installing sound generation into a navigation system by using signal processing and ultrasonic echolocation. Their system has been applied successfully with a 3D sound-generation technique for mobile robots. Other research discussed in [3] is the Electronic Travel Authority (ETA). An ETA is similar to Mihajlik's device in that both use ultrasonic waves to detect obstacles, but ETAs aim to identify objects specifically for visually impaired users. Later research undertaken by [8] considered a vision sensor camera for capturing images and then processing these images to convert them to sound. Most of this research has employed a grey-level technique to identify objects in images, and the NAVI system [8] is a well-known example of this approach. Our proposed system has been described in detail in papers [12–14].

3   Planning the Usability Tasks

The usability testing required participants to undertake a variety of tasks, ranging from a simple task such as walking from point 2 towards point 3 along the same line as shown in part (A) in Fig. 5, to more complex tasks, all shown in Fig. 5 below.

For instance, navigating from point 9 to point 2, is shown as (E) in Fig. 5 and is the most complex task. This overall concept was designed to give the participants the opportunity to become more familiar with the system, as we believed that training on the system was a necessary requirement for new users to enjoy its full benefits.

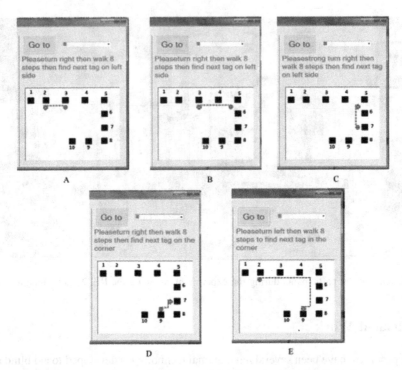

Fig. 5. The test routes from the simple 'A' to more complex 'E'.

Participants were asked to undertake the following tasks:

- Identify their destination. As shown in Fig. 5(A), low-vision people may be able to indicate their destination by clicking the 'Go To' button, but a voice recognition feature was added to the system so that blind people could communicate their desired destination via verbal commands;
- Make an error. The participants were asked to deliberately commit an error, such as turning right instead of following instructions from the system to turn left. The purpose of this was to evaluate the error-detection feature shown in Fig. 6(C). This tested the ability of the system to calculate an alternative path to guide the user from their current incorrect location to their target destination successfully.
- Recognise when they have arrived. This is to test whether or not the participant could see or hear the message shown in Fig. 6(B).
- Apply the QR-code navigation system alone. Each participant was asked to walk to five destinations using the QR-codes alone and pointing the camera in the general direction.
- Apply the RFID navigation system alone. Each participant was asked to do the test again just using the RFID technology, where pointing was unnecessary, but locations were slightly more error prone.
- Apply the integrated system of RFID plus QR-codes to do the test again and navigate towards a variety of destinations.
- Answer eight questions regarding usability of the system.

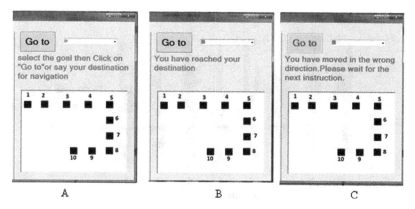

Fig. 6. Interface of the mobile navigation program. Part (A) represents the start interface, Part (B) represents the final stage when the user reaches the destination successfully, and Part (C) represents the error-detection feature.

4   Results

As soon as each participant completed their requested navigational tasks, they were asked to answer the questions explained in the following sections.

4.1   Trust in the System

The average confidence in reaching destinations by using the navigation system with QR-codes alone was 3.875 out of 5. This increased using the RFID system to 4.25 out of 5 while the average trust for using the integrated system was 4.75 out of 5, as shown in Fig. 7. Half of the participants were more trusting of the RFID system to help them reach their destination. Three participants trusted the RFID and QR-code systems

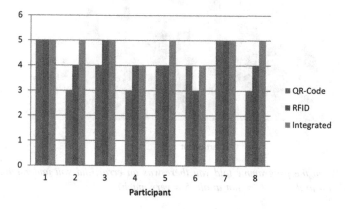

Fig. 7. *Q1: Do you feel that you were guided well to reach the destinations? Answers ranged from 1 (Unsatisfactory) to 5 (Excellent).*

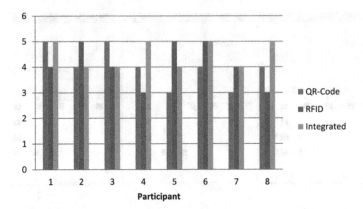

Fig. 8. *Q2: Do you believe you reached each waypoint on time, according to the program?*

equally and only one participant preferred the QR-code over the RFID system. An integrated system was more trusted by most participants.

4.2 User Tracking During the Trip

The system estimates the time required to reach each waypoint on the trip. This enables it to track the user for error-detection purposes. The required time is calculated based on a standard blind walking speed of approximately 1 m per second. The average satisfaction with the required time calculation method was similar for the QR-codes, RFID and the integrated system where the average overall was $\sim$ 4 out of 5, as shown in Fig. 9.

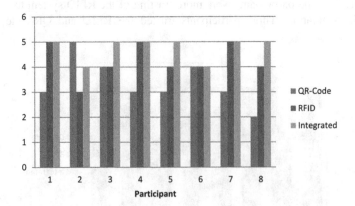

Fig. 9. *Q3: When the programme told you there was an error, did you understand what the system asked you to do next (1 = not at all, 5 = very much)?*

4.3   Error Detection and Path Recalculation

This question relates to the error-detection feature and enabled an examination of the degree to which participants believed that the system was able to recalculate an alternative path to guide them to their destination. As shown in Fig. 8, the average satisfaction of participants regarding the QR-code system was 3.375 out of 5 and the average level of satisfaction increased with the RFID system to 4.25 of 5. Using the integrated system, satisfaction increased to 4.75 out of 5 for error detection and successful re-routing of participants to their destinations.

4.4   The Importance of Training

Almost every participant gave a score of 4 or 5 out of 5 for considering the benefit of training on the system. All participants believed that training is required and helpful for the systems (QR-code, RFID and integrated) so they gave the same scores for all systems regarding this question, as shown in Fig. 10.

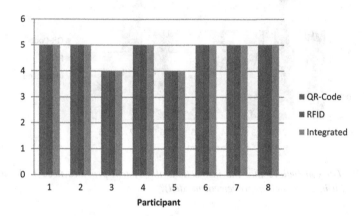

Fig. 10. *Q4: Do you feel you got more confident using the system over time (1 = not at all, 5 = very much)?*

4.5   Requirements for Improvement

After participants performed all tasks they were asked: '*Can you suggest any improvements?*' Most suggestions were with respect to voice instructions, in terms of language and volume level. Around one-third of the participants preferred to hear Arabic instructions, and three-quarters of participants found it difficult to hear the instructions because of the background noise in the school.

4.6   Satisfaction Regarding Mode of Instruction

The instructions were the same for all designs of the system (QR-code, RFID and integrated) so all participants gave the same score for their levels of satisfaction regarding the way in which the instructions were delivered to them: only two participants gave 1 of 5 regarding the way of instructions as shown in Fig. 10, which means that participants were relatively dissatisfied with the mode of instruction. It is believed that language and volume level were mainly responsible for this lack of satisfaction.

4.7   Perspectives of Participants Regarding RFID, QR-Code and the Integrated System

Three of the participants preferred to use the RFID navigation system. In contrast, all other participants stated that the integrated system (RFID + QR-code) was more beneficial and useful for them (see Fig. 11). All participants reported that using QR-code system by itself was difficult compared with the integrated system, so none of

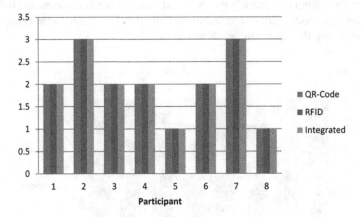

Fig. 11. *Q6: Do you believe that the instructions the system provides need to be improved (1 = Happy with it, 5 = Much improvement needed)?*

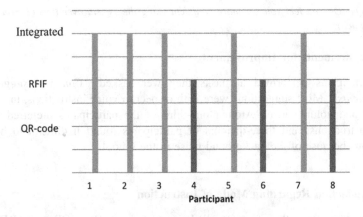

Fig. 12. *Q7: With which of the systems are you more comfortable: the QR-code system or the RFID system? Or do you prefer both of them? Why?*

them preferred the QR-code navigation system. Also, from the responses to Q1 we found participants trusted the RFID and the integrated systems more than QR-code system. Therefore, circles have been added around the QR-codes to make them easier to detect from a greater distance (Fig. 12).

4.8   Preferred Application Method

As can be seen in Fig. 13, two of the participants would prefer to use this navigation system and receive the navigational instructions via spectacles or headphones. The other participants preferred to have this navigation system installed as an application on their smartphones.

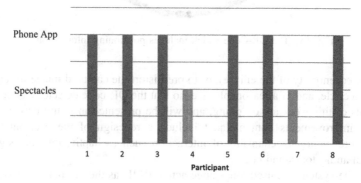

Fig. 13. *Q8: If we turned this system into a product that you can buy, would you prefer it as a mobile phone app or as spectacles that can speak into your ears?*

5   Further Work

Subsequent to this research, we have made a number of changes to the system, in order to improve its performance. One of the changes was in the presentation of the QR code.

We found that the binary hit-and-miss nature of QR-code detection was a problem, in that there was sense of getting closer to or further away from a QR-code, and being able to adapt based on distance. In other words, if a user was too far away for adequate code detection, they may not even have a clue that a QR-code exists.

To improve on this, we adapted the QR-code detector as in Fig. 14 to allow a more distant measure of it, by having the system say "There may be a QR code ahead. Please move closer so that it can be read".

The system would first look for circles within the captured image, with the line-width matching the figure, (which may be colored to further reduce the likelihood of false matches). In addition, it would require a monochrome dual-tone color-set within the circle which is the QR-code itself and the background color.

Unless presented normally to the user camera (which is unlikely), this circle would appear as an ellipse, and the major axis, eccentricity and orientation of the ellipse would provide clues for either repositioning the user to be more normal (and hence

Fig. 14. The QR-Code which includes positioning information

reduce the eccentricity of the ellipse), or to pre-distort the captured image to render the ellipse as a circle, and of a reasonable size, so that the QR-code detector can do its job. The results of this work are on-going, and will be presented in future papers.

Other improvements contemplated include a redesign of the user interface to employ more natural mechanisms of interaction such as haptic, pressure signals or non-verbal audio tones and cues.

While the system has used long-range active RFID as the mechanism, we are also exploring other approaches such as WiFi signal strength detection, although with this technology, we lose the advantage of a portable transmitter to do the ranging.

6   Conclusion

The chapter presents a user testing of a navigational system based on QR-codes integrated with active RFID technology. The system has been tested in two stages: firstly by sighted people for debugging purposes and secondly by blind people for usability. With respect to the results of the usability test, the majority of blind participants preferred to use an integrated system of RFID and QR-codes. Because the active RFID system works independently, its accuracy is less than 2 m and its range is up to 70 m, to increase precision of positioning information the user needs to start scanning in that 1-m area to detect QR-codes, which are very difficult for the blind to detect without the assistance of RFID. Therefore, from a blind user's perspective, RFID has the advantage that it works independently while the advantage of QR-code is that it makes users more confident and gives them trust in the system which includes QR-codes. Hence, most participants believed that the integrated system provided higher precision navigational instructions to them.

References

1. Science Daily 2007, viewed 10 April 2014
2. http://www.sciencedaily.com/releases/2007/02/070216221522.htm
3. Dijkstra, E.W.: A note on two problems in connexion with graphs. Numer. Mathe. 1(1), 269–271 (1959)
4. Balakrishnan, G., Sainarayanan, G., Nagarajan, R., Yaacob, S.: Stereo image to stereo sound methods for vision based ETA. In: 1st International Conference on Computers, Communications, & Signal Processing with Special Track on Biomedical Engineering, pp. 193–196, IEEE (2005)
5. Calder, D.J.: Travel aids for the blind—the digital ecosystem solution. In: 7th IEEE International Conference on Industrial Informatics, pp. 149–154. IEEE (2009)
6. Choudhury, M.H., Aguerrevere, D., Barreto, A.B.: A pocket-PC based navigational aid for blind individuals. In: IEEE Symposium on Virtual Environments, Human–Computer Interfaces and Measurement Systems, pp. 43–48. IEEE (2004)
7. Nagarajan, R., Yaacob, S., Sainarayanan, G.: Fuzzy clustering in vision recognition applied in NAVI. In: Proceedings of the Annual Meeting of the North American Fuzzy Information Processing Society, pp. 261–266. IEEE (2002)
8. Nagarajan, R., Yaacob, S., Sainarayanan, G.: Role of object identification in sonification system for visually impaired. In: TENCON 2003, Conference on Convergent Technologies for the Asia–Pacific Region, vol. 2, pp. 735–739. IEEE (2003)
9. Nagarajan, R., Sainarayanan, G., Yacoob, S., Porle, R.R.: An improved object identification for NAVI. In: TENCON 2004, IEEE Region 10 Conference, pp. 455–458. IEEE (2004)
10. Xia, L., Chen, C.-C., Aggarwal, J.: Human detection using depth information by Kinect. In: IEEE Computer Society Conference on Computer Vision and Pattern Recognition Workshops, pp. 15–22. IEEE (2011)
11. Wong, F., Nagarajan, R., Yaacob, S.: Application of stereovision in a navigation aid for blind people. In: Proceedings of the 2003 Joint Conference of the Fourth International Conference on Information, Communications and Signal Processing, vol. 2, pp. 734–737. IEEE (2003)
12. Mihajlik, P., Guttermuth, M., Seres, K., Tatai, P.: DSP-based ultrasonic navigation aid for the blind. In: Proceedings of the 18th IEEE Instrumentation and Measurement Technology Conference, vol 3, pp. 1535–1540. IEEE (2001)
13. Alghamdi, S., van Schyndel, R., Khalil, I.: Accurate positioning using long range active RFID technology to assist visually impaired people. J. Netw. Comput. Appl. 41, 135–147 (2014)
14. Alghamdi, S., van Schyndel, R.: Accurate positioning based on a combination of power attenuation and a signal strength indicator using active RFID technology. In: Third International Conference on Indoor Positioning and Indoor Navigation (IPIN), Nov 2012, pp. 1–4. Sydney, Australia (2012)
15. Alghamdi, S., van Schyndel, R., Alahmadi, A.: Indoor navigational aid using active RFID and QR-code for sighted and blind people. In: Eighth International Conference on Intelligent Sensors, Sensor Networks and Information Processing (ISSNIP), Apr 2013, pp. 18–22. Melbourne, Australia (2013)
16. Alghamdi, S., van Schyndel, R., Hamilton, M.: Blind user response to a navigational system to assist blind people using active RFID and QR-code. In: Proceedings of the 8th International Conference on Pervasive Computing Technologies for Healthcare (PervasiveHealth 2014). ICST (Institute for Computer Sciences, Social-Informatics and Telecommunications Engineering), ICST, pp. 313–316. Brussels, Belgium (2014) DOI=10.4108/icst.pervasivehealth.2014.255354, http://dx.doi.org/10.4108/icst.pervasivehealth.2014.255354

Smart Garment Design for Rehabilitation

Qi Wang, Wei Chen, and Panos Markopoulos[✉]

Eindhoven University of Technology,
Den Dolech 2, 5612 AZ Eindhoven, The Netherlands
p.markopoulos@tue.nl

Abstract. During rehabilitation training posture monitoring is very important for enhancing training effectiveness. This article presents the design and implementation of a smart rehabilitation garment (SRG) to support posture correction. The garment the design and implementation of a smart rehabilitation garment (SRG) to support posture correction. The garment has been designed to supports posture monitoring feedback, during training. The garment consists of accelerometers in various positions with smart textile integration, controlled by a Lilypad Arduino processor which also controls vibrator motors that provide tactile feedback to patients. The SRG is driven by a software application running on a smartphone or personal computer by Bluetooth, which presents fine grain feedback, and training results and reminders to patients. In this paper we focus on the sensing modules' placements and embedded design based on the integration of smart textiles. This work places particular emphasis on having a practical, wearable, and aesthetic device, as these are crucial elements for making the device useful in context and accepted by its users.

Keywords: Wearable technology · Arm-hand rehabilitation · Smart garment design · Smart textiles

1 Introduction

There is a growing need for rehabilitation for patients with neurological and musculoskeletal conditions, some of which are age related (e.g., stroke, Parkinson, multiple sclerosis) [1] and others that are chronic (low back pain, cerebral palsy). For a variety of reasons, the most important of which is the aging of the population, there is a growing need to support rehabilitation training with technology in order to provide more efficient and effective therapy, and to support patients to reach their full potential for recovery.

In this context there is particular interest for technologies that can reduce the requirements upon direct involvement and supervision by health professionals. For example, in stroke rehabilitation technology can support training through providing interactive exercises and even games, designed to help the patient practice tasks, to improve their strength, and control, see for example [2, 3]. Due to the long duration of such rehabilitation processes, the prospect of using rehabilitation technologies at home offers the promise of cost-efficiency and of increase in the amount of training, which can in turn improve training outcomes.

© Springer-Verlag Berlin Heidelberg 2015
H.M. Fardoun et al. (Eds.): REHAB 2014, CCIS 515, pp. 260–269, 2015.
DOI: 10.1007/978-3-662-48645-0_22

One of the most important tasks currently requiring attention and efforts by therapists concerns the correct execution of exercises. For example, neurological patients who have a diminished capability to control their arm and hand, tend to develop compensatory strategies where they use alternative movements and muscle groups to compensate for the diminished capability in their upper extremities: rather than reaching out to grasp an object they are likely to bend forward to get closer to it and then grasp it. Applying such compensatory strategies can be necessary for getting by in daily life, but during training it reduces training effectiveness and prevents patients from reaching their full potential. It is typically the task of therapists to supervise the correct execution of exercises and, when necessary to remind patients to keep the right posture or to provide corrective feedback when the patient moves outside a specific range. Having to do this limits the ability of therapists to supervise multiple patients at any time or even the ability of patients to train unsupervised. This observation suggests the potential utility of posture monitoring and feedback technology for rehabilitation training.

Earlier research provides ample examples of how posture monitoring and training could be used for rehabilitation. For example, Timmermans et al. used sensors on the arm and torso of stroke patients during training with the Philips stroke exerciser [4], in order to ensure the correct execution of exercise. Beursgens et al., developed a vest for monitoring the patient posture while playing a serious game intended to support arm-hand rehabilitation [5, 6]. These systems suggest how wearable sensor technology can be used in combination with other rehabilitation technologies in the specific context of neurological rehabilitation of upper extremities.

Posture correction can have a much wider applicability than upper extremity rehabilitation. For example, Wong et al. show how trunk posture monitoring can support scoliosis patients and can prevent further pain and deterioration of their condition [7]. In the context of a research study Seo et al. [8] showed how monitoring the trunk position could help assess risks imposed by asymmetric posture at workplaces using detectors that consisted of gyroscopes and accelerometers.

Here, we present the design of a prototype wearable device for supporting posture monitoring and correction during rehabilitation training - an earlier description of this prototype can be found in [9]. The device is a stand alone system that is designed to be used independently as well as in combination with exercises or gaming systems supporting rehabilitation. We focus especially on improving the engineering and design qualities of this smart rehabilitation garment.

Paralleling the advances in wearable application in rehabilitation and miniaturization in particular, a number of SRG's aiming at support arm-hand training have been developed [10, 11]. Although wearable technology shows great promise and provides many technical benefits in these systems [12], other aspects like wearability, comfort and aesthetics are often neglected [13]. A potential explanation could lie in the novelty of this technological field, where most effort is still directed towards the development of sensors and establishing their measuring accuracy rather than in their integration into complete systems. For example, a recent literature survey [1] of wearable sensor systems to support upper extremity rehabilitation, could only find 27 articles reporting the development of systems beyond the proof of concept, only 4 of which were integrated into a complete exercise system that could support training and another 5 in gaming applications. We note however that particularly when aiming to support tele-rehabilitation it is important to consider more practical aspects of the garments, how easy they are to wash, how flexible and light they are, whether they are aligned with current style trends, etc., all issues that directly influence the wearer's experience.

We describe in this research how sensor – based wearable technologies can be used for posture monitoring and correction during rehabilitation training. We propose an interactive wearable system that consists of: a sensing garment integrated with wearable acceleration sensors and conductive networks; an android-based application that communicates with the garment by Bluetooth that can control the garment and can provide visual feedback. We expect this system has great potential to be an associated therapy contributing to the rehabilitation training.

2 Related Work

In recent years, systems and applications for motion capture for training has attracted a lot of attention. For example, in 2011 Lee et al. [14] proposed a wearable limb monitoring system using integrated accelerometers that do not constrain human movement and were easy to wear. Although the system does not provide feedback to subjects, the accurate results during measurements showed its potential for rehabilitation systems. Markopoulos et al. [15] developed a wrist-worn system to support the monitoring of relative movement of the two limbs through the day, with the aim to motivate stroke patients with a unilateral deficit to keep moving their damaged arm.

3 System Concept and Requirements

We propose a monitoring system that aims to improve motor training quality by sensing the compensation movement with shoulder and torso, as shown in Fig. 1. While wearing the garment during rehabilitation exercises, the patient or the therapist can set a goal range. Further to continuous feedback regarding posture, notifications for wrong movements can be provided. When the detected compensation movement exceeds the set values, the user can receive some vibration or audio notification, which can be turned off when not desirable.

Following the guidance from therapist and earlier investigations [6, 16], we identified the design of the garment system for arm-hand rehabilitation should consider the following requirements for both the function and user experience aspects:

- It should be easy to put on and take off and should be worn with normal clothes on.
- It should be light, comfortable, and appropriate for long term monitoring.
- Sensors should always be close to the user's body for data accuracy.
- It should provide feedback for monitoring result and system's functioning.
- It should be scalable for other modular functions.
- It should be adjustable for different sizes.

Currently our prototype system consists of two parts: a smart sensing jacket and a smartphone application that controls the system and provides graphical feedback. The

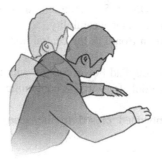

Fig. 1. Example of compensation movement

sensor position is shown in Fig. 2, two accelerometers (S1, S2) are placed on the T1 and T5 of spinal column for monitor trunk movement [17]. While the other one placed on the shoulder of the patients affected side (S3 or S4).

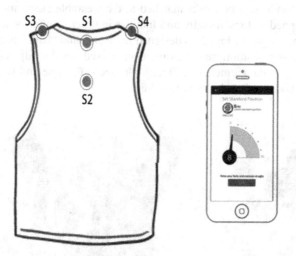

Fig. 2. System Overview

4 Prototype and Architecture

We provide a description of the prototype design and application development in this section.

4.1 Components in Detail

The system contains three sensor nodes that communicate to two Lilypad Arduinos. The sensor comprises the following components:

- 2 LilyPad Accelerometer ADXL335 sensing unit; these sensors were preferred over other possibilities because of their wearability.
- 2 LilyPad Arduino 328 Main Board as the central node read sensor data from the 3 accelerometer separately,
- a small and inconspicuous LilyPad Power Supply with input battery from 1.2v–5v,
- a Bluetooth Mate Silver module for wireless communication between the jacket and smartphone,
- LilyPad Vibe Board embedded closed to the accelerometer provide vibration feedback.

4.2 Garment Design

The whole system is designed to be modular, allowing the hard electronic parts to be easily detached and reattached for washing. The removable design of the wearable electronics, potentially allows users to have garments made of different material or for various scenarios during their rehabilitation exercise at home. The sensing garments have the same conductive networks matched to the wearable electronics. The sensing garment is designed to look friendly and familiar in order to offer better engagement.

The garment, shown in Fig. 3, is designed in "front" and "back" parts for ensuring the accurate sensor position and measurement. Based on the adjustable design on shoulder and wrists, the garment can fit multiple sizes of people and keeps the sensors close to users' body and at the right location.

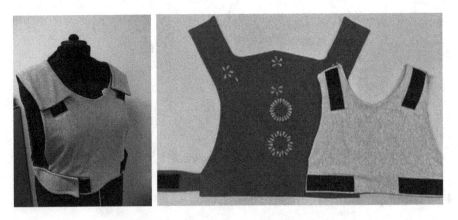

Fig. 3. Prototype of Smart Rehabilitation Garment

4.3 Conductive Textiles Integration

Conductive textiles in health care garment applications show a great potential, can help users who wear them feel more free and monitoring posture all day for home-based rehabilitation. In this system, a conductive network was applied to enhance the aesthetics of the design without adding the original resistances.

We designed conductive fabric pattern for the removable design of wearable sensor and conductive path for the connection between the electronic modules, shown in Figs. 4 and 5. The sensors can easily connect to the garment by attached snaps.

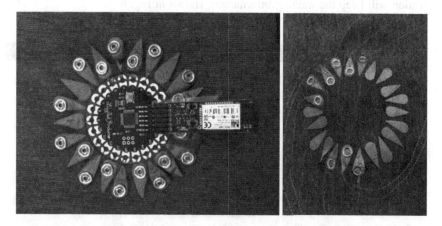

Fig. 4. Conductive fabric pattern for Lilypad Arduino.

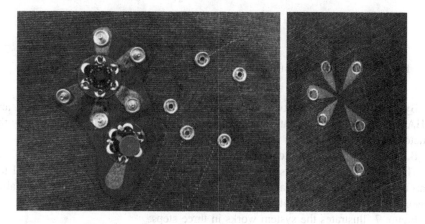

Fig. 5. Conductive fabric pattern for Accelerometer.

Furthermore, as the cut pieces are small and need to match exactly, a laser cutter is effective for this process.

4.4 Application Implementation

'SmartSuit' is our application supported the garment that runs on android-based smart phone and tablet computer. The application is implemented using the MIT App Inventor (see www.appinventor.mit.edu) that is an online open-source and block-based programming tool. The main functions and interface design of 'SmartSuit' are described below.

A. Enabling the garment

Before enabling the garment, user needs to login 'SmartSuit', in this way the application will keep the training information, shown in Fig. 6.

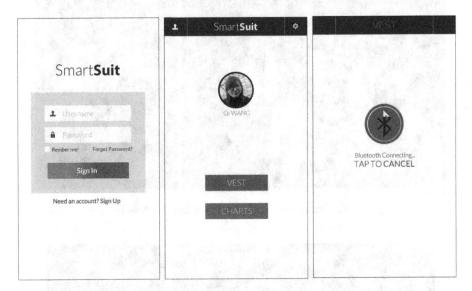

Fig. 6. Interface design. (a) Login Page. (b) Navigation (c) Bluetooth Connection.

By now, we developed two functions: 'VEST' provide real-time feedback and 'CHARTS' goes to history data. 'SmartSuit' connects with the sensing garment by the Bluetooth module plugged in the Lilypad arduino.

B. Control the training process

The 'VEST' page consists of 3 items: personal information on top; graphical fan chart and pointer; instruction and control button. Key point is the pointer will visualize sensor data in real-time by rotation and value in circle.

Figure 7 illustrates the system works in three steps:

(1) Setting the start value while they relax their body and maintain straight their body;
(2) Setting the target value that is suggested by therapist and based on training difficulty and history data;
(3) The pointer will rotate as the user moving forward and upward, while the pointer is out of range, the dark circle shown in Fig. 7, garment will vibrate on the special place (torso or shoulder sensor).

C. Dashboard

Figure 8 illustrates the dashboard design. This interactive page is an interactive tool that lets you explore your historic progress by selecting the buttons on the right side to see the process obtained yearly/monthly/daily. We also offer the complete situation in

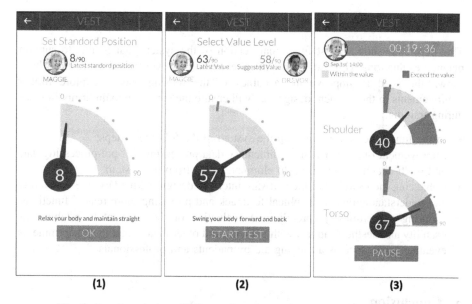

Fig. 7. Interface design. (1) Start value. (2) Target value (3) Training value

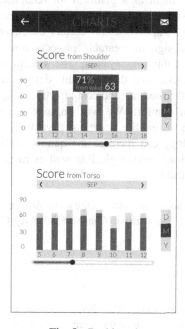

Fig. 8. Dashboard

the bar graph that when the user is nearing the goal and when they achieved them. So both the user and therapist can see the positive result of long-term home rehabilitation and adjust the training project.

5 Future Work

This paper has shown a fist functional version of the system that is able to support planned evaluations with users and clinical experts. However, initial evaluations have shown the need to improve the accuracy of the sensing and to explore further improvements in the garment design that will ensure the sensors remain firmly in place during training.

- In the future we plan to develop the system in the following steps:
- Improvement of the currently rudimentary data processing, for pre-processing data and multi-channel data fusion to eliminate noise from the system.
- Enhancing the usability of the software interface design, particularly the readability and understandability of graphical feedback and providing more related functions.
- Carrying a preliminary (pre-clinical) evaluation of the garment to establish its usability and aesthetic appeal with patients, and other factors that may determine its eventual acceptance as a training aid by patients and professionals.

6 Conclusion

We set out to design a garment as a platform for rehabilitation research. We have proposed a design of the smart rehabilitation garment system, providing feedback of compensation movement to improve users' correct execution of exercise. The integration of smart textiles design to wearable projects contributes to implement the reliable and comfortable monitoring system. The system can be used in different context and training approaches and the adjustable design ensures the sensors stay in the right positions. Due to the modular and cost-effective design, the system has a good potential for accuracy and comfort. We will improve the system to become more applicable and easy-to-use to real-life situations. Eventually we aspire that wearable posture correction technology can increase the quality of living for patients with a variety of conditions requiring neurological as well as musculoskeletal rehabilitation for upper extremities and trunk.

Acknowledgments. We acknowledge with gratitude to Annick A.A. Timmermans for the sensing position guidance. We also thanks to Chinese Scholarship Council support the research.

References

1. Wang, Q., Markopolous, P., Chen, W.: Literature review on wearable systems in upper extremity rehabilitation. In: International Conference on Biomedical and Health Informatics (BHI), pp. 551–555 (2014)
2. Langhorne, P., Bernhardt, J., Kwakkel, G.: Stroke rehabilitation. Lancet **377**(9778), 1693–1702 (2011)

3. Alankus, G., Lazar, A., May, M., Kelleher, C.: Towards customizable games for stroke rehabilitation. In: Proceedings of the SIGCHI Conference on Human Factors in Computing Systems, pp. 2113–2122 (2010)
4. Timmermans, A.A.A., Saini, P., Willmann, R.D., Lanfermann, G., te Vrugt, J., Winter, S.: Home stroke rehabilitation for the upper limbs. In: Engineering in Medicine and Biology Society, 29th Annual International Conference of the IEEE, pp. 4015–4018 (2007)
5. Beursgens, L., Timmermans, A.A.A., Markopoulos, P.: Playful arm hand training after stroke. In: CHI 2012 Extended Abstracts on Human Factors in Computing Systems, pp. 2399–2404 (2012)
6. Delbressine, F., Timmermans, A.A.A., Beursgens, L., de Jong, M., van Dam, A., Verweij, D., Janssen, M., Markopoulos, P.: Motivating arm-hand use for stroke patients by serious games. In: Engineering in Medicine and Biology Society (EMBC), Annual International Conference of the IEEE, pp. 3564–3567 (2012)
7. Wong, W.Y., Wong, M.S.: Smart garment for trunk posture monitoring: A preliminary study. Scoliosis 3(7), 1–9 (2008)
8. Seo, A., Uda, S.: Trunk rotation monitoring using angular velocity sensors. Ind. Health 35, 222–228 (1997)
9. Wang, Q., Markopolous, P., Chen, W.: Smart rehabilitation garment design for arm-hand training. In: Proceedings of the 8th International Conference on Pervasive Computing Technologies for Healthcare (PervasiveHealth 2014). ICST (Institute for Computer Sciences, Social-Informatics and Telecommunications Engineering), ICST, pp. 328–330. Brussels, Belgium (2014)
10. Dunne, L., Walsh, P., Smyth, B. Caulfield, B.: A system for wearable monitoring of seated posture in computer users. In: 4th International Workshop on Wearable and Implantable Body Sensor Networks (BSN), pp. 203–207 (2007)
11. Nguyen, K.D., Chen, I.-M., Luo, Z., Yeo, S.H., Duh, H.-L.: A wearable sensing system for tracking and monitoring of functional arm movement. IEEEASME Trans. Mechatron. 16(2), 213–220 (2011)
12. Patel, S., Park, H., Bonato, P., Chan, L., Rodgers, M.: A review of wearable sensors and systems with application in rehabilitation. J. Neuroengineering Rehabil. 9(1), 21 (2012)
13. Li, L., Au, W.M., Hua, T., Feng, D.: Smart textiles: a design approach for garments using conductive fabrics. Des. J. 17(1), 137–154 (2014)
14. Lee, G.X., Low, K.S., Taher, T.: Unrestrained measurement of arm motion based on a wearable wireless sensor network. IEEE Trans. Instrum. Meas. 59(5), 1309–1317 (2010)
15. Markopoulos, P., Timmermans, A.A., Beursgens, L., van Donselaar, R., Seelen, H.A.: Us' em: the user-centered design of a device for motivating stroke patients to use their impaired arm-hand in daily life activities. In: Engineering in Medicine and Biology Society, EMBC, pp. 5182–5187 (2011)
16. Timmermans, A.A., Lemmens, R.J., Geers, R.P., Smeets, R.J., Seelen, H.A.: A comparison of treatment effects after sensor-and robot-based task-oriented arm training in highly functional stroke patients. In: Engineering in Medicine and Biology Society, EMBC, Annual International Conference of the IEEE, pp. 3507–3510 (2011)
17. Claus, A.P., Hides, J.A., Moseley, G.L., Hodges, P.W.: Different ways to balance the spine: subtle changes in sagittal spinal curves affect regional muscle activity. Spine 34(6), E208–E214 (2009)

Design Principles for Hapto-Virtual Rehabilitation Environments: Effects on Effectiveness of Fine Motor Hand Therapy

Cristina Ramírez-Fernández[1], Eloísa García-Canseco[1(✉)],
Alberto L. Morán[1], and Felipe Orihuela-Espina[2]

[1] Facultad de Ciencias, Universidad Autónoma de Baja California,
Km. 103 Carretera Tijuana-Ensenada, 22860 Ensenada, Mexico
{cristina_ramirez,eloisa.garcia,alberto.moran}@uabc.edu.mx
[2] Depto. de Ciencias Computacionales,
Instituto Nacional de Astrofísica, Óptica y Electrónica,
Luis Enrique Erro 1, 72840 Tonantzintla, Puebla, México
f.orihuela-espina@inaoep.mx

Abstract. We propose a set of principles to facilitate the design of haptic feedback virtual environments, which is expected to contribute to the effectiveness of the fine motor hand therapy. Firstly, we conducted a contextual study in a rehabilitation center to identify preliminary design elements using grounded theory. Based on these results, we defined a set of principles aiming to aid in the design of haptic feedback virtual environments to favour therapy effectiveness and patient's safety. Secondly, in order to evaluate the proposed design principles, we developed a haptic feedback virtual environment based on them and conducted a formative evaluation with five patients and three therapists. Preliminary results provided promising evidence, indicating a high perception of usefulness, ease of use and intention of use of the proposed environment and principles. Finally, to validate the impact of the design principles in therapy effectiveness, we carried out a second study with thirty participants, from which fifteen elderly had hand motor impairments. We found no significant differences in task execution time between healthy adults and elders with hand motor impairments. We found significant differences in precision or accuracy of the exercise. We confirmed the importance of key principles to facility the design of hapto-virtual environments that contribute to the effectiveness of the fine motor hand therapy. Further evaluations are needed to validate our results from a clinical viewpoint. We confirmed the importance of key principles to contribute to the effectiveness of the fine motor hand therapy. Further evaluations are needed to validate our results from a clinical viewpoint.

Keywords: Virtual rehabilitation · Haptics · User-centered design · Design principles · Neurorehabilitation

This work was partially funded by the Mexican Council for Science and Technology (CONACYT) under grant 218709 and CONACYT scholarship number 97753 for the first author.

© Springer-Verlag Berlin Heidelberg 2015
H.M. Fardoun et al. (Eds.): REHAB 2014, CCIS 515, pp. 270–284, 2015.
DOI: 10.1007/978-3-662-48645-0_23

1   Introduction

In the recent years, several innovative strategies have been developed for improving post-stroke upper extremities motor recovery such as constraint induced movement therapy, electromyographic biofeedback, electromechanical assisted training, electrostimulation, high intensity therapy, robotics, repetitive task training, splinting and physical fitness training, among others [14,36,39]. The incorporation of emerging technologies such as virtual reality and haptic feedback in the rehabilitation therapy has attracted the attention of researchers and therapists because of its potential benefits, namely its capability to comply with neurorehabilitation principles [15,21] such as repetition, feedback, motivation, early intervention, and task oriented training—see for instance [36] and references therein.

As pointed out by [34,37], virtual reality allows for the design, creation and control of multi-dimensional simulated and interactive valid stimulus environments within which behavioral responding can be measured and recorded, providing in this way clinical assessments and rehabilitation tools that are usually not available in traditional therapy methods. Furthermore, when haptic feedback is also incorporated into the virtual environment, additional benefits such as force-feedback and tactile or kinesthetic input/output that are essential in many rehabilitation tasks are also provided [20].

Although there have been several proposals concerning the implementation of different kinds of hapto-virtual rehabilitation systems i.e., haptic-enhanced virtual reality environments, e.g., [20,23–25,28,40], there is still a gap between the design phase of those systems and their usage with real patients due to the lack of design principles that take into account both the needs of patients and therapists [30]. Most research works rely on the patient point-of-view to identify criteria (mainly for visual-based virtual environments) either focusing on the patient motivation, entertainment and engagement [4–8,13,16,18,19,22,33,36] or on the therapy usefulness [11,27,29,35,38]. However, ensuring therapy effectiveness and patient safety while providing the therapist with the adequate parameters to track patients performance and progress in hapto-visual rehabilitation environments are among the questions that remain yet to be answered [17]. To this end, we present in this work the preliminary results that allows us to identify designing principles for hapto-visual rehabilitation environments in fine motor hand therapy. We also present the evaluation results that allowed us to iterate these design principles, as well as to explore their effects on therapy effectiveness.

The remainder of the paper is organized as follows: Sect. 2 describes the contextual case study performed at the regional rehabilitation center. Section 3 explains the preliminary design principles that were identified during the study. We describe in Sect. 4 the methodology carried out to obtain feedback regarding the design principles with patients and therapists. Section 5 presents the evaluation results of the design principles, with emphasis on therapy effectiveness. In Sect. 6 we discuss the identified key design principles. We conclude with final remarks and future work in Sect. 7.

2   Contextual Case Study

A qualitative study was carried out during three months at the regional rehabilitation center located in Ensenada, Baja California, México, to gain an initial
understanding regarding traditional fine motor hand therapy. Twelve specialists (e.g. rehabilitation medical specialist, occupational therapists, psychologists,
among others.) took care of approximately 80 patients with motor and cognitive
impairments in this center. We performed structured and unstructured interviews with 5 of the 12 specialists, from which 1 rehabilitation medical specialist, 1 occupational therapist, 2 physical therapists and 1 psychologist. All of
them answered a 5-point Likert scale questionnaire of 40 items. Additionally, 8
non-participative direct observation sessions (30 min each, 4 h total) involving 5
patients with different conditions such as carpal tunnel surgery, cerebrovascular
accidents, and brain lesions were performed (Fig. 1).

Interviews and observation sessions were recorded, transcribed and analyzed
using grounded theory [9]. As a result, we have identified the different stages of
a traditional occupational therapy session (Fig. 2). On average, an occupational
therapy session lasts 30 min. During the first session, occupational therapists create an individual treatment program based on the initial patient assessment. In

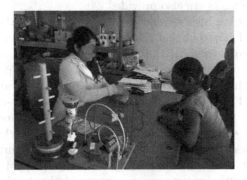

Fig. 1. Non-participative direct observation of a traditional occupational therapy session.

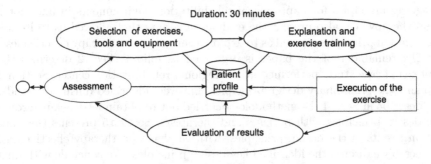

Fig. 2. The different stages of a traditional occupational therapy session.

subsequent sessions, occupational therapists select the tools and equipment that will be used by patients in each therapy session. Then, therapists explain and show the patient how to perform the exercises, review the treatments periodically, evaluate patient's progress and make changes to the treatment as needed. The whole therapy session is carried out under therapists supervision and assistance. Finally, occupational therapists analyze patient's performance and write it down on his medical record.

We have further identified the main characteristics of the occupational therapy for improving fine motor hand skills (Table 1). For instance, ludic activities are among the strategies used by occupational therapists to motivate the patients. Depending on the function to be enhanced, the exercises are selected as: exercises to improve muscle strength (e.g., pulling or moving objects of different weight and size, or pressing dough), exercises to improve eye-hand coordination (e.g., solving puzzles, mazes and dot-to-dot pictures), exercises to increase range of motion (e.g., stretching rubber) and exercises to increase sensitivity (e.g., touching objects with different textures).

3 Preliminary Design Principles

A design principle is used by interaction designers to guide them when designing user-centered applications [11,31]. From the contextual study described in Sect. 2, we have identified a preliminary set of designing principles that incorporates the therapists viewpoint. These design principles are classified in two categories: principles that aim (a) to guarantee therapy effectiveness, and (b) to ensure patient's safety when designing the interaction with hapto-visual environments.

With respect to *therapy effectiveness* we distinguish the following design principles:

- Adaptability. According to occupational therapists, this principle is important to assess the range of motion and strength of the patient, to thereby adapt therapy.
- Therapy tasks tailored according to the patient's motor impairment.
- Motivation based on recreational activities to engage and entertain the patient during the therapy.
- Suitable selection of the haptic interface.

Concerning *patient's safety*, the design principle involves the careful selection of the range of motion and strength of the therapy tasks according to the patient's physical ability.

4 Evaluation of the Design Principles

In this section we describe the virtual environment we developed taking into account the design principles explained in Sect. 3. We also present a formative evaluation conducted with 5 patients, as well as a refined version of the design principles.

Table 1. Characteristics of traditional occupational therapy.

Category	Property	Dimension
Fine motor skills hand therapy	Feature	Based on formal or ludic activities
		Goal-based movements
		Exercises for specific movements
	Tools	Everyday toys, textures, mirror
	Equipment	Mechanotherapy
		Electromyography
	Exercise	Move and press divers artifacts
	Movement	Fingers, palm and wrist flexion or extension
		Fingers and wrist abduction or adduction
		Tip, palmar, lateral
		Wrist supination or pronation
		Cylindrical, spherical or hook grasp
	Function to be enhanced	Strength
		Sensation
		Range of motion
		Precision (eye-hand coordination)
	Etiology	Birth defect
		Injury or accident
		Degenerative disease
	Problem	Patient's absenteeism
		Lack of motivation
		Subjective assessment
		Lack of technology that motivates to exercise
	Strategy	Ludic or formal activities according to patient's skills

4.1 Hapto-Virtual Environment

As a proof-of-concept of the preliminary design principles, we have developed a haptic maze environment. Haptic feedback is provided with the Novint Falcon haptic device [2]. The Novint Falcon is a 3 degrees-of-freedom (dog) parallel robot that provides users with haptic feedback. It has a workspace of approximately $10.6\,cm^3$. Open-source three-dimensional (3D) computer graphics software Blender [1] as well as the cross-platform game creation system Unity [3] were used to develop the virtual environment. The user in the virtual environment is represented by a proxy (or avatar) that moves in a 3D space. The

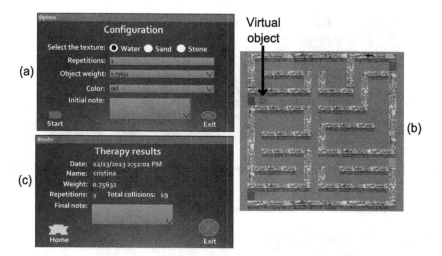

Fig. 3. Haptic-enhanced virtual environment: (a) therapy configuration; (b) exercise in the haptic maze for wrist therapy; (c) therapy results.

collision detection algorithm is carried out with Unity libraries as well as with penalty-based methods [26,32].

Our main objective in developing the haptic maze was to enhance the strength and wrist-movement accuracy of the patient. In the virtual environment (Fig. 3) we distinguish three main components: (a) a configuration screen where the occupational therapist selects not only the visual features of the virtual environment, but also the number of task repetitions and the simulated weight of the haptic proxy; (b) the haptic maze; and (c) the results screen where patient performance is displayed.

4.2   Formative Evaluation

In order to evaluate the design principles that were used for the development of the virtual environment, we conducted two therapy sessions with 5 patients (Fig. 4). These sessions were supervised by two occupational therapists and one physical therapist. After each therapy session a Technology Acceptance Model (TAM) [10] Likert scale 5 questionnaire regarding perception of usefulness, ease of use and intention of use of the haptic virtual environment was answered by patients and therapists. Evaluation results are shown on Table 2. These results provide evidence about patients and therapists having a high perception about the proposed environment's usefulness, although the latter perceived a higher usefulness (i.e. completely agree) than the former (i.e. agree). Also, therapists perceived the environment as having a high ease of use (agree), although it was not the case for patients which were neutral. Finally, intention of use was projected as high (i.e. completely agree) by both kinds of users.

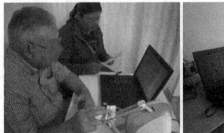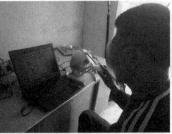

Fig. 4. Patients conducting therapy sessions during the formative evaluation of the design principles.

Table 2. Perceived usefulness, ease of use and intention of use.

Aspect analyzed	Patients	Therapists	Total
Perceived usefulness	4.0/5	4.5/5	4.2/5
Perceived ease of use	3.0/5	4.2/5	3.6/5
Intention of use	4.5/5	4.6/5	4.5/5

Based on the lessons learned during the development and evaluation of the haptic virtual environment, the preliminary design principles described in Sect. 3 were modified (others were added) as follows.

Therapy Effectiveness

– *Patient's data accessibility:* Store the patient's data according to the clinical record requirements; allow for data access according to the specialist's role; display a performance record of the patient.
– *Therapy adaptability:* Execute a task that allows to determine objectively the level of difficulty of the exercise for the patient (for instance, number of repetitions, weight of the virtual object); automatically suggest the difficulty level according to the patient's performance record; learning level of the exercise that does not add excessive difficulty to the patient's motor rehabilitation.
– *Ludic activity based motivation:* Gain the patient's attention by including game-based visual and auditory elements combined with strength feedback.
– *Goal-oriented movements for skill generalization:* Repetitive and intense basic movements (such as finger and wrist flexion and extension, finger adduction and abduction, fine pincer grasp) for motor re-learning.
– *Suitable selection of the haptic interface for movement execution:* Careful selection of the haptic interface according to the movement to be enhanced (e.g., exoskeleton or haptic device with end effector).
– *Mechanisms for determining success of the therapy:* Establish mechanisms that allow to identify patients' improvements based on quantifiable results (for example speed, position, weight of the virtual objects).

Table 3. Biomechanical properties of the hand [12].

Movement	Value
Hand opening maximum range	15 cm
Wrist rotation maximum range	180 deg
Thumb mean orientation	45 deg
Maximum grasping force, measured for one finger	40 N
Maximum wrist torque	0.5 Nm

– *Continuous interactions:* Guarantee the synchronization between the visual, auditory and haptic feedback according to the virtual objects' characteristics.

Patient's Safety

– *Regarding the range of movement and hand's maximum strength:* Limit the range of movement of the exercise and the maximum weight of the virtual objects according to the biomechanical properties of the patient's hands (see Table 3.

– *In case of failure, stop communication with the device at an appropriate time:* Provide simple mechanisms that allow for stopping the activity in case of failure of the haptic device.

5 Evaluating Therapy Effectiveness

In order to further evaluate the proposed design principles, as well as to gather additional evidence regarding their influence in therapy effectiveness based on patient's performance, we conducted a second study that is briefly described next. A second version of the haptic maze was also developed, which integrates the design principles (for instance: data accessibility, ludic elements and auditory feedback) described in previous sections.

5.1 Participants

2 groups of 15 participants each were recruited. In the control group, 15 healthy adults (8 women and 7 men, average age 55.73 ± 7.56 years) who live an independent life and have no apparent motor impairment problems served as participants. In the intervention group, 15 elders (8 women and 7 men, average age 78.80 ± 11.30 years) with hand motor impairments, e.g., rheumatoid arthritis, were recruited from the home for elderly "Casa Hogar del Anciano" and "Casa del Abuelo", both located in Ensenada, Baja California, Mexico.

5.2   Experiment Design and Procedure

The experiment followed was a within subjects paradigm, i.e., both groups performed the task under the same following condition:

C1. Virtual environment with auditory, visual and haptic feedback using the Novint Falcon haptic interface (Fig. 5).

Participants of both groups performed one task consisting of moving an object through the maze to virtually "touch" three doors of different colors in the indicated order—red, green and blue—(Fig. 6) with a simulated proxy weight of 100 gr. While moving the object through the labyrinth, if the participant collides the avatar with any wall, he gets auditory, visual and haptic feedback. We formulated the following hypotheses:

H1. The task execution time of healthy adults is shorter than the task execution time of elderly with motor impairments.
H2. The number of collisions detected for healthy adults is smaller than the number of detected collisions for elderly with motor impairments.

5.3   Evaluation Results

The exercises were evaluated using objective performance data from the virtual environment, namely, the task execution time (efficiency) and the number of collisions detected with the virtual walls (precision of movement or accuracy). Table 4 presents a summary of the scores obtained by each participant.

We analyzed the results of the therapy effectiveness in terms of performance of both groups (see Table 5). As can be seen in Table 5, we found no significant difference in task execution time between healthy adults and elders with hand motor impairments (H1), we found significant difference in precision of the exercise (H2). These results confirms the importance of provide adaptability in the exercise. The balance between exercise and challenge should be appropriate to

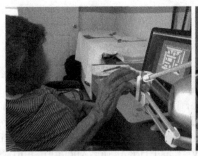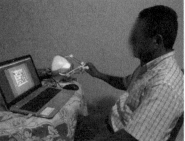

Fig. 5. Participants conducting the exercise with the Novint Falcon haptic interface during the therapy effectiveness evaluation of design principles: (a) elder with motor impairment, (b) adult with no motor impairment.

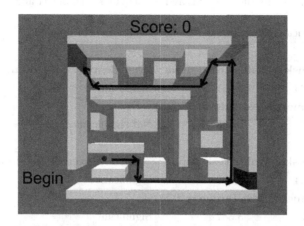

Fig. 6. Exercise in the haptic maze. The ideal trajectory motion is depicted in black. The proxy (red dot) changes its color to indicate the wall color that the user has to touch in the indicated order (red, green and blue) (Color figure online).

Table 4. Evaluation results of the exercise in terms of task execution time and number of collisions. G1: group of healthy adults, G2: group of elderly with hand motor impairments. SD: Standard Deviation.

Participant	Outcome			
	Time (sec)		Number of collisions	
	G1 (SD = 23.63)	G2 (SD = 28.93)	G1 (SD=15.63)	G2 (SD = 12.56)
1	46.13	74.74	14	51
2	51.35	109.74	15	21
3	31.12	57.68	13	21
4	43.87	84.48	19	36
5	44.03	58.39	13	34
6	94.37	79.57	19	17
7	64.41	47.37	22	30
8	26.94	27.26	18	13
9	33.88	46.33	8	14
10	69.34	89.51	18	33
11	110.24	130.48	76	55
12	35.32	52.13	8	25
13	26.47	44.74	16	21
14	46.32	84.56	13	26
15	38.30	21.25	16	11

Table 5. Summary of Kruskal-Wallis and Nemenyi test [41] on H1 and H2 hypotheses.

Critical value	Statistical value	Significance of difference
H1		
Kruskal-Wallis test (alpha = .1, 1 degree of freedom)		
2.706	3.561	Significant
Nemenyi test (alpha = .025)		
3.17	2.668	Not significant
H2		
Kruskal-Wallis test (alpha = .025, 1 degree of freedom)		
5.024	5.160	Significant
Nemenyi test (alpha = .025)		
3.17	3.387	Significant

ensure a successful and effective therapy. In addition, it is important that the selection of exercises and level of challenge be a simple task for both therapists and patients. Moreover, it is important to gradually modify the difficulty level of the exercise to out ongoing progress. This can be done either automatically by means of a decision algorithm or manually with the help of a therapist during the execution of the exercise [36]. For instance, the properties of the virtual objects within the hapto-virtual rehabilitation environment such as weight, size and quantity, among others, can be adjusted during the exercise to ensure an appropriate level of force and range of movements, while providing and adequate level of challenge and engagement to the patient.

6   Discussion

The results of the conducted formative evaluation allowed, on the one hand for gathering preliminary evidence towards the perception of participants about the usefulness, ease of use and intention of use of the developed environment, and on the other hand for obtaining a refined version of the principles for the design of haptic virtual environments for fine motor hand rehabilitation.

Regarding participants' perceptions, although this perception was high on usefulness and intention of use for both patients and therapists, this was not the case for ease of use. In the latter case, therapists perceived it high, but patients were neutral about it. This could be due to the challenge imposed to patients by the indirect manipulation required to interact with/through the haptic device. In this sense, it is necessary to further investigate principles to balance this challenge, to try to increase the patient's ease-of-use perception. Concerning the design principles, these aim at achieving *therapy effectiveness* and *patient's safety*. Although other research works have proposed similar principles for therapy effectiveness (e.g. [38] considers principles about goal-based movements, ludic activity based motivation, and patient's performance), our proposal includes principles regarding accessing patient's information according to the specialist's role for decision making, and the appropriate selection of the haptic interface according to the movement to be enhanced. To the best of our knowledge, none of these principles have been included in previous efforts. Additionally, and also to the best of our knowledge, no other proposal have considered the inclusion of design principles for patient's safety, such as the importance of having a simple mechanism for stopping the haptic device in case of failure.

Moreover, the results from the second study allowed us firstly, to further scrutinize therapy effectiveness based on performance, and secondly, to iterate the preliminary design principles. Although we found no significant difference in task execution time between healthy adults and elders with hand motor impairments, we found significant difference in precision of the exercise. These results suggests that the elderly, having visual and hand motor disabilities, find more motivating finishing the task rather than completing the exercise with accuracy. It is worth mention that only 2 of the 15 elders had experience on the use of the computer, compared to 7 from 15 of the healthy adults. In addition, the auditory feedback enhanced the user experience of participants with visual disabilities from both groups. We also found that 80 % of participants were interested in comparing their performance with that of the others. This suggest the inclusion of elements in the virtual environment that promote motivation and engagement such as different kinds and level of challenges, and incentives.

7   Conclusions and Future Work

We have reported the evaluation results of a preliminary set of principles for the design of hapto-virtual rehabilitation environments for fine motor hand therapy, with an emphasis on effectiveness of the therapy. With this we aim at supporting developers to facilitate their understanding of key principles to include in the design of hapto-virtual rehabilitation environments for upper limb rehabilitation. Our main findings suggest that although the elements introduced through the principles (e.g. the inclusion of haptic force feedback) are well appreciated by both the patients and the therapists regarding usefulness and intention of use, additional work should be conducted to overcome some of the challenges introduced by them regarding ease of use (e.g. the use of a haptic device to provide force feedback introduces indirect manipulation, which imposes an additional challenge to patients, whom need to "map" their movements in the physical to the actions on the objects in the virtual environment). In addition, the results from the evaluation of the effectiveness in terms of performance, suggest the importance of the design principles and the identification of new ones such as sharing information among participants to increase motivation. So far we have not evaluated the safety design principles. Nevertheless, it is important to take into account the maximum range of motion and strength of the hand, according to the participant assessment. We believe that the principles may reduce development times, and increase chances of therapeutic validity of hapto-virtual rehabilitation environments in terms of therapy effectiveness and patient's safety.

Further studies are needed not only to iterate and evaluate the safety design principles, but also to evaluate the design principles impact from the clinical point of view.

Acknowledgments. The authors would like to thank the specialists and patients from "Centro Integral de Rehabilitación", and the elderly from "Casa Hogar de Anciano" and "Casa del Abuelo" in Ensenada, Baja California, México, for their valuable support and participation in this research work. We are also grateful to undergraduate students who have participated in the development of the haptic maze application.

References

1. Blender. http://www.blender.org. Accessed 15 Aug 2014
2. Novint Falcon. http://www.novint.com. Accessed 15 Aug 2014
3. Unity game engine. http://unity3d.com. Accessed 15 Aug 2014
4. Alankus, G., Lazar, A., May, M., Kelleher, C.: Towards customizable games for stroke rehabilitation. In: Proceedings of the 28th International Conference on Human Factors in Computing Systems - CHI 2010, pp. 2113–2122, no. 2113 (2010)
5. Annema, J., Verstraete, M., Abeele, V., Desmet, S., Geerts, D., Leuven, I.: Videogames in therapy: a therapist's perspective. In: International Conference on Fun and Games, pp. 94–98 (2010)
6. Boulanger, C., Boulanger, A., de Greef, L., Kearney, A., Sobel, K., Transue, R., Sweedyk, Z., Dietz, P., Bathiche, S.: Stroke rehabilitation with a sensing surface. In: Proceedings of the SIGCHI Conference on Human Factors in Computing Systems-CHI 2013, pp. 1243–1246. ACM Press (2013)
7. Burke, J., McNeill, M., Charles, D., Morrow, P., Crosbie, J., McDonough, S.: Optimising engagement for stroke rehabilitation using serious games. Vis. Comput. **25**(12), 1085–1099 (2009)
8. Chen, Y., Lehrer, N., Sundaram, H., Rikakis, T.: Adaptive mixed reality stroke rehabilitation: system architecture and evaluation metrics. In: Proceedings of the First Annual ACM SIGMM Conference on Multimedia Systems, pp. 293–304 (2010)
9. Corbin, J., Strauss, A.: Grounded theory research: procedures, canons, and evaluative criteria. Qual. Sociol. **13**(1), 3–21 (1990)
10. Davis, F.: Perceived usefulness, perceived ease of use, and user acceptance of information technology. MIS Q. **13**(3), 319–340 (1989)
11. Dix, A., Finlay, J., Abowd, G., Beale, R.: Human-Computer Interaction, 3rd edn. Pearson/Prentice-Hall, Harlow (2004)
12. Dovat, L., Lambercy, O., Ruffieux, Y., Chapuis, D., Gassert, R., Bleuler, H., Teo, C., Burdet, E.: A haptic knob for rehabilitation of stroke patients. In: 2006 IEEE/RSJ International Conference on Intelligent Robots and Systems, pp. 977–982, October 2006
13. Flores, E., Tobon, G., Cavallaro, E., Cavallaro, F., Perry, J., Keller, T.: Improving patient motivation in game development for motor deficit rehabilitation. In: International Conference on Advances in Computer, pp. 381–384 (2008)
14. Henderson, A., Korner-Bitensky, N., Levin, M.: Virtual reality in stroke rehabilitation: a systematic review of its effectiveness for upper limb motor recovery. Top. Stroke Rehabil. **14**(2), 52–61 (2007)

15. Holden, M., Dyar, T.: Virtual environment training-a new tool for neurorehabilitation. Neurol. Rep. **26**(2), 62–71 (2002)
16. Ines, D., Abdelkader, G.: Mixed reality serious games: the therapist perspective. In: International Conference on Serious Games and Applications for Health, pp. 1–10, no. V (2011)
17. Jones, C.: Design Methods. Wiley, New York (1982)
18. Jung, Y., Yeh, S., Stewart, J.: Tailoring virtual reality technology for stroke rehabilitation: a human factors design. In: Computer Human Interaction, pp. 929–934 (2006)
19. Kaber, D., Zhang, T.: Human factors in virtual reality system design for mobility and haptic task performance. Rev. Hum. Factors Ergon. **7**(1), 323–366 (2011)
20. Kayyalil, R., Shirmohammadil, S., Saddik, A., Lemaire, E.: Daily-life exercises for haptic motor rehabilitation. In: IEEE International Workshop on Haptic Audio Visual Environments and their Applications, pp. 12–14, no. October (2007)
21. Kleim, J., Jones, T.: Principles of experience-dependent neural plasticity: implications for rehabilitation after brain damage. J. Speech Lang. Hear. Res. JSLHR **51**(1), S225–S239 (2008)
22. Lewis, G., Woods, C., Rosie, J., McPherson, K.: Virtual reality games for rehabilitation: perspectives from the users and new directions. In: 2011 International Conference on Virtual Rehabilitation, pp. 1–2. IEEE, June 2011
23. Li, Y., Kaber, D., Tupler, L., Lee, Y.: Haptic-based virtual environment design and modeling of motor skill assessment for brain injury patients rehabilitation. Comput.-Aided Des. Appl. **8**(2), 149–162 (2011)
24. Mali, U., Goljar, N., Munih, M.: Application of haptic interface for finger exercise. IEEE Trans. Neural Syst. Rehabil. Eng. **14**(3), 352–360 (2006)
25. McLaughlin, M., Rizzo, A., Jung, Y., Peng, W., Yeh, S., Zhu, W., USC/UT Consortium for Interdisciplinary Research: Haptics-enhanced virtual environments for stroke rehabilitation. In: Proceeding of IPSI (2005)
26. Moore, M., Wilhelms, J.: Collision detection and response for computer animation. Comput. Graph. **22**(4), 289–298 (1988)
27. Morán, A.L., Orihuela-Espina, F., Meza-Kubo, V., Grimaldo, A.I., Ramírez-Fernández, C., García-Canseco, E., Oropeza-Salas, J.M., Sucar, L.E.: Borrowing a virtual rehabilitation tool for the physical activation and cognitive stimulation of elders. In: Collazos, C., Liborio, A., Rusu, C. (eds.) CLIHC 2013. LNCS, vol. 8278, pp. 95–102. Springer, Heidelberg (2013)
28. Mullins, J., Mawson, C., Nahavandi, S.: Haptic handwriting aid for training and rehabilitation. In: IEEE International Conference on Systems, Man and Cybernetics, vol. 3, pp. 2690–2694. IEEE (2005)
29. Nielsen, J.: Usability Enginnering. Academic Press, Inc., Boston (1994)
30. Ramírez-Fernández, C., García-Canseco, E., Morán, A.L.: Towards a set of design principles for hapto-virtual rehabilitation environments: preliminary results in fine motor therapy. In: Proceedings of the 8th International Conference on Pervasive Computing Technologies for Healthcare (PervasiveHealth 2014). ICST (Institute for Computer Sciences, Social-Informatics and Telecommunications Engineering), Oldenburg, 20 May 2014. http://dx.doi.org/10.4108/icst.pervasivehealth.2014.255359
31. Rogers, Y., Sharp, H., Preece, J.: Interaction Design: Beyond Human-Computer Interaction. Wiley, New York (2011)
32. Saddik, A.E.: Computer haptics (Chap. 5). In: Saddik, A.E., Orozco, M., Eid, M., Cha, J. (eds.) Haptics Technologies. Springer Series on Touch and Haptic Systems, pp. 105–143. Springer, Heidelberg (2011)

33. Saini, S., Rohaya, D., Rambli, A., Sulaiman, S., Zakaria, M.N., Rohkmah, S., Shukri, M., Iskandar, B.S.: A low-cost game framework for home-based stroke rehabilitation system. In: 2012 International Conference on Computer & Information Science (ICCIS), pp. 55–60 (2012)
34. Schultheis, M., Rizzo, A.: The application of virtual reality technology in rehabilitation. Rehabil. Psychol. **46**(3), 296–311 (2001)
35. Seo, K., Kim, J., Lee, J., Jang, S., Ryu, H.: Serious games for stroke patients: attending to clinical staff's voices. In: The 5th International Congress of International Association of Societies of Design Research, pp. 1–11 (2013)
36. Sucar, L., Orihuela-Espina, F., Velazquez, R., Reinkensmeyer, D., Leder, R., Hernandez-Franco, J.: Gesture therapy: an upper limb virtual reality-based motor rehabilitation platform. IEEE Trans. Neural Syst. Rehabil. Eng. **22**(3), 634–643 (2014)
37. Sveistrup, H.: Motor rehabilitation using virtual reality. J. Neuroeng. Rehabil. **1**(1), 1–8 (2004)
38. Timmermans, A., Seelen, H., Willmann, R., Kingma, H.: Technology-assisted training of arm-hand skills in stroke: concepts on reacquisition of motor control and therapist guidelines for rehabilitation technology design. J. Neuroeng. Rehabil. **6**(1), 1–18 (2009)
39. Woldag, H., Hummelsheim, H.: Evidence-based physiotherapeutic concepts for improving arm and hand function in stroke patients: a review. J. Neurol. **249**(5), 518–528 (2002)
40. Xu, Z., Yu, H., Yan, S.: Motor rehabilitation training after stroke using haptic handwriting and games. In: Proceedings of the 4th International Convention on Rehabilitation Engineering & Assistive Technology (2010)
41. Zar, J.H.: Biostatistical Analysis. Prentice Hall, New Jersey (2010)

Impact of a NFC-Based Application
with Educational Purposes on Children
Affected by Language Disorders

Emilia Biffi[✉], Maria Luisa Lorusso, and Gianluigi Reni

IRCCS E. Medea, Bosisio Parini, LC, Italy
{emilia.biffi,marialuisa.lorusso,
gianluigi.reni}@bp.lnf.it

Abstract. In the past few years, new devices for children and disabilities has proliferated thanks to the development of more and more inexpensive mobile technology and to the availability of free-downloadable software applications. In this work we describe the design, development and testing of an integrated system which combines the use of a tablet, a group of toys (e.g. small plastic animals), Near Field Communication (NFC) technology and a software application with educational purposes. The goals of the device are to improve the structural knowledge and the semantic competences of typically developing and disabled children while offering an entertaining environment.

Keywords: Software application · Children · NFC · Learning · Language disorder

1 Introduction

The proliferation of inexpensive mobile technology is dramatically changing the landscape for both typically developing subjects and individuals with complex communication needs and learning difficulties. Indeed, software application, or "apps" as they are commonly called, are readily adopted by people even when a disability or a cognitive disorder is present [1]. In the past few years, programmers in the Android community have come up with varied applications for education, development, communication and rehabilitation for children with different disabilities, most notably autism [2]. Some apps have been used to improve basic speech/language capabilities as a support for traditional, impairment-based treatments. Others are available to convey spoken, written or visual messages to other people, to facilitate communication attempts [3].

Recently, efforts have been made to use electronic media to promote healthy eating, physical activity and weight control among children [4]. Often, the goal of many developed apps is to facilitate communication between children and the outside world using pictures, applications that help form sentences, or online resources. The process has proved successful and popular among both parents and children. However, to our knowledge, it still lacks an application developed to speed learning and to improve the structural knowledge and the semantic competence of children while offering an

© Springer-Verlag Berlin Heidelberg 2015
H.M. Fardoun et al. (Eds.): REHAB 2014, CCIS 515, pp. 285–293, 2015.
DOI: 10.1007/978-3-662-48645-0_24

entertaining environment. Moreover, few apps specifically address the needs of children with mild linguistic or cognitive impairments that affect semantic organization (and therefore lexical and conceptual comprehension and expression abilities) rather than gross motor and communication skills. Children with language impairments or delays and mild cognitive deficits represent instances of such needs [5, 6]. Any device addressing such subtle communication impairments may, in addition, be seen as a precious aid to support and enhance communication abilities in typically developing individuals as well.

In this work we describe the development and testing of an integrated system which combines the use of a tablet, a group of toys (e.g. small plastic animals), Near Field Communication (NFC) technology and a software application with educational purposes. A preliminary design of the system has been already presented in [7]. In this application, each toy connected to a NFC tag, calls different activities when it passes close to the NFC reader, embedded into the tablet. These activities allow the user to read information, or a tale, or to listen to a song or to look at a picture, all describing the subject (animal or object) represented by that specific toy. These contents are taken from specific websites, that we filtered for children. Further, the user can choose to listen to the content of the webpages by means of a text-to-speech tool. The system was proposed to pre-school children with speech disorders to evaluate its ease of use and understanding, and the interest it raises. Our app reverses the standard model of communication with the outside world through pictures and text-to-speech functions, and uses images and audio to instruct. The application uses auditory, visual, and tactile information to improve the speed of learning and entertainment value for users. Finally, it uniquely uses NFC to incorporate physical objects outside of the tablet.

2 Materials and Methods

The system integrates a tablet, equipped with a NFC reader, the custom software application and some NFC tag stickers (NTAG203) that are placed on hypoallergenic plastic animals, making possible the unique recognition of each toy (currently three animals: lion, zebra and giraffe; Fig. 1).

2.1 Device Choice

A Nexus 10 tablet was chosen to run the custom application. It features a Samsung Exynos 5250 system on chip, a dual-core 1.7 GHz Cortex A15 central processing unit and a quad-core ARMMali T604 graphics processing unit. It provides a front NFC reader, required to recognize the toys with attached NFC tags, a micro USB port, used for charging or connecting the device to a PC or other USB-compatible device, and a micro HDMI port to connect the system to a larger screen if necessary. The tablet's screen is large enough (263.9 × 177.6 mm) for children to view images puzzles and videos clearly as well as to easily pass toys over. It is widely sold and available on the web for about 260 USD. The tablet was tested to ensure it worked correctly before programming the custom education and rehabilitation software. Specifically, the Nexus

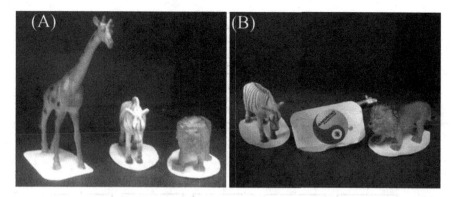

Fig. 1. Example of three plastic animals (left) each one equipped with an NFC tag below their paws (right)

10 had the NFC tags passed over it to check if its sensor was operational, before the custom application was successfully loaded onto the tablet.

2.2 Development of the Software

The custom application was developed in Eclipse by using a series of public access methods developed by the Android community, modifying them and integrating them into one application. The architecture of the main application is designed as follows (Fig. 2). First an application to read and write onto NFC tags was created to recognize the toys as children pass them over the screen of the tablet. When a specific toy, with a recognized NFC tag is passed over the tablet a second method calls that toy's activity, a navigational page. The navigational page is unique for each NFC tag and allows the user to access a unique web-view activity, introducing a series of dynamic websites providing stories, interactive games and puzzles, information and songs. If the user wishes to access an activity with a written description in the website (e.g. information, tale), the application uses a JSOP HTML parser method to retrieve the website's text, or uses a prewritten script, and uses a text-to-speech method to convert the writing into speech.

2.3 Preliminary Tests

Five children (age 4–6) with mild language disorders or delays were asked to play with the integrated device during one 45 min speech therapy session. Table 1 shows demographic data of the patients. A structured observation grid and a questionnaire about the positive and negative reactions of the children was filled by the therapist at the end of every session to evaluate the interest raised by the educational app and the usability of the integrated system. Median values $\pm \Delta$IQ (difference between the 3rd and the 1st quartiles) were computed and a non-parametric statistical analysis (Kruskal-Wallis test and Mann-Whitney test) was performed on the number of accesses to each activity. All the sessions were video recorded for further observations.

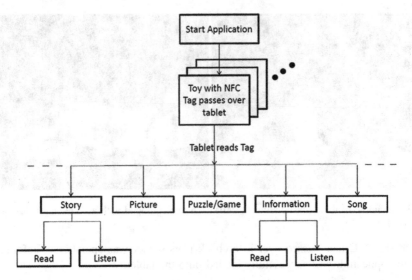

Fig. 2. Architecture of the main application. A toy with a NFC tag passes over the tablet and it is recognized, thus calling different activities. These activities allow the user to read a tale (*story*), or to look at a picture (*picture*), or to make a game (*puzzle*), or to read didactic information (*information*) describing that specific toy. These contents can be read or listened by means of a text-to-speech method.

Table 1. Demographic data of the patients. Legend: LD = Language Disorder; PMR = Psycho-motor Retardation.

Patient	Age (months)	Gender	Diagnosis
S1	74	M	LD
S2	70	M	LD
S3	66	F	LD
S4	51	M	LD and PMR
S5	60	M	LD

3 Results

3.1 Hardware Testing

The functionality of the Nexus 10 Tablet and NFC Tags (NTAG203) was verified. A separate application, TagWriter, was downloaded onto the tablet to write plain text files onto the NFC tags to distinguish them in the custom application. Each NFC tag was programmed to activate the menu pertaining the specific animal.

3.2 Custom Application

The application awaits a recognized NFC tag before it displays a menu offering a puzzle activity, a story, pictures, multimedia information and a song associated with that NFC tag and thus the specific animal. Both the story and information pages can be read aloud, by a text-to-speech function that reads a predetermined script. Extra punctuation was added and some words were spelled phonetically in the script to render the speech easier to understand.

Figure 3 displays an example of the app functionality when the plastic giraffe passes over the NFC reader embedded into the Nexus 10 tablet. The app (Fig. 3B) recognizes the NFC Tag and prompts the application to display a menu screen (Fig. 3A). From here the user can choose to access:

- "Puzzle" where games based on puzzles (where number and shape of the pieces can be varied) can be played (Fig. 3C)
- "Story" which opens one or more websites where tales about the animal can be read (or can be listened by means of the text-to-speech tool),
- "Information" which opens one or more webpages giving scientific information about the animal that can be read or listened by means of the text-to-speech tool,

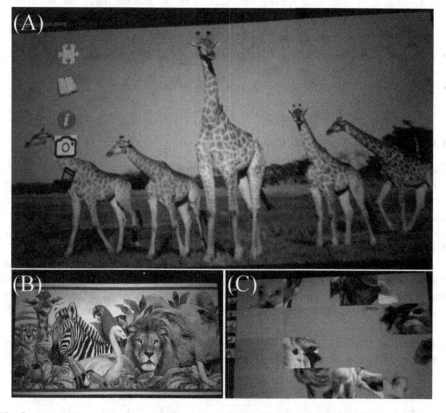

Fig. 3. (a) Initial menu that appears when the plastic giraffe passes over the NFC reader. (b) App initial view: the user can interact with it only by means of NFC-tagged animals. (c) An example of the puzzle activity (giraffe menu).

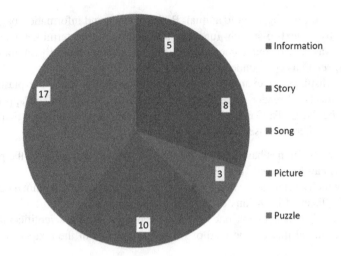

Fig. 4. Number of times each activity was accessed by the children during the observation session (Color figure online).

- "Picture" that returns different webpages showing pictures and photos about the target animal,
- "Song" which allows the user to play a song about the target animal.

3.3   Preliminary Tests with Children

The five children (age: 66 ± 10 months) spent 1866 ± 264 s (approximately 31 ± 4 min) playing with the animals and the tablet. The times each kind of activity was accessed were recorded and compared (see Fig. 4). Significant differences in the number of accesses were observed (Kruskal-Wallis test, $p < 0.05$) between the activity "Puzzle" and both the activity "Information" ($p = 0.0238$) and the activity "Songs" ($p = 0.0317$). All the data about the use of the device are reported in Table 2.

To evaluate the interest raised by the educational app and the usability of the integrated system, the speech therapist filled an observation grid about the positive and negative reactions of the children. Moreover, each child was asked at the end of every session to give a feedback, expressing his/her level of satisfaction (on a 4-level scale

Table 2. Data about the use of the device: consecutive time spent by playing with the app, number of accesses to the app by using different animals, number of entries to every activity

Patient	Played time (s)	Number of entries	Puzzle	Story	Info	Picture	Song
S1	2155	1	3	0	1	1	0
S2	1866	3	3	5	0	1	0
S3	2058	10	5	1	2	4	0
S4	1794	4	4	1	2	3	3
S5	1627	4	2	1	0	1	0

from 0 to 3) and indicate his/her preferred activity. The median scores obtained were 3 ± 0 and 3 ± 1 in terms of level of autonomy in the use of the device and motivation, respectively. The children gave a median score of 3 ± 0 to the session, that is a positive feedback and their level of satisfaction was high (3 ± 0). They mainly preferred the puzzle activity, thus confirming the statistics. All the data about the results of the structured observation grid and the questionnaire are reported in Table 3.

Table 3. Results about the structured observation grid and the questionnaire. Legend: 0 none/absent; 1 negative/poor; 2 neutral/moderate; 3 positive/high. Pu puzzle; St Story, Pic pictures, So Song

Patient	Autonomy level	Motivation	Feedback	Satisfaction	Preferred activity
S1	3	3	3	3	Pu
S2	3	2	3	3	Pu St
S3	3	2	2	3	Pu
S4	1	3	3	3	Pic So
S5	3	3	3	3	Pu

4 Discussion

In the past few years, technology for children and disabilities has proliferated thanks to the development of more and more inexpensive mobile technology and to the availability of free-downloadable software applications. Apps for autism [2], speech and language disorders [1, 3], and health promotion [4] are only few examples of the huge amount of software application currently available on the web. However, to our knowledge a multisensory teaching application for both typically developing and disabled children still lacks in this landscape. In this work we describe the design and development of an integrated system which combines the use of a tablet, a group of toys (e.g. small plastic animals), Near Field Communication (NFC) technology and a software application with educational purposes aimed at improving the speed of learning in an entertaining environment.

The application recognizes the NFC tags placed below the animals' paws and lets the user choose one activity among reading/listening to information webpages, playing a puzzle, reading/listening to a tale, looking at a picture or listening to a song. The user's choice of one of the menu options randomly opens one of a list of predetermined websites. This list is only limited by the number of children-appropriate learning websites on the internet associated with each subject, which are assumed to be increasing.

The choice of the activities to be included into the app was guided by four specific goals that neuropsychiatries and speech therapists usually have in mind during a rehabilitation program. Specifically, pictures and puzzles are instruments to improve structural knowledge and mental representations, respectively. Information can help in improving semantic knowledge while songs and stories enrich conceptual networks. Finally, the text-to-speech tool allows to overcome specific decoding deficits in accessing written information.

The integrated system was proposed to 5 pre-school children with speech disorders. All of them used the device with a good autonomy level, were motivated and expressed high levels of satisfaction. The device was easy to understand and to learn, it was engaging and rewarding. Even if the sample is small and has to be increased in the future, our data attest that the device was successful likely because of the integration of smart and well-known technology, such as a tablet, and real and tangible objects.

This prototype offered only a limited number of activities; however the number of activities that can be embedded into the custom software application is not limited and the system can be easily extended. The number of objects can also be increased (more animals with a NFC tag) and even the number of subjects (currently only animals) can be expanded by using a variety of topics, essentially any tangible object that is appropriate for a child. This would exponentially increase the number of learning sources and domains.

One of the features of the system is the possibility of converting a text into speech by means of a text-to-speech function that reads either text taken directly from the webpage, by a JSOUP Parser, or a predetermined script. The JSOUP parser is more dynamic and allows a larger variety of websites to be programmed into the application, however, a script can be programmed into the application to make the text-to-speech application sound more natural. It was determined that for the prototype in Italian the text-to-speech tool would use a script rather than the JSOUP Parser. However for the full application the JSOUP parsing method may be used instead, because the stories and information could be read and displayed in different languages which may more easily fit a text-to-speech program.

The text-to-speech feature gives the possibility of reading a website also to those children whose language and reading skills are minimal or to subjects with complex communication needs or other disabilities.

In conclusion, the integration of different elements can provide a rich spectrum of new education and research benefits. Moreover, the device is not specifically designed only for disabled people and it can represent an educational tool for both able and disabled children. The application can have a large pool of information on a topic and also provide an element of variety to keep the child's attention over a longer period. This would offer a child a tangible encyclopedia and also entertaining stories and games.

Taken together the integrated system we described in this work is a learning and educational environment with possible benefits that incorporates auditory, visual and kinesthetic processes.

Acknowledgments. Authors would like to thank Matteo Cavalleri for his initial help and Peter Taddeo for his support in app development.

References

1. Light, J., McNaughton, D.: Supporting the communication, language, and literacy development of children with complex communication needs: state of the science and future research priorities. Assist. Technol. **24**(1), 34–44 (2011)

2. Stephan, J., Limbrick, L.: A review of the use of touch-screen mobile devices by people with developmental disabilities. J. Autism. Dev. Disord. **43**, 7 (2013)
3. Holland, A.L., Weinbeg, P., Dittelman, J.: How to use apps clinically in the treatment of aphasia. Semin. Speech Lang. **33**(3), 223–233 (2012)
4. Baranowski, T., Frankel, L.: Let's get technical! gaming and technology for weight control and health promotion in children. Child Obes. **8**(1), 34–37 (2012)
5. McGregor, K.K., et al.: Semantic representation and naming in children with specific language impairment. J. Speech Lang. Hear. Res. **45**, 998–1014 (2002)
6. Bishop, D.V.M., Nation, K., Patterson, K.: When words fail us: insights into language processing from developmental and acquired disorders. Philos. Trans. Roy. Soc. B Biol. Sci. **369** (1634), 20120403 (2014)
7. Biffi, E., Taddeo, P., M.aria Luisa Lorusso, Reni, G.: NFC-based application with educational purposes. In: Proceedings of the 8th International Conference on Pervasive Computing Technologies for Healthcare (PervasiveHealth 2014), pp. 370–372. ICST (Institute for Computer Sciences, Social-Informatics and Telecommunications Engineering), Brussels (2014). doi:10.4108/icst.pervasivehealth.2014.255350

Consonantal Phonation: Appling ICTs for Diagnosis and Treatment of Vocalization Problems

Habib M. Fardoun[1(✉)], Abdullah S. AL-Malaise ALGhamdi[1],
and Antonio Paules Cipres[2]

[1] Information Systems Department, King Abdulaziz University (KAU),
Jeddah, Saudi Arabia
{hfardoun, aalmalaise}@kau.edu.sa
[2] European University of Madri, Madrid, Spain
apcipres@gmail.com

Abstract. Speech and language therapists assess and treat speech, language and communication problems in people of all ages to help them communicate better. In this case, technology is a tool that can support therapy. However, related resources presentation and utilization for these vocalization difficulties are limited to pictograms and static web pages developed by speech therapists. This chapter describes a prototype based on mobile devices (tablets) and cloud computing aiming at supporting speech therapists and teachers towards the diagnosis and treatment of vocalization problems with particular interest in consonantal phonemes. The proposal have been designed and evaluated for therapist's sessions. It provides an initial diagnosis, creation word's composition, phonemes histories generation and management, lips positioning, and phonetic exercises tables. This process is conducted by the speech therapists or the system as such, and, at the same time, prepares the exercises collection in order to provide with the therapeutic a sequence to support the patient's treatment. Cloud technologies provide the appropriate place to host a platform supporting the system with the associated features due to the wider development and distribution for tablets cloud computing provided.

1 Introduction

According to the Real Academy of Spanish Language [1], sound is: the *oral realization of a phoneme, which is constituted by pertinent and non-pertinent features*. Sound is also a mental representation of a phoneme in the brain. The language sounds are innumerable, as many as the speakers and even more as many as a speaker uses them. This physic realization of the *t* or the *r* is what we call sound. For example, there is only one *t* or one *r* in the speaker's mind; however, later on, there are indeed a lot of forms to pronounce them. This ideal and unique *t* or *r* is what we call *phoneme*.

For example, if several people pronounce the word *train*, more or less clear differences in the pronunciation can be noticed; the *t* would sound more or less energetic; the *r* would vibrate more or less. Even if the same person pronounces a word in

© Springer-Verlag Berlin Heidelberg 2015
H.M. Fardoun et al. (Eds.): REHAB 2014, CCIS 515, pp. 294–305, 2015.
DOI: 10.1007/978-3-662-48645-0_25

different situations there will be noticeable variations. These variations, perceptible to the ear, are much clearer when we use special equipment.

Consequently, when we classify consonants, attention is attached not only to the place where they are pronounced, but also consideration is needed on the manner they are pronounced. These two elements are known as 'the articulation's point' (the place inside of the mouth cavity where it is used) and the articulation's mode (elements involved in the pronunciation).

This chapter is a complement to a publication presented in the workshop of the 8th International Conference on Pervasive Computing Technologies for Healthcare (Per-vasiveHealth '14) [9] taking into consideration the previous work, we describe in detail the system functionality in order to help the reader to design similar systems focusing on speech rehabilitation.

2   Consonantal Phonemes Classification

The sound produced by de vocal cords is a "raw" sound and does not differentiate with the animal sounds. When reaches the mouth, this "noise" is modified so to be converted into sound; this modification is what we call articulation.

Articulation is the position adopted by the mouth's organs when producing a sound. The sound articulation organs are classified in actives (lips, tongue, inferior teeth, palate) and passives (superior teeth, superior alveolus, palate) [2, 3]. As for the consonantal sounds articulation, there is always a bigger or smaller barrier blocking the air from the lungs to the exterior space. Depending on the circumstances around this exit of the air, there are diverse factors need to be taken into account for their classification [4, 5]:

Articulation's point or Articulation's zone. This is the place where the organs, which participate in the sound production, make contact. It can be classified into features depending on the previous fact (Table 1).

Table 1.   Articulation's point classification

Feature	Organs	Examples (Spanish)
Bilabial	The lips	/p/,/b/,/m/
Dental Lip	Inferior lip and superior teeth.	/f/
Inter dental	The tongue among the teeth.	/z/
Dental	The tongue behind of superior teeth.	/t/,/d/
Alveolar	The tongue over the superior teeth's root.	/s/,/l/,/r/,/rr/,/n/
Palatal	Tongue and palate.	/ch/,/y/,/ll/,/ñ/
Velar	Tongue and palate's veil.	/k/,/g/,/j/

Articulation's mode: This is the posture that the organs, which produce the sounds, adopt (Table 2).

Table 2. Articulation's point classification

Feature	Organs	Examples (Spanish)
Occlusive	Total and momentary air closure.	/p/,/b/,/t/,/d/,/k/,/g/ ,/n/,/m/
Fricative	Narrowing by where the air is passing through.	/f/,/z/,/j/,/s/
Affricate	An occlusion is produced and after that a frication.	/ch/,/ñ/
Lateral	The air grazes the laterals of the mouth cavity while passes through.	/l/,/ll/
Vibrant	The air makes to vibrate the point of the tongue when it passes through.	/r/,/rr/

Vocal cords activity: When we produce sounds, the vocal cords may vibrate or not. If the vocal cords do not vibrate, the sounds are called deaf; when the opposite happens, and the vocal cords vibrate, the sounds are called sonorous (Table 3).

Table 3. Vocal cords activity

Feature	Organs	Examples (Spanish)
Deaf	The vocal cords don't vibrate.	/p/,/t/,/k/,/ch/,/z/,/s/,/j/,/f/
Sonorous	The vocal cords vibrate.	/b/,/z/,/d/,/l/,/r/,/rr/,/m/,/n/,/ll/,/y/,/g/

Nasal cavity activity: When humans produce sounds, part of the air passes through the nasal cavity; these sounds are called nasals. When the air passes through the mouth cavity, these sounds are called orals (Table 4).

Table 4. Nasal cavity activity classification

Feature	Organs	Examples (Spanish)
Nasal	Part of the air passes through the nasal cavity.	/m/,/n/,/ñ/
Oral	All the air passes through the mouth.	The rest.

Based upon this classification, the consonantal phonemes classification summary is presented in the following table (Table 5).

There are mechanisms that a speech therapist performs during such problems detection related to the phonemes' vocalization and pronunciation due to the dysarthria. The target is to detect and evaluate the functionality of the organs so to validate the functionality degree following the previous attributes. These mechanisms are connected to checking and evaluating the lips positioning, teeth's positioning, tongue's movement, palate's veil or sonorous glottis. These are all parts of the human's speech system and are the most commonly described for a speech therapist so to treat and comment on treatment upon, as referred previously.

Table 5. Consonant phonemes classification

Bilabial		Dental Lip		Inter dental		Dental		Alveolar		Palatal		Velar		
Deaf	Sonorous	Deaf	Sonorous	Deaf	Sonorous	Deaf	Sonorous	Deaf	Sonorous	Deaf	Sonorous	Deaf	Sonorous	
p	b					t	d					k	g	Occlusive
										ch				Affricate
		f		z				s			y	j		Fricative
									l		ll			Lateral
									r, rr					Vibrant
	m								n		ñ			Nasal

3 Objectives

This paper presents a cloud-based system aiming at helping speech therapists, teachers and parents in the identification, prevention, diagnosis and rehabilitation of patients with problems on pronouncing consonants. After seeing a speech therapist and attending therapy sessions with a pronunciation problems patient, the consonants for clinic motives were chosen for this study. These problems were due to serious clinic motives such as an ear infection with hearing loss so the patient recovers very slowly. In this case, a primary school teacher noticed that a student could not pronounce the consonants properly; so he suggested to his parents to go and see a speech therapist so the student can get specific phonetic exercises targeting at avoiding the delay in his learning. The patient has completely recovered; there were no delays in his educational process in acquiring his normal hearing functionality after only a year.

Therefore, the research target is to design and develop an application so to detect whether a school student appears to have any type of hearing problems so to start his/her treatment as soon as possible avoiding both hearing organs functionality difficulties as well as educational problems.

4 Study Case

In this case study, a prototype is presented within four therapist's sessions. Just as a note, in one of the sessions the patient rejected to perform any of the exercises proposed by the speech therapist due to the known environment available for this task.

First, a prototype environment was designed; the system uses pictograms with added text to facilitate the speech therapist at creating words' composition so that a

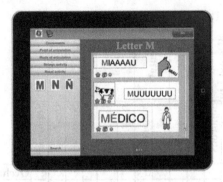

Fig. 1. Phonemes histories generation screen

child can watch his/her process with his/her parents or tutor targeting at providing an initial diagnosis.

In Fig. 1, the speech therapist compares the phonemes necessary to support diagnosis. As such, the therapist accesses a pictographic database with words selection representing the phonemes.

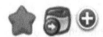

Fig. 2. Application buttons

The buttons, as in Fig. 2, perform the following actions:

Add the information to favorites.
Go directly to patient's history.
Add minimum text required to complete the pictogram and associated information.

When the book button is pressed (as in Fig. 3), the speech therapist sees an identified patient's history on the device's screen and can fill it in and complete the information needed. The usual process is that, depending on the child's age, there are minimum actions required to add words associated to images the child is able to pronounce.

Fig. 3. Book button

In Fig. 4, the speech therapist accesses to the patient's histories and pictograms on a day-to-day basis. Based upon the personalized library, the therapist may perform the necessary modifications for every diagnosis and/or treatment. Therefore, the interface

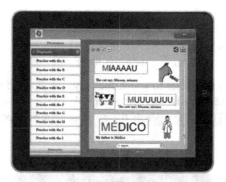

Fig. 4. Generated histories collection

provides options for 'search' and 'edit' at the top screen section, where the user can pre-visualize, add, remove or share a patient's history.

The "share history" button allows the speech therapist to send a patient's history to the child's parents so to support the student in performing the suggested exercises in an easier way; thus, the number of entries is increased so to support and confirm the exact diagnosis.

The teacher or parent receives the suggested exercise/s the child has to perform in his/her terminal so to support and finalize the diagnosis. These exercises can be repeated several times in many different histories targeting at detecting the phonemes the child has difficulties in pronouncing them properly. In Fig. 5, the child pronounces the phonemes; the application stores the data and finally the data is sent to the server.

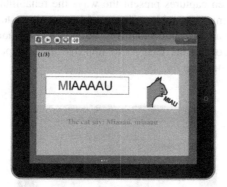

Fig. 5. Diagnosis screen

The speech therapist indicates the specific steps to perform towards a complete exercise so to support the child's diagnosis. In this example, a child articulates the phoneme without the needed larynx's vibrations replacing /b/ by the phoneme /p/. The correction is as follows:

– In front of a mirror the parents suggest him/her to observe the correct position in articulating the phoneme 'b'.
– Perform lip massages.
– Articulate several words starting with the letter 'b'.

First, the child uses the tablet to watch the ways the lips are positioned when they are moving, pronouncing words with the letter 'b'. These video records are stored in the system platform. Then, the speech therapist generates specific exercises for the child as in Fig. 6.

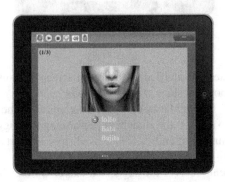

Fig. 6. Lips positioning

The parent or teacher can click on the "mirror" button, so to aid the child to compare the image of his/her lips, captured by the tablet's webcam, with the ones on the video. Below, screen captures present the ways the rehabilitation exercises of the phoneme/b/are represented on tables. These tables are consisted of several written words with the consonantal sound /b/. In Fig. 7, the child pronounces the words and watches both the video and his face so to improve the lips positioning during the pronunciation of the phoneme /b/.

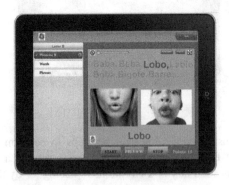

Fig. 7. Phonetic exercises tables

5   Architecture

This section presents the proposed system's architecture. Consideration was taken towards automating the tasks in order to recognize the phonemes, one in each diagnosis phase. This process can be conducted by the speech therapists or the system as such, and, at the same time, prepares the exercises collection in order to provide with the therapeutic sequence so to support the patient's treatment.

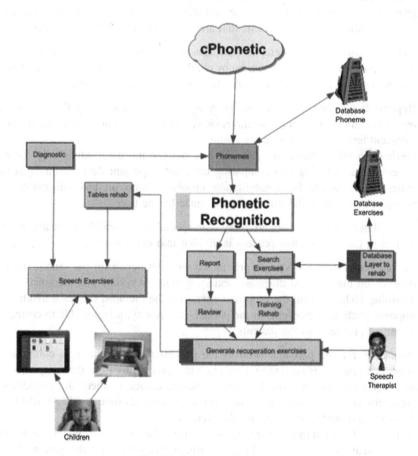

Fig. 8. System architecture

The speech therapist performs the phonetic rehabilitation exercises by filtering and testing. The platform also analyzes the diagnosis exercises suggested by the speech therapist or the system as such for the children to do. Thus, the therapist receives a report with the phonemes and the rehabilitation exercises processing and in result, analyses the platform selects and the child later completes on the mobile device.

The architecture is divided into two parts. On the one hand we have the rehabilitation and detection tools. It allows detect problems in children. Teachers and therapist can save data and analyze it to improve the sessions with the children.

On the other hand, there is a tool that provides specific exercises for children and teachers.

- **Speech Exercises**: This section stores all exercises, i.e., it is the presentation logic of the system. From this part users interact with the system and can send the data to the diagnostic system.
- **Rehab Tablets**: The tablets set exercises that patients should perform; the specialists from the analysis of the last exercises generate these.
- **Diagnostic**: This module links the activities with phonics; it is as a bridge of communication for audio streams that are sent to the cloud from the exercises.

The tool used by the therapist performs the following steps: First generate a diagnosis based on performed exercises by children. From this information the therapist can create a personalized treatment and directed to different children.

- **Report:** It generates a report on the analysis of information by the system, this report contains data specific to the review, analysis of audio, the required parameters and text associated with the audio file.
- **Review**: In this section, the therapist can analyze the data individually for each patient. After studying and comparing the most important data the therapist generates the treatment for rehabilitation process. Based on this information, the therapist may follow the improvements made by the user.

The following functions are advisory. The specialist can search the treatment to be performed in the session; this process is divided into two parts:

- **Search Exercises**: The system provides a workout bench for the search. This set depends on the detected diagnosis and symptoms by system and therapist.
- **Training Rehab**: From the proposed exercises, the therapist creates a treatment to improve phonation problems in the patient. In this way, it is possible to correct the identified problems in the patients.

Phonemes are the part that controls the processing of sound. It is composed of phonemes and packages needed to carry out audio processing from the symptoms. The central server contains the required packages, the database where the phonemes in different languages are stored (phonemes are stored in fields such as CLOB, BLOB...), it allows to store audio file in binary data format.

This type of system must have the management of the identified patients associated with a medical history number. In this form, we can have all the patient data in compliance with safety regulations in medical records.

The following diagram (Fig. 8) shows the next components: A model about the architecture diagram for cloud environments. In this case, we can highlight the part of the system for the distribution of audio and video, since it is the main resource that this system works.

We can see in the Fig. 9 the difference between the input data (streams format). These are derived from diagnostic tests conducted by therapists and output streams for the proposed treatment. We have two packages; one of them has presentation logic where the interface performs the basic operation and another package containing the logic necessary for broadcast or storage of streams. In this way, the application interacts

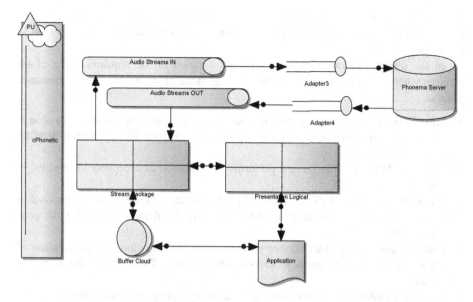

Fig. 9. System architecture, streams

directly with the streams. This requires a component with parameters is able to communicate with the corresponding stream.

This system provides load balancing capabilities, exclusively for audio and video streams requests, our system provides a tool for the daily work of professionals. For this reason we have put specific buses for streams (audio and video). These are run as independent processes. This makes it possible to better control the resolution of conflicts.

The processes' priority can be increased depending on where the system load is located inside the cloud.

In order to guarantee delivery of data with integrity and quality, we establish a queue in services, cloud buffer, set this intermediate buffer and compensate speeds transmission and reception systems input and output. We send the tests when they have been completed. In other words, the recording is performed at the intermediate buffer and sent, that is, our goal is to create a buffer system for the cloud or the cloud itself.

In order to perform this buffer in the cloud, you need to have the following information:

- **Stream to store**: Frame of complete data where the audio and video necessary for analysis is stored, this can be done through the socialization of objects.
- **Data Type**: Specify the file format of the file to be saved.
- **Data source**: This is the source data needed to identify who is the source of information, these data are generated by the application requesting the buffer and will be processed by the server knowing that information to be treated.

The system knows who needs the information, it will be consumed system who seek the necessary data through the generation, the system generates a unique number as a primary key that is stored by the consumer system and allow access to contents of the buffer with the data requested, giving direct access to the information to improving the speed in searches.

In the diagram below we have found the location of the required buffer cloud services where streams and input are stored. It is made up of services and a consumer process.

- **Start Service**: This service connects customers to initialize the session, thus able to identify the values required for receiving stream. Then, the user can start to sending or receiving stream.
- **Streams IN/OUT**: This service performs the emission or reception of streams, is activated once logged.
- **Flags/Streams**: That package adds and prepares data to create an access channel to stream. Moreover, it generates an XML file with the data necessary for the consumer process.
- **Distribution service**: This service performs operations to cloud the distribution of streams and send the signals to the systems that need the buffer of the receiving stream.
- **Storage Cluster**: The cluster service that stores video and audio streams in the system. We can see directly how it interacts with system processes consumed.

The cloud CPhonetic receives signals service end and through consumers and generating processes streams sent to customers. That is, through of the new service in the cloud buffer (Fig 10).

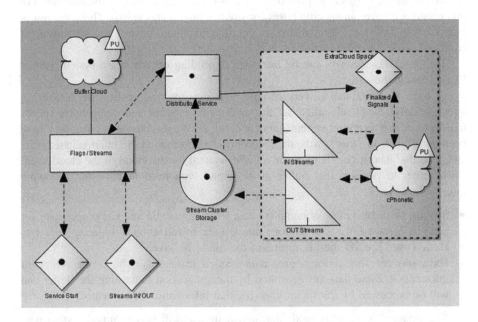

Fig. 10. Buffer cloud streams.

6 Conclusions

This paper presents the initial work on the documentation of sessions so to assist speech therapists and associated support centres. This research was due to the fact that any improvement in a child's phonation process is actually based upon a rehabilitation technique. Therefore, risks exist related to this new form of understanding the speech therapy, by utilising the new generation of computer applications as an extension of a users' diagnosis and therapy necessities.

More research work is needed on children with phonation problems and the rehabilitation processes related to designing new hardware. This is due to the fact that the speech therapists need to be involved in the early stages of tools design and equipment built by them. A possible extension of this line of research may focus upon the use of phonetics and associated techniques therapists use, in order to support the foreign languages learning processes. As such, improving the students' expression capacity in a foreign language can be a major target in future research.

Buffer system on the cloud is a part necessary to allow communication between clients and cloud systems. This component sends and receives audio and video allowing a significant improvement in the system performance and quality of the service.

References

1. Diccionario de la Real Academia (Dictionary of the Real Academy). http://lema.rae.es/drae/?val=sonido
2. Arandiga, A.V.: Prueba de articulación de fonemas: Evaluación de la dislalia, CEPE. Ciencias de la educación preescolar y especial. ISBN: 9788478690176
3. de Fonética Española, M.: Eugenio Martínez Celdrán, Ana Fernández. Ed Ariel. ISBN: 9788434482722
4. Martínez Celdrán, E. Fonología general y española, Ed. Teide. ISBN: 9788430773442
5. Antonio, Q.: Tratado de fonología y fonética españolas. Gredos. ISBN: 9788424922474
6. Fardoun, H.M., Altalhi, A.H., Cipres, A.P., Castillo, J.R., Albiol-Pérez, S.: CRehab: a cloud-based framework for the management of rehabilitation processes. In: 7th International Conference on Pervasive Computing Technologies for Healthcare (PervasiveHealth), pp. 397–400 (2013) E-ISBN: 978-1-936968-80-0
7. Fardoun, H., Montero, F., Jaquero, V.L.: eLearniXML: towards a model-based approach for the development of e-learning systems considering quality. In: Advances in Engineering Software, pp. 1297–1305 (2009) DOI: http://dx.doi.org/10.1016/j.advengsoft.2009.01.019
8. Fardoun, H.M., Ciprés, A.P., Alghazzawi, D.M.: CSchool: DUI for educational system using clouds. In: Proceedings of the 2nd Workshop on Distributed User Interfaces: Collaboration and Usability, in conjunction with CHI 2012, pp. 684–695
9. Fardoun, H.M., Al-Malaise Al-Ghamdi, A.S., Cipres, A.P.: Consonantal phonation rehabilitation. In: Proceedings of the 8th International Conference on Pervasive Computing Technologies for Healthcare (PervasiveHealth 2014). ICST (Institute for Computer Sciences, Social-Informatics and Telecommunications Engineering), ICST, Brussels, Belgium, Belgium, pp. 381–385 (2014). DOI: 10.4108/icst.pervasivehealth.2014.255391, http://dx.doi.org/10.4108/icst.pervasivehealth.2014.255391

Detection of Interaction with Depth Sensing and Body Tracking Cameras in Physical Rehabilitation

Lubos Omelina[1,2,3(✉)], Bart Jansen[1,2], Bruno Bonnechère[4],
Milos Oravec[3], and Serge Van Sint Jan[4]

[1] Department of Electronics and Informatics,
Vrije Universiteit Brussel, Pleinlaan 2, 1050 Brussels, Belgium
{lomelina, bjansen}@etro.vub.ac.be
[2] Department of Future Health, iMinds, Ghent, Belgium
[3] Institute of Computer Science and Mathematics, Slovak University
of Technology in Bratislava, Slovakia Ilkovičova 3, 812 19 Bratislava, Slovakia
milos.oravec@stuba.sk
[4] Laboratory of Anatomy, Biomechanics and Organogenesis,
Université Libre de Bruxelles, Lennik Street 808, 1070 Brussels, Belgium
{bbonnech, sintjans}@ulb.ac.be

Abstract. Body tracking sensors have become an integral part of the physical therapy not only as a motivational tool used by games but also as a diagnostic instrument. Skeletal tracking helps to analyze and quantify human motion and thus can provide tangible results from therapy sessions. Markerless skeletal tracking with depth sensing cameras represents currently the most popular approach mainly due to low cost cameras that use a model based approach to recognize a human skeleton. The model based approach works in many scenarios but faces limitations as well. This paper presents a method for identifying the patient and detecting interactions between the patient and the therapist. Identifying interactions helps to discriminate between active and passive motion of the patient as well as to estimate the accuracy of the skeletal data. Our experiments show the state-of-the-art performance of real-time face recognition from a low resolution images that is sufficient to use in adaptive systems. We also compare the performance of our interaction detection method with two other approaches (markerless and marker based approach) and shows its superior performance.

Keywords: User identification · Interaction detection · Rehabilitation · Face recognition

1 Introduction

A 3D camera combined with serious games (SG) for physical rehabilitation seems to be a perspective tool in advanced rehabilitation sessions. Several systems use markerless skeletal tracking with low cost cameras not only to control the games but also as a measuring tool or to provide feedback to the patient and the therapist [1–3].

© Springer-Verlag Berlin Heidelberg 2015
H.M. Fardoun et al. (Eds.): REHAB 2014, CCIS 515, pp. 306–317, 2015.
DOI: 10.1007/978-3-662-48645-0_26

Although the use of markerless systems (MLS) for gaming purposes has gained popularity, there are still problems related to these technologies. Current low cost MLS can provide reliable recognition and tracking of human skeletons when only a single player or two clearly separated people are in the scene. However, the occurrence of another person in front of the camera who is interacting with the player(s) leads to problems; e.g. switching between tracked users, tracking of wrong people or significant decrease in the quality of the recognized skeletons. For instance, the first version of the Microsoft Kinect camera can track only two skeletons simultaneously and needs approximately 2.5 m clear space in between players and the sensor[1]. The presence of more than 2 people leads to unstable user selection for skeletal tracking, especially when they are interacting. The second version of the Kinect camera can track up to six skeletons but stability of the skeletal tracking remains low when more people are in the scene.

Problems related to skeletal tracking are even more frustrating in serious games for physical therapy due to the frequent occurrence of a therapist in the scene. Therapists need to intervene and help a patient in case of problems or difficulties to play. This intervention leads to skeletal detection defects and thus the ability to detect this interaction would help to increases ergonomics of SG, and its relevancy in a rehabilitation context.

There are two approaches to tackle the problems:

Creating constraints – creating a set of rules on how to use the SG system in order to avoid situations that are causing problems, e.g. people should not stand closer than a specific distance. This solution significantly decreases usability and ergonomics of the system since it limits ways of using the systems and users need to learn additional rules on how to use it.

Improving system intelligence – additional processing that can identify and track the right person and can identify whether the people in the scene are interacting or not, e.g. the system can notify people about problematic poses. This may increase computational complexity, but does not decrease usability and ergonomics.

Detection of interactions between a patient and a therapist has also several advantages in modern SG applied to physical rehabilitation. For instance, discriminating between active and passive motion or the identification of unreliable and inaccurate skeletal measurements would be helpful to the therapist in order to assess the patient's compliance to planned therapy (i.e., a typical physical therapy scheme must be adapted to the patient's problems in order to be efficient). In addition, modern SG systems in physical rehabilitation should not only motivate the patient, but also reliably recognize the quality of skeletons for simultaneous biomechanical (medical) analysis.

We propose a simple, fast and robust approach for detecting human interactions in the RGBD (RGB + depth) video stream and an increased system intelligence, in order to improve the serious gaming experience in therapeutic practice. In our method, we employ continuous face recognition to detect, recognize and track the patient with other people in the scene (e.g. the therapist, or a clinician). We use a method based on local binary patterns (LBP) that is considered to be state-of-the-art in facial recognition [4].

---

[1] Kinect Quick Setup Guide & Kinect Sensor Manual.

After identifying users in the scene we identify interactions between the patient and other people in the scene. We use a depth map/point cloud for estimating the distance between two people. Our method uses association of depth regions to user identities provided by the underlying framework and computes the minimal distance between the regions. The same method for user disambiguation and for interaction detection can also be integrated in home based rehabilitation systems.

The presented method is used within the context of rehabilitation system that is using serious games in order to capture movement data. During a rehabilitation session, the patient is playing a game and the therapist assists him with the exercise. In this scenario skeletal tracking faces difficulties due to occluding bodies and interactions. The skeleton recognition algorithm does not recover the joint positions correctly and thus the skeletal data become corrupted. We detect the intervals when this corruption occurs in order to exclude such data from further processing. On the other hand, skeletal data may be corrected (e.g. by using accelerometers to improve positions and rotation of body segments) in which case the detected interaction could be a valuable source of information in order to analyze passive range of motion of different joints.

2   Related Work

Topics covered in face recognition are very broad. We focus only on feature based methods as they are reaching state-of-the-art performance and have the ability to run in real-time in unconstrained environments. M. Turk & A. Pentland [5] introduced the first successful approach for recognition faces, capable of running in real time called eigenfaces. Although a lot of approaches were proposed since then, there are still open problems related mostly to changes in poses and lighting [6]. To address this problem current approaches use light-invariant features like LBP, HOG or Gabor features [7, 8]. Especially the method based on LBP proposed by T. Ahonen [4] gained a lot of attention and belongs to state-of-the-art in face recognition [8]. A strong advantage of LBP features in contrast to other (e.g. Gabor) features is its low computational complexity.

For matching features a hand-crafted distance metric with nearest neighbor classifier or a learning algorithm may be used. Methods based on eigenfaces typically use Euclidean or Mahalanobis distance [5]. T. Ahonen used Chi-square distance with the nearest neighbor (NN) classifier in order to match LBP features. Although machine learning approaches (e.g. neural networks or support vector machines) reach better performance than nearest neighbor matching, they need time consuming training that makes them unusable for some use-cases.

A significant part of the current research in human interactions is devoted to recognizing actions [9]. Yun et al. [10] proposed a method for recognizing different types of interactions from RGBD sources using Support Vector Machines and Multiple Instance Learning. However, in automated therapy sessions, we need to detect in real time whether the therapist is helping the patient, without a need to classify the type of interaction.

3   Method

Our method works as a preprocessing step for any motion analysis system that is tracking/analyzing movements of a particular patient and where support by the therapist needs to be detected. An overview of the approach is shown in Fig. 1. The patient is at first recognized based on his face in the color image and afterwards the positions of people close by are detected from the depth map. The method assumes also labeled regions in the depth-map that specify clusters of points where each cluster represents a human body in the scene. Based on the depth map and labeled regions we identify whether the therapist is supporting or interacting with the patient.

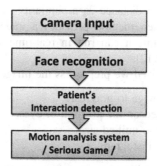

Fig. 1. Schematic overview of detection.

3.1   Environment and Use-Case Constraints

The general unconstrained face recognition is still an open problem mainly due to varying illumination, different facial expressions and poses. However, we can avoid some of the open problems by considering constraints of the environment in which the real system is used. Our approach (assuming its use in therapy and serious games) contains several inherited constraints (i.e. constraints given by the use-case and environment in which users interact with the system) that help us improve the face recognition accuracy and thus make the overall system more reliable.

Playing a video game requires users to face the screen in order to interact with the game. In our system we assume that the user's head is oriented towards the screen what significantly limits the poses performed during the game-play. Occasional cases when the patient's pose exceeds the tolerance can be easily filtered out by temporal filtering. A longer lasting change of facial pose means that the patient does not look to the camera and is not paying attention to instructions on the screen (and thus not following the exercises). In this case, the system does not collect data because the movement is not result of the exercise, but rather a free motion that should be excluded from exercise analysis.

Current gaming MLSs are made exclusively for indoor environments and are hence faced with limited variability in lighting. In addition, the games are played in the therapist's practice or at patients' home making the position of the camera rather static (i.e. no large lateral displacements will occur). Most popular MLSs are using depth cameras based on the time-of-flight (ToF) principle. These cameras illuminate the scene uniformly with near infra-red light. The source of the NIR light is typically placed near the sensor and thus all acquired facial images are lightened under the same condition.

In our approach we also assume that the user is located in the center of the field of view of the camera and thus the probability of appearing at the sides is rather low.

3.2   Recognition of a Patient

Facial recognition is a well-studied area and there are many different methods with varying accuracy based on the specific use cases. We decided to use a method based on LBP features with Chi-square distance as a similarity metric which is described in details in [4, 11]. The chosen method provides a trade-of between accuracy and computational complexity; thus it can run in real-time while maintaining state-of-the-art recognition accuracy [12].

Before the face is recognized we preprocess the image as follows:

- conversion of the color image to grayscale,
- alignment of the face based on the position of eyes,
- scaling of the face image to unified size,
- equalization of the image histogram.

In order to compute the LBP histogram features, the image is segmented into several non-overlapping regions and from each of these regions a histogram of uniform LBP patterns is computed (Fig. 2). Histograms are concatenated from left to right and from top to bottom.

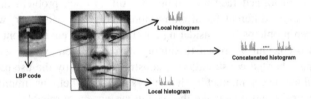

Fig. 2. Process of creating concatenated LBP histograms.

The method requires training of the patient's face. In this step the camera captures multiple images of the patient's face and creates a training set. Training needs to be done in advance and requires to perform 5 different poses in front of the camera. For each pose the subject needs to keep the pose for one second. The camera captures 30 frames per second and thus the captured image set contains around 150 samples per view. In order to choose the most representative images per view, we use the k-means clustering algorithm [13].

3.3   Recognition of the Interaction

Physical interactions between the patient and the physical therapist (PT) are the essence
of physical rehabilitation. The PT can, for example, perform the motion (together) with
the patient in order to show him the right way to do it, can stabilize the trunk in order to
avoid compensatory movement, can palpate some muscles during exercises to be sure
that the patient is recruiting the right muscles, can evaluate passive range of motion of a
particular joint by helping the patient to perform this motion, etc. Therefore, it is
important that the games are robust to the presence of the therapist in the scene and that
the games can detect when the therapist is interacting with the patient.

In this section we describe the method for detecting interaction from a depth map
camera stream. In our method we assume that part of the preprocessing, i.e. the
detection of humans from a depth-map, is done by the camera itself or the underlying
framework[2]. The input to our method is the set of points associating people with depth
regions.

Let I be a depth map acquired from a camera and $I(x, y)$ a point from the depth
map. We define a set of points $U \subset I$, such that U contains points representing the
detected human bodies. We say that two different bodies U_1 and U_2, $U_1 \cap U_2 = \{\}$ are
interacting when there exist such points $p_1 \in U_1$ and $p_2 \in U_2$ that $\|p_1 - p_2\| < \lambda$, where
the threshold λ represents a critical distance (aka comfort zone). The comfort zone
represents a parameter of our model.

Since the depth map I is represented as a grid/matrix of depth points, we assume
uniform distances in the X and Y axes. In order to detect collisions, we explore a
circular neighborhood $(N, f(\lambda))$ of each point $p \in U$ where N is the number of points
being explored and f a function mapping metric space to pixel space (Fig. 3). Exploring
only a limited amount of points in the neighborhood provides only an approximation of
the intersection between U_1 and U_2, but is computationally less expensive and can run
in real-time, leaving resources for other tasks (the game and actual skeleton
processing).

$$G_{neighbor}(p_c) = \sum_{n=1}^{N} s(p_c, p_n) max(0, \|p_c - p_n\| - \lambda) \qquad (1)$$

Where $s(p_1, p_2)$ is defined as follows

$$s(p_1, p_2) = \begin{cases} 1 & \text{if } id(p_1) ! = id(p_2) \\ 0 & \text{otherwise} \end{cases} \qquad (2)$$

The resulting image $G_{neighbor}$ that describes the local neighborhood of every pixel,
may still contain misdetections caused by the noise of the depth sensor. In contrast to
positive areas caused by noise, interaction areas occur in blobs. We detect these
interaction blobs by applying a Laplacian of Gaussian filter of an appropriate size:

---

[2] An example of the underlying framework is the Kinect for Windows SDK,
More information: http://www.microsoft.com/en-us/kinectforwindows.

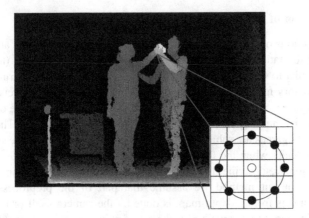

Fig. 3. An example of a circular (8,2) neighborhood that is explored for a particular point in the depth map.

$$LoG(x, y) = -\frac{1}{\pi\sigma^4}\left[1 - \frac{x^2 + y^2}{2\sigma^2}\right]e^{-\frac{x^2+y^2}{2\sigma^2}} \tag{3}$$

The result is an image containing positive values in blobs that correspond to the interaction points.

4 Experiments

In our method we test the face recognition and detection interaction as two separate aspects. We integrated the proposed method to a previously developed gaming system used in rehabilitation of children suffering from cerebral palsy [14]. This system is using the Microsoft Kinect sensor as the MLS and thus no additional hardware is necessary. By proper placement of the camera we can limit poses of the face that occur while the patient is performing the exercises. From our preliminary experiments where patients played the games, we observed that the variance of the horizontal head movement is 42 degrees and 33 degrees for vertical head movement (See Fig. 4. Although the facial pose variation is limited, it decreases the face recognition accuracy. In order to reduce negative influence of the pose variability we collect training images for each face under different poses (see Fig. 5).

Each patient needs to enroll to our system. In enrollment we collected facial images from 10 different people using a Kinect camera. The images are scaled to a size of 36 × 48 pixels. The system requires users to pass the training procedure in which they demonstrate 5 different facial poses in order to make face recognition pose invariant (see Fig. 5). From each facial image we compute the LBP code image that is divided into 12 non-overlapping regions (3 divisions vertically and 4 regions horizontally) – these are used to compute the resulting concatenate LBP histograms. Features are clustered with k-means algorithm to 5 different canonical centers that are stored in the database as templates for a user. The face recognition performance is shown in the Fig. 6.

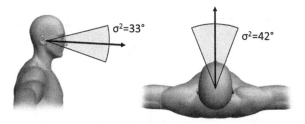

Fig. 4. Average direction of a head with respect to the camera while using a SG system, mean and variance in up/down rotation - left, and in left to right rotation - right.

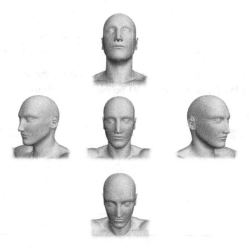

Fig. 5. 5 different facial poses required in enrolment for the face recognition subsystem.

To test interaction detection, we used a MLS (MS Kinect) together with a marker-based stereophotogrammetry system (MBS) (Vicon) to capture the patient's skeleton. The MBS was using 8 calibrated NIR cameras. Both systems recorded the scene simultaneously while the patient was interacting with a therapist. In Fig. 7 measurements are shown from one session. During this session the therapist approached the patient 3 times and left the scene afterwards.

In order to demonstrate the performance of our method, we compared events from our method (start/stop of the interaction) with stability of the skeletal segment lengths over time as the frames become available. We used the following measures to evaluate this stability:

Confidence value of the skeleton tracker – The Kinect SDK provides 3-state confidence information about the tracking state for each joint. A joint can be (i) tracked, (ii) inferred or (iii) not tracked. Our observations show that while two people are interacting in the scene, the quality of the recognized skeletons slightly decreases. It is important to note that the decreased quality does not relate only to interactions but also to the pose, occlusions. In order to compute the cumulative confidence value we simply sum values for each joint while the tracked state has weight 0.06, the inferred state has

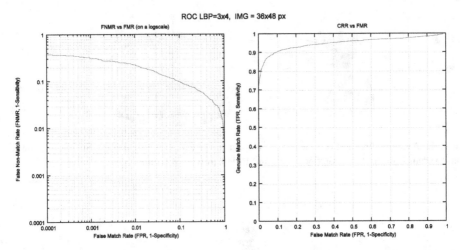

Fig. 6. ROC curves of the face recognition system tested on the dataset collected with MS Kinect v.1 containing 1464 facial images of 10 people in 2 sessions.

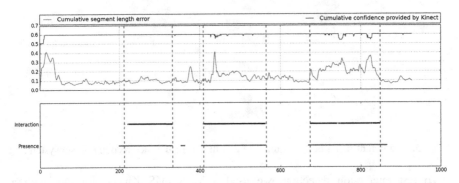

Fig. 7. Evolution of skeletal stability and detection of interactions. The top part shows the variability of segment lengths measured by the MLS (in red) together with cumulative confidence based on the tracking state of each joint (in blue). The bottom part shows 3 detected interaction periods (in black) and periods when the therapist was present in the scene (in green) (Color figure online).

weight 0.015 and the not tracked state has weight 0. The influence of an interaction between a patient and a therapist on Kinect's confidence values is shown in Fig. 7. We can see that the confidence values are rather stable even during the interaction when the skeleton segments are unstable.

Stability of segment lengths – a common problem of skeleton detecting cameras is that segment lengths are varying over time. Since there is no prior knowledge about the skeleton, the camera continuously makes new hypotheses about poses and segment lengths [15]. We know that the lengths should remain the same and their increased variability indicates low skeleton stability. For the comparison purpose, we compute a cumulative error from all segments as a sum of absolute differences of all segments between the first frame (the T pose of the patient while faces the camera provides accurate measurements) and the current frame.

Stability of segment lengths measured with MBS – we tracked the skeleton of the patient with a MLS and MBS simultaneously in order to compare their performance when two people are interacting. It is important to note that although the MBS is considered to be the gold standard for human motion tracking, this system might also experience errors due to the lack of visibility of markers while interacting (Fig. 8). We used the MBS to track only the patient, not the therapist.

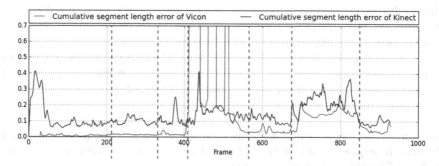

Fig. 8. Comparison of cumulative segment length errors for MBS (Vicon, in red) and MLS (Kinect, in blue) (Color figure online).

A part of the data processed during the experiments is shown in Fig. 7. This recording contains three separate interactions and in-between the therapist leaves the scene. We can see that the segment length variability is increasing in each interaction. This is caused by the decreasing distance between the therapist and the patient. In the third interaction, the segments vary the most. Although there is a significant error, the Kinect reports confident results about the tracked joints and thus doesn't provide reliable identification of the skeleton's accuracy.

Figure 8 shows that the MBS provides accurate results when only a single person is in the scene. Segment lengths are stable even during the first interaction when the therapist approached the patient from a side. In the second and third interaction the therapist occluded several markers – the MBS reported significantly worse results. We can see that in case of close interaction, the stability of both systems decreases. In case of close interactions the MBS loses track of markers and thus cannot provide any information about joints connected to those markers. Results also demonstrate that MLS can even provide more stable results due to the presence of all joints inferred from the depth map.

5 Conclusion

The use of SGs still faces a lot of problems in physical rehabilitation. Interaction between people negatively influences the accuracy of the sensory devices and thus makes further analysis more challenging.

However, based on the used technology, SGs could be used for more than performing exercises. Since data of the patients can be recorded during the rehabilitation (games), this data can be used to follow the patients' evolution and to be sure that they are doing the right exercises [16]. In order to have a precise follow up of the patient, the clinician must be sure that the patient was playing alone and was not helped by friends, parents or others (therapist, clinicians).

We proposed to improve automated rehabilitation systems by detecting the identity of the patient as well as the therapist and by tracking both over time. The presented approach allows to detect interactions between the patient and other people, and also helps to discriminate between active and passive motion. We show that during an interaction, the precision of the capturing devices decreases and a good detection for these interactions can help to filter out erroneous measurements.

A possible extension of this work might be more detailed segmentation of the scene in order to detect other supporting objects. Games played with balance boards could also benefit from recognizing users standing on the board and thus tracking the authenticity of the measured data.

Acknowledgments. Research described in the paper was done within the RehabGoesHome and ICT4REHAB projects (www.ict4rehab.org) funded by Innoviris and within the grant No. 1/0529/13 of the Slovak Grant Agency VEGA.

References

1. Chang,C.Y., Lange, B., Zhang, M., Koenig, S., Requejo, P., Somboon, N., Sawchuk, A.A., Rizzo, A.A.: Towards pervasive physical rehabilitation using Microsoft Kinect. In: 2012 6th International Conference on Pervasive Computing Technologies for Healthcare (PervasiveHealth), pp. 159–162 (2012)
2. Chang, Y.J., Chen, S.F., Da Huang, J.: A kinect-based system for physical rehabilitation: a pilot study for young adults with motor disabilities. Res. Dev. Disabil. **32**(6), 2566–2570 (2011)
3. Clark, R.A., Pua, Y.H., Bryant, A.L., Hunt, M.A.: Validity of the Microsoft Kinect for providing lateral trunk lean feedback during gait retraining. Gait Posture **38**(4), 1064–1066 (2013)
4. Ahonen, T., Hadid, A., Pietikäinen, M.: Face recognition with local binary patterns. Comput. Vision ECCV 2004 **3021**, 469–481 (2004)
5. Turk, M., Pentland, A.: Eigenfaces for recognition. J. Cogn. Neurosci. **3**(1), 71–86 (1991)
6. Grother, P.J., Quinn, G.W., Phillips, P.J.: Report on the evaluation of 2D still-image face recognition algorithms. In: NIST Interagency Report 7709, Multiple-Biometric Evaluation (MBE) 2010 (2010)
7. Zhu, Z., Luo, P., Wang, X., Tang, X.: Deep learning identity-preserving face space. In: 2013 IEEE International Conference on Computer Vision (ICCV), pp. 113–120 (2013)
8. Chen, D., Cao, X., Wen, F., Sun, J.: Blessing of dimensionality: high-dimensional feature and its efficient compression for face verification. In: CVPR 2013 Proceedings of the 2013 IEEE Conference on Computer Vision and Pattern Recognition Pages, pp. 3025–3032 (2013)

9. Poppe, R.: A survey on vision-based human action recognition. Image Vis. Comput. **28**(6), 976–990 (2010)

10. Yun, K., Honorio, J., Chattopadhyay, D., Berg, T.L., Samaras, D.:Two-person interaction detection using body-pose features and multiple instance learning. In: 2012 IEEE Computer Society Conference on Computer Vision and Pattern Recognition Workshops, pp. 28–35 (2012)

11. Ban, J., Pavlovicova, J., Feder, M., Omelina, L., Oravec, M.: Face recognition methods for multimodal interface. In: 2012 5th Joint IFIP Wireless and Mobile Networking Conference (WMNC), pp. 110–113(2012)

12. Oravec, M., Pavlovičová, J., Mazanec, J., Omelina, Ľ., Féder, M., Ban, J.: Efficiency of recognition methods for single sample per person based face recognition. Rev. Refinements New Ideas Face Recogn. Rijeka : InTech **2011**, 181–206 (2011)

13. Ban, J., Feder, M., Jirka, V., Loderer, M., Omelina, L., Oravec, M., Pavlovicova, J.: An automatic training process using clustering algorithms for face recognition system. In: Proceedings ELMAR-2013: 55th International Symposium. Zadar, Croatia, pp. 15–18 (2013)

14. Omelina, L., Jansen, B.: Serious games for physical rehabilitation: designing highly configurable and adaptable games. In: Proceedings 9th International Conference Disability, Virtual Reality & Associated Technologies, pp. 195–201 (2012)

15. Shotton, J., Fitzgibbon, A., Cook, M., Sharp, T., Finocchio, M., Moore, R., Kipman, A., Blake, A.: Real-time human pose recognition in parts from single depth images. In: CVPR 2011 Proceedings of the 2011 IEEE Conference on Computer Vision and Pattern Recognition, pp. 1297–1304 (2011)

16. Bonnechère, B., Jansen, B., Omelina, L., Da Silva, L., Mouraux, D., Rooze, M., Van Sint Jan, S.: Patient follow-up using serious games. a feasibility study on low back pain patients. In: Proceedings of the 3rd European Conference on Gaming and Playful Interaction in Health Care, pp. 185–195 (2013)

Author Index

Printed in the United States
by Bookmasters

Printed in the United States
By Bookmasters